Third Edition

Psychiatric–Mental Health Nurse Practitioner Review Manual

CONTINUING EDUCATION SOURCE
NURSING CERTIFICATION REVIEW MANUAL
CLINICAL PRACTICE RESOURCE

Kathryn Johnson, MSN, PMHNP-BC, PMHCNS-BC
Dawn Vanderhoef, PhD, DNP, PMHNP-BC, PMHCNS-BC

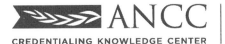 | Conferences.
Consultation.
Education.

Library of Congress Cataloging-in-Publication Data

Johnson, Kathryn, 1947- author.
  Psychiatric-mental health nurse practitioner review manual / by Kathryn Johnson and Dawn Vanderhoef. – 3rd edition.
      p. ; cm.
  Preceded by Psychiatric-mental health nurse practitioner review and resource manual / Karen Guess. 2nd ed. 2008.
  ISBN 978-1-935213-42-0
  I. Vanderhoef, Dawn, author. II. Guess, Karen. Psychiatric-mental health nurse practitioner review and resource manual. Preceded by (work): III. American Nurses Credentialing Center, publisher. IV. Title.
  [DNLM: 1. Psychiatric Nursing–methods–Outlines. WY 18.2]
  RC438
  616.89'0231–dc23
                        2013043878

The American Nurses Credentialing Center (ANCC), a subsidiary of the American Nurses Association (ANA), provides individuals and organizations throughout the nursing profession with the resources they need to achieve practice excellence. ANCC's internationally renowned credentialing programs certify nurses in specialty practice areas; recognize healthcare organizations for promoting safe, positive work environments through the Magnet Recognition Program® and the Pathway to Excellence ® Program; and accredit providers of continuing nursing education. In addition, ANCC's Credentialing Knowledge Center provides leading-edge information and education services and products to support its core credentialing programs.

ISBN 13: 9781935213628

© 2013 American Nurses Credentialing Center.
8515 Georgia Ave., Suite 400
Silver Spring, MD 20910
All rights reserved.

PSYCHIATRIC–MENTAL HEALTH NURSE PRACTITIONER REVIEW MANUAL, 3RD EDITION

DECEMBER 2013

Please direct your comments and/or queries to: revmanuals@ana.org

The healthcare services delivery system is a volatile marketplace demanding superior knowledge, clinical skills, and competencies from all registered nurses. Nursing autonomy of practice and nurse career marketability and mobility in the new century hinge on affirming the profession's formative philosophy, which places a priority on a lifelong commitment to the principles of education and professional development. The knowledge base of nursing theory and practice is expanding, and while care has been taken to ensure the accuracy and timeliness of the information presented in the **Psychiatric–Mental Health Nurse Practitioner Review Manual,** clinicians are advised to always verify the most current national guidelines and recommendations and to practice in accordance with professional standards of care used with regard to the unique circumstances that apply in each practice situation. In addition, every effort has been made in this text to ensure accuracy and, in particular, to confirm that drug selections and dosages are in accordance with current recommendations and practice, including the ongoing research, changes to government regulations, and the developments in product information provided by pharmaceutical manufacturers. However, it is the responsibility of each nurse practitioner to verify drug product information and to practice in accordance with professional standards of care. In addition, the editors wish to note that provision of information in this text does not imply an endorsement of any particular products, procedures or services.

Therefore, the authors, editors, American Nurses Association (ANA), American Nurses Association's Publishing (ANP), American Nurses Credentialing Center (ANCC), and the Institute for Credentialing Innovation cannot accept responsibility for errors or omissions, or for any consequences or liability, injury, and/or damages to persons or property from application of the information in this manual and make no warranty, express or implied, with respect to the contents of the **Psychiatric–Mental Health Nurse Practitioner Review Manual.** Completion of this manual does not guarantee that the reader will pass the certification exam. The practice examination questions are not a requirement to take a certification examination. The practice examination questions cannot be used as an indicator of results on the actual certification.

PUBLISHED BY

American Nurses Credentialing Center
Credentialing Knowledge Center
8515 Georgia Avenue, Suite 400
Silver Spring, MD 20910-3402
www.nursecredentialing.org

INTRODUCTION TO THE CONTINUING EDUCATION (CE) CONTACT HOUR APPLICATION PROCESS FOR *PSYCHIATRIC–MENTAL HEALTH NURSE PRACTITIONER REVIEW MANUAL, 3RD EDITION*

The Credentialing Knowledge Center now offers the continuing education contact hours for this manual online at www.NursingWorld.org, the American Nurses Association's Web site. This process involves answering approximately 25–30 questions that test knowledge of the information contained within this manual. The continuing education contact hours can be completed at any time and a certificate can be printed from the Web site immediately upon successful completion of the test.

After studying the manual and given an online multiple-choice test, the exam candidate will be able to:

1. Pass the posttest with at least 75% of the answers correct.

2. Select responses to test questions based on key principles, standards of practice, and theoretical basis of nursing practice.

3. Choose accepted therapeutic interventions in answering questions related to quality nursing practice.

4. Utilize direct and indirect professional role responsibilities and applications regarding nursing practice in answering test questions.

Upon completion of this manual *and* the online CE test, a nurse can receive a total of 24.09 continuing education contact hours at a price of $46. (ANA members receive a discount on CEs.) **The entire process—online test and evaluation form—must be completed by December 31, 2016 in order to receive credit.** To begin the process, please e-mail **revmanuals@ana.org.** Your patience with this process is greatly appreciated.

Inquiries or Comments

If you have any questions about the CE contact hours, please e-mail the Credentialing Knowledge Center at revmanuals@ana.org. You may also mail any comments to Editorial Project Manager, at the address listed below.

Duplicate CE Certificates

Once you have successfully passed the CE test, you may go back and re-print your certificate as often as you wish.

Conflicts of Interest

A conflict of interest occurs when an individual has an opportunity to affect educational content about health-care products or services of a commercial company with which she/he has a financial relationship.

The planners and presenters of this CNE activity have disclosed no relevant financial relationships with any commercial companies pertaining to this activity.

Credentialing Knowledge Center
American Nurses Credentialing Center
Attn: Editorial Project Manager
8515 Georgia Avenue, Suite 400
Silver Spring, MD 20910-3492
Fax: (301) 628-5342

A maximum of 24.09 contact hours may be earned by learners who successfully complete this continuing nursing education activity.

ANA's Center for Continuing Education and Professional Development is accredited as a provider of continuing nursing education by the American Nurses Credentialing Center's Commission on Accreditation.

ANCC Provider Number 0023.

ANA's Center for Continuing Education and Professional Development is approved by the California Board of Registered Nursing, Provider Number CEP6178 for a maximum of 12.56 contact hours (50 minute contact hour).

The ANA Center for Continuing Education and Professional Development includes ANCC's Credentialing Knowledge Center.

Note About the *Fifth Edition of the Diagnostic and Statistical Manual of Mental Disorders (DSM-V)*

The ANCC *Psychiatric–Mental Health Nurse Practitioner Review Manual, 3rd Edition* was written to help nurses prepare for the ANCC Psychiatric–Mental Health Nurse Practitioner certification exam that is based on the test content outline effective August 6, 2013. This current exam, which will be used through 2016, incorporates the *DSM-IV-TR*. Because this is the manual referenced in the test, we continue to reference *DSM-IV-TR* in this review manual.

CONTENTS

INTRODUCTION TO THE CONTINUING EDUCATION (CE) . . . . **V**
CONTACT HOUR APPLICATION PROCESS

NOTE ABOUT THE FIFTH EDITION OF THE DIAGNOSTIC . . . . **VII**
AND STATISTICAL MANUAL OF MENTAL DISORDERS

CHAPTER 1. Taking the Certification Examination **1**

General Suggestions for Preparing for the Exam

About the Certification Exams

CHAPTER 2. Psychiatric–Mental Health Nurse Practitioner Role,
Scope of Practice, and Regulatory Process **11**

Nurse Practitioner Advanced Practice Core Content

Nurse Practitioner Advanced Practice Specialized Content

History of the NP Role

Health Policy

Public Health Principles

Cultural Competency

Research

CHAPTER 3. Theoretical Basis of Care **41**

Biopsychosocial Framework of Care

Classification of Psychiatric Disorders: *DSM-IV-TR*, *DSM-V*

Therapeutic Relationship

Developmental Theories

Fundamental Theories Supporting PMHNP Role

Nursing Theories

CHAPTER 4. Neuroanatomy, Neurophysiology, and Behavior **55**

The Nervous System

Neuroanatomy and the Brain

Neurophysiology and the Brain

Neuroimaging Assessment and Diagnostic Procedures

Genomics

CHAPTER 5. Assessment of Acute and Chronic Disease States **71**

Statistics for Psychiatric Disorders

Assessment of Psychiatric Disorders

Therapeutic Communication Considerations

Assessment of Spiritual Needs

Nature of Symptom Presentation of Psychiatric Disorders

Components of the PMHNP Assessment Process

Mental Status Examination (MSE)

Mini-Mental Status Exam (MMSE)

Montreal Cognitive Assessment (MoCA) and Short Portable Mental Status Questionnaire (SPMSQ)

Gender-Based Medical Testing and Screening Recommendations for the General Public

Developing and Prioritizing a Differential Diagnosis List

Health Behavior Guidelines

Therapeutic Communication Principles

Assessment Tools

CHAPTER 6. Pharmacological Principles **133**

Concepts in Pharmacological Management

PMHNP Role of Pharmacological Management

CHAPTER 7. Nonpharmacological Treatment **143**

Individual Therapy

Interpersonal Therapy

Group Therapy

Family Therapies

Complementary/Alternative Therapies (CAMs)

CHAPTER 8. Depressive Disorders, Grief and Bereavement States, and Bipolar Disorders.................................... **157**

Sadness as a Common Emotional State

Major Depressive Disorder

Dysthymic Disorder

Grief and Bereavement

Bipolar Disorder

Cyclothymic Disorder

CHAPTER 9. Anxiety Disorders **211**

Normal Emotion of Anxiety

Anxiety Disorders

Panic Disorder

Agoraphobia

Specific Phobias (Simple Phobias)

Social Anxiety (Phobia) Disorder

Obsessive–Compulsive Disorder

Posttraumatic Stress Disorder

Generalized Anxiety Disorder

CHAPTER 10. Schizophrenia and Other Psychotic Disorders **247**

General Description of Psychotic Disorders

Schizophrenia

Schizophreniform Disorder

Schizoaffective Disorder

Delusional Disorder

Brief Psychotic Disorder

Shared Psychotic Disorder (Folie á Deux)

CHAPTER 11. Delirium, Dementia, and Other Cognitive Disorders **283**

Cognitive Disorders

Delirium

Dementia

Traumatic Brain Injury Associated With Military Action

CHAPTER 12. Substance-Related Disorders **305**

CHAPTER 13. Personality Disorders **327**

Personality

Personality Disorders

CHAPTER 14. Disorders of Childhood and Adolescence **341**

          Assessment and Care Planning for Children and Adolescents

          Oppositional Defiant Disorder

          Conduct Disorder

          Attention-Deficit Hyperactivity Disorder

          Asperger Syndrome

          Rett Syndrome

          Autism Spectrum Disorder

          Eating Disorders

          Mental Retardation

CHAPTER 15. Sleep **375**

CHAPTER 16. Violence **385**

          Domestic Violence

          Sexual Assault and Abuse

          Lethality Assessment

APPENDIX A. Case Studies Discussion **397**

APPENDIX B: Review Questions **409**

APPENDIX C: Answers to the Review Questions **421**

INDEX **425**

ABOUT THE AUTHORS **443**

CHAPTER 1

TAKING THE CERTIFICATION EXAMINATION

When you sign up to take a national certification exam, you will be instructed to go online and review the testing and review handbook (http://www.nursecredentialing.org/CertificationHandbook.aspx). Review it carefully and be sure to bookmark the site so you can refer to it frequently. It contains information on test content and sample questions. This is critical information; it will give you insight into the nature of the test. The agency will send you information about the test site; keep this in a safe place until needed.

GENERAL SUGGESTIONS FOR PREPARING FOR THE EXAM

Step One: Control Your Anxiety
Everyone experiences anxiety when faced with taking the certification exam.

- ► Remember, your program was designed to prepare you to take this exam.
- ► Your instructors took a similar exam, and have probably talked to students who took exams more recently, so they know how to help you prepare.
- ► Taking a review course or setting up your own study plan will help you feel more confident about taking the exam.

Step Two: Do Not Listen to Gossip About the Exam

A large volume of information exists about the tests based on reports from people who have taken the exams in the past. Because information from the testing facilities is limited, it is hard to ignore this gossip.

▶ Remember that gossip about the exam that you hear from others is not verifiable.

▶ Because this gossip is based on the imperfect memory of people in a stressful situation, it may not be very accurate.

▶ People tend to remember those items testing content with which they are less comfortable; for instance, those with a limited background in women's health may say that the exam was "all women's health." In fact, the exam blueprint ensures that the exam covers multiple content areas without overemphasizing any one.

Step Three: Set Reasonable Expectations for Yourself

▶ Do not expect to know everything.

▶ Do not try to know everything in great detail.

▶ You do not need a perfect score to pass the exam.

▶ The exam is designed for a beginner level—it is testing readiness for *entry-level* practice.

▶ Learn the general rules, not the exceptions.

▶ The most likely diagnoses will be on the exam, not questions on rare diseases or atypical cases.

▶ Think about the most likely presentation and most common therapy.

Step Four: Prepare Mentally and Physically

▶ While you are getting ready to take the exam, take good physical care of yourself.

▶ Get plenty of sleep and exercise, and eat well while preparing for the exam.

▶ These things are especially important while you are studying and immediately before you take the exam.

Step Five: Access Current Knowledge

General Content

You will be given a list of general topics that will be on the exam when you register to take the exam. In addition, examine the table of contents of this book and the test content outline, available at www.nursecredentialing.org/cert/TCOs.html.

▶ What content do you need to know?

▶ How well do you know these subjects?

Take a Review Course

► Taking a review course is an excellent way to assess your knowledge of the content that will be included in the exam.

► If you plan to take a review course, take it well before the exam so you will have plenty of time to master any areas of weakness the course uncovers.

► If you are prepared for the exam, you will not hear anything new in the course. You will be familiar with everything that is taught.

► If some topics in the review course are new to you, concentrate on these in your studies.

► People have a tendency to study what they know; it is rewarding to study something and feel a mastery of it! Unfortunately, this will not help you master unfamiliar content. Be sure to use a review course to identify your areas of strength and weakness, then concentrate on the weaknesses.

Depth of Knowledge

How much do you need to know about a subject?

► You cannot know everything about a topic.

► Remember that the depth of knowledge required to pass the exam is for entry-level performance.

► Study the information sent to you from the testing agency, what you were taught in school, what is covered in this text, and the general guidelines given in this chapter.

► Look at practice tests designed for the exam. Practice tests for other exams will not be helpful.

► Consult your class notes or clinical diagnosis and management textbook for the major points about a disease. Additional reference books can be found online at http://www.nursecredentialing.org/Publications.aspx.

► For example, with regard to medications, know the drug categories and the major medications in each. Assume all drugs in a category are generally alike, and then focus on the differences among common drugs. Know the most important indications, contraindications, and side effects. Emphasize safety. The questions usually do not require you to know the exact dosage of a drug.

Step Six: Institute a Systematic Study Plan

Develop Your Study Plan

▶ Write up a formal plan of study.

- ▸ Include topics for study, timetable, resources, and methods of study that work for you.

- ▸ Decide whether you want to organize a study group or work alone.

- ▸ Schedule regular times to study.

- ▸ Avoid cramming; it is counterproductive. Try to schedule your study periods in 1-hour increments.

▶ Identify resources to use for studying. To prepare for the examination, you should have the following materials on your shelf:

- ▸ A good pathophysiology text.

- ▸ This review book.

- ▸ A physical assessment text.

- ▸ Your class notes.

- ▸ Other important sources, including: information from the testing facility, a clinical diagnosis textbook, favorite journal articles, notes from a review course, and practice tests.

- ▸ Know the important national standards of care for major illnesses.

- ▸ Consult the bibliography on the test blueprint. When studying less familiar material, it is helpful to study using the same references that the testing center uses.

▶ Study the body systems from head to toe.

▶ The exams emphasize health promotion, assessment, differential diagnosis, and plan of care for common problems.

▶ You will need to know facts and be able to interpret and analyze this information utilizing critical thinking.

Personalize Your Study Plan

▶ How do you learn best?

- ▸ If you learn best by listening or talking, attend a review course or discuss topics with a colleague.

▶ Read everything the test facility sends you as soon as you receive it and several times during your preparation period. It will give you valuable information to help guide your study.

▶ Have a specific place with good lighting set aside for studying. Find a quiet place with no distractions. Assemble your study materials.

Implement Your Study Plan

You must have basic content knowledge. In addition, you must be able to use this information to think critically and make decisions based on facts.

► Refer to your study plan regularly.

► Stick to your schedule.

► Take breaks when you get tired.

► If you start procrastinating, get help from a friend or reorganize your study plan.

► It is not necessary to follow your plan rigidly. Adjust as you learn where you need to spend more time.

► Memorize the basics of the content areas you will be required to know.

Focus on General Material

► Most of what you need to know is basic material that does not require constant updating.

► You do not need to worry about the latest information being published as you are studying for the exam.

Pace Your Studying

► Stop studying for the examination when you are starting to feel overwhelmed and look at what is bothering you. Then make changes.

► Break overwhelming tasks into smaller tasks that you know you can do.

► Stop and take breaks while studying.

Work With Others

► Talk with classmates about your preparation for the exam.

► Keep in touch with classmates, and help each other stick to your study plans.

► If your classmates become anxious, do not let their anxiety affect you. Walk away if you need to.

► Do not believe bad stories you hear about other people's experiences with previous exams.

► Remember, you know as much as anyone about what will be on the next exam!

Consider a Study Group

► Study groups can provide practice in analyzing cases, interpreting questions, and critical thinking.

 ► You can discuss a topic and take turns presenting cases for the group to analyze.

 ► Study groups can also provide moral support and help you continue studying.

Step Seven: Strategies Immediately Before the Exam

Final Preparation Suggestions

▶ Use practice exams when studying to get accustomed to the exam format and time restrictions.

- Many books that are labeled as review books are simply a collection of examination questions.

- If you have test anxiety, such practice tests may help alleviate the anxiety.

- Practice tests can help you learn to judge the time it should take you to complete the exam.

- Practice tests are useful for gaining experience in analyzing questions.

- Books of questions may not uncover the gaps in your knowledge that a more systematic content review text will reveal.

- If you feel that you don't know enough about a topic, refer to a text to learn more. After you feel that you have learned the topic, practice questions are a wonderful tool to help improve your test-taking skill.

▶ Know your test-taking style.

- Do you rush through the exam without reading the questions thoroughly?

- Do you get stuck and dwell on a question for a long time?

- You should spend about 45 to 60 seconds per question and finish with time to review the questions you were not sure about.

- Be sure to read the question completely, including all four answer choices. Choice "a" may be good, but "d" may be best.

The Night Before the Exam

▶ Be prepared to get to the exam on time.

- Know the test site location and how long it takes to get there.

- Take a "dry run" beforehand to make sure you know how to get to the testing site, if necessary.

- Get a good night's sleep.

- Eat sensibly.

- Avoid alcohol the night before.

- Assemble the required material—two forms of identification, pencil, and watch. Both IDs must match the name on the application, and one photo ID is preferred.

- Know the exam room rules.

  ▷ You will be given scratch paper, which will be collected at the end of the exam.

  ▷ Nothing else is allowed in the exam room.

▷ You will be required to put papers, backpacks, etc., in a corner of the room or in a locker.

▷ No water or food will be allowed.

▷ You will be allowed to walk to a water fountain and go to the bathroom one at a time.

The Day of the Exam

▶ Get there early. You must arrive at the test center at least 15 minutes before your scheduled appointment time. If you are late, you may not be admitted.

▶ Think positively. You have studied hard and are well-prepared.

▶ Remember your anxiety reduction strategies.

Specific Tips for Dealing With Anxiety

Test anxiety is a specific type of anxiety. Symptoms include upset stomach, sweaty palms, tachycardia, trouble concentrating, and a feeling of dread. But there are ways to cope with test anxiety.

▶ There is no substitute for being well-prepared.

▶ Practice relaxation techniques.

▶ Avoid alcohol, excess coffee, caffeine, and any new medications that might sedate you, dull your senses, or make you feel agitated.

▶ Take a few deep breaths and concentrate on the task at hand.

Focus on Specific Test-Taking Skills

To do well on the exam, you need good test-taking skills in addition to knowledge of the content and ability to use critical thinking.

Exam Format

This exam includes multiple choice questions.

▶ Multiple-choice tests have specific rules for test construction.

▶ A multiple-choice question consists of three parts: the information (or stem), the question, and the four possible answers (one correct and three distracters).

▶ Careful analysis of each part is necessary. Read the entire question before answering.

▶ Practice your test-taking skills by analyzing the practice questions in this book and on the ANCC Web site.

Analyze the Information Given

► Do not assume you have more information than is given.

► Do not overanalyze.

► Remember, the writer of the question assumes this is all of the information needed to answer the question.

► If information is not given, it is not relevant and will not affect the answer.

► Do not make the question more complicated than it is.

What Kind of Question Is Asked?

► Are you supposed to recall a fact, apply facts to a situation, or understand and differentiate between options?

  ▸ Read the question thinking about what the writer is asking.

  ▸ Look for key words or phrases that lead you (see Figure 1–1). These help determine what kind of answer the question requires.

FIGURE 1–1. EXAMPLES OF KEY WORDS AND PHRASES

► avoid	► initial	► most
► best	► first	► significant
► except	► contributing to	► likely
► not	► appropriate	► of the following
		► most consistent with

Read All of the Answers

► If you are absolutely certain that answer "a" is correct as you read it, mark it, but read the rest of the question so you do not trick yourself into missing a better answer.

► If you are absolutely sure answer "a" is wrong, make a note on your scratch paper and continue reading the question.

► After reading the entire question, go back, analyze the question, and select the best answer.

► Do not jump ahead.

► If the question asks you for an assessment, the best answer will be an assessment. Do not be distracted by an intervention that sounds appropriate.

► If the question asks you for an intervention, do not answer with an assessment.

► When two answer choices sound very good, the best one is usually the least expensive, least invasive way to achieve the goal. For example, if your answer choices include a physical exam maneuver or imaging, the physical exam maneuver is probably the better choice provided it will give the information needed.

▶ If the answers include two options that are the opposite of each other, one of the two is probably the correct answer.

▶ When numeric answers cover a wide range, a number in the middle is more likely to be correct.

▶ Watch out for distracters that are correct but do not answer the question, combine true and false information, or contain a word or phrase that is similar to the correct answer.

▶ Err on the side of caution.

Only One Answer Can Be Correct

▶ When more than one suggested answer is correct, you must identify the one that best answers the question asked.

▶ If you cannot choose between two answers, you have a 50% chance of getting it right if you guess.

Avoid Changing Answers

▶ Change an answer only if you have a compelling reason, such as you remembered something additional, or you understand the question better after rereading it.

▶ People change to a wrong answer more often than to a right answer.

Time Yourself to Complete the Whole Exam

▶ Do not spend a large amount of time on one question.

▶ If you cannot answer a question quickly, mark it and continue the exam.

▶ If time is left at the end, return to the difficult questions.

▶ Make educated guesses by eliminating the obviously wrong answers and choosing a likely answer even if you are not certain.

▶ Trust your instinct.

▶ Answer every question. There is no penalty for a wrong answer.

▶ Occasionally a question will remind you of something that helps you with a question earlier in the test. Look back at that question to see if what you are remembering affects how you would answer that question.

ABOUT THE CERTIFICATION EXAMS

The American Nurses Credentialing Center Computerized Exam

The ANCC examination is given only as a computer exam, and each exam is different.

The order of the questions is scrambled for every test, so even if two people are taking the same exam, the questions will be in a different order. The exam consists of 200 multiple-choice questions.

▶ 175 of the 200 questions are part of the test and how you answer will count toward your score; 25 are included to refine questions and will not be scored. You will not know which ones count, so treat all questions the same.

▶ You will need to know how to use a mouse, scroll by either clicking arrows on the scroll bar or using the up and down arrow keys, and perform other basic computer tasks.

▶ The exam does not require computer expertise.

▶ However, if you are not comfortable with using a computer, you should practice using a mouse and computer beforehand so you do not waste time on the mechanics of using the computer.

Know what to expect during the test.

▶ Each ANCC test question is independent of the other questions.

  ▹ For each case study, there is only one question. This means that a correct answer on any question does not depend on the correct answer to any other question.

  ▹ Each question has four possible answers. There are no questions asking for combinations of correct answers (such as "a and c") or multiple-multiples.

▶ You can skip a question and go back to it at the end of the exam.

▶ You cannot mark key words in the question or right or wrong answers. If you want to do this, use the scratch paper.

▶ You will get your results immediately, and a grade report will be provided upon leaving the testing site.

Internet Resources:

▶ ANCC Web site: www.nursecredentialing.org

▶ ANA Bookstore: www.nursesbooks.org. Catalog of ANA nursing scope and standards publications and other titles that may be listed on your test content outline

▶ National Guideline Clearinghouse: www.ngc.gov

CHAPTER 2

PSYCHIATRIC–MENTAL HEALTH NURSE PRACTITIONER ROLE, SCOPE OF PRACTICE, AND REGULATORY PROCESS

Starting in the 1950s with the seminal work of two psychiatric nurses, June Mellow (1951) and Hildegard Peplau (1952), psychiatric nursing has been a well-established, well-recognized subspecialty of nursing. The emergence of the psychiatric–mental health nurse practitioner (PMHNP) role reflects the growth of the advanced practice role, the acceptance of a brain-based etiology of psychiatric disorders, and an awareness of the need to provide holistic nursing care that does not artificially separate mind and body (Stuart & Laraia, 2001).

The PMHNP role is built on fundamental, core advanced practice knowledge common to all nurse practitioners. This base of knowledge is expanded to include the very specific knowledge of the subspecialty of psychiatry. This chapter reviews the role of the PMHNP, the scope of practice, and the regulatory process.

Advanced practice nurses specializing in psychiatry are educationally prepared at the master's or doctoral level, possess in-depth knowledge and skills in the specialty area, and provide primary psychiatric care to individuals or families at risk for or currently experiencing a psychiatric disorder.

NURSE PRACTITIONER ADVANCED PRACTICE CORE CONTENT

All nurse practitioners upon graduation are expected to meet a set of core competencies (National Organization of Nurse Practitioner Faculties, 2006). Specialty competencies, such as the *Psychiatric-Mental Health Nurse Practitioner Competencies*, are then built upon these core competencies (National Organization of Nurse Practitioner Faculties, 2007).

Nurse Practitioner Core Competencies

Management of Health Status

▶ Health assessment

▶ Health history

▶ Physical exam

▶ Screening and diagnostic testing

▶ Diagnosing

▶ Prescribing meds and other treatment modalities

▶ Evaluating care outcomes

Maintenance of Nurse–Patient Relationship

▶ Displaying environment of trust and respect

▶ Maintaining healthy boundaries

▶ Engaging in therapeutic communication

Teaching and Coaching

▶ Health promotion and disease prevention

▶ Risk reduction

▶ Coaching toward behavioral change

Professional Role

▶ Serving as patient advocate

▶ Using information and technology in health care

▶ Using interdisciplinary collaboration and consultation

▶ Works within and across organizations to foster collaboration and improve health care

▶ Practicing ethically

▶ Showing leadership

▶ Undertaking professional development

▶ Participating in policy-making

Managing and Negotiating Healthcare Delivery Systems

▶ Decision-making with regard to cost, access, and efficacy

▶ Applying business strategies to practice

▶ Negotiating legislative change when needed

Monitoring Quality of Care

▶ Evaluating quality of care

▶ Incorporating continuous quality improvement into practice

Providing Culturally Sensitive Care

▶ Remaining culturally sensitive when assessing a patient's symptoms and his or her perceptions of symptoms

NURSE PRACTITIONER ADVANCED PRACTICE SPECIALIZED CONTENT

The specialty competencies are specifically designed for entry-level psychiatric–mental health nurse practitioners. These specialty competencies are to be used with the NP Core Competencies. The specialty competencies address the life span PMHNP focus, with families and populations. As changes occur within the healthcare system, these competencies will also change (National Organization of Nurse Practitioner Faculties, 2003).

▶ Health promotion, health protection, disease prevention, and treatment

  ▹ *Assessment*: Physical and mental health assessment; psychiatric evaluation including mental status evaluation; differentiating normal and abnormal symptomology; family system assessment

▶ Reasons for conducting a physical assessment in psychiatry:

  ▹ To identify general health status of patient

  ▹ To screen for general, nonpsychiatric disorders or problems

  ▹ To ascertain differential diagnoses

  ▹ To identify primary psychiatric disorder

▶ *Diagnosis of health status:* Ordering and interpreting diagnostic tests, differential diagnoses; diagnosing psychiatric disorders, applying taxonomy systems to the diagnosis

▶ Neurobiological and associated taxonomies:

  ▹ *International Classification of Diseases* (*ICD-9;* World Health Organization, 2007)

  ▹ *Diagnostic and Statistical Manual of Mental Disorders* (*DSM-IV-TR;* American Psychiatric Association, 2000)

  ▹ Health Insurance Portability and Accountability Act (HIPAA, P.L. 104-191) code sets

  ▹ *Nursing Interventions Classification* (*NIC;* McCloskey & Bulechek, 2000)

- *Nursing Outcomes Classification* (*NOC*; Johnson, Maas, & Moorhead, 2003)
- North American Nursing Diagnosis Association (NANDA, 2000)

▶ *Plan of care and implementation of treatment:* Applying etiological models to care of patients (e.g., neurobiological, psychosocial); using evidence-based standards of care and practice guidelines; using psychotherapy; prescribing psychotropic meds; managing psychiatric emergencies

▶ NP–patient relationship

- Using therapeutic communication
- Promoting trust
- Maintaining professional boundaries

▶ Teaching and coaching function

- Psychopharmacological education
- Psychoeducation

▶ Professional role

- Interdisciplinary collaboration
- Consultation
- Coordination of referrals
- Participation in professional organizations
- Research involvement and utilization
- Use of ethical and legal standards

▶ Managing and negotiating healthcare delivery systems

- Using ethical principles to advocate for patients
- Participating in health policy

▶ Monitoring and ensuring the quality of healthcare practice

- Consulting with others to improve quality of care
- Engaging in continuing education
- Staying current with research

▶ Cultural competence

- Remaining culturally sensitive when assessing patient's symptoms and his or her perceptions of symptoms

HISTORY OF THE NP ROLE

The NP role was introduced in 1965 by Dr. Loretta C. Ford and Henry K. Silver, MD, at the University of Colorado (Mirr Jansen & Zwygart-Stauffacher, 2006). They identified new roles in which experienced registered nurses with advanced education and skills were performing clinical duties traditionally reserved for physicians. Universities were slow to implement NP programs at the master's level. However, RNs embraced the new role and rushed into continuing education programs of varying lengths, quality, and focus to accomplish the necessary educational preparation for this new role.

▶ Proven competence brought an acceptance of the NP role in the healthcare system

▶ Acceptance and recognition of the title and role by patients and other health professionals

▶ NP programs are accredited by one of two organizations to achieve standardization and control over quality: the Commission on Collegiate Nursing Education (CCNE; AACN, 2013) and the Accredited Commission for Nursing Education (ACNE, 2013).

▶ NPs are recognized providers under many third-party insurance coverage plans (e.g., Medicare, Medicaid, CHAMPUS, federal programs funding school-based clinics, U.S. military, Veterans Administration).

Growth of the NP Role

▶ Facilitating factors for growth

  ▹ Patient demand for services

  ▹ Acceptance of the advanced practice nursing role

  ▹ Emergence of the PMHNP role

  ▹ Decreasing stigmatization

  ▹ Emphasis on integrated healthcare services

▶ Constraining factors for growth

  ▹ Growing competition in job market in general for NPs

  ▹ Reduction in salaries because of NP oversupply

  ▹ Reimbursement struggles with Medicare and private insurance companies

  ▹ Issue of overlapping scope of practice with other NPs

  ▹ Increased concerns over reimbursement fraud and abuse (e.g., issues of coding and billing for services)

  ▹ Mandatory supervisory/collaborative agreements with physicians

Regulatory and Statutory Dimensions of the NP Role

▶ State legislative statutes

  ▹ Grant *legal authority* for NP practice

  ▹ Are the *Nurse Practice Act* of every state

▷ Provide title protection (who may be called a nurse practitioner)

▷ Define advanced practice

▷ Are prevailing state laws that define scope of practice (what NPs may do)

▷ Place restrictions on practice

▷ Sets NP credentialing requirements (e.g., educational requirements, certification)

▷ State grounds for disciplinary action:

  ▸ Practicing without valid license

  ▸ Falsification of records

  ▸ Medicare fraud

  ▸ Failure to use appropriate nursing judgment

  ▸ Failure to follow accepted nursing standards

  ▸ Failure to complete accurate nursing documentation.

▷ May specifically require that an NP develop a collaborative agreement with a physician

  ▸ *Collaborative agreement:* Also known as a protocol that describes what types of drugs might be prescribed and defines some form of oversight board for NP practice

► Statutory law

  ▸ Rules and regulations differ for each state

  ▸ May further define scope of practice and practice requirements

  ▸ May provide restrictions in practice unique to specific state

► Licensure

  ▸ A process by which an agency of state government grants permission to individuals accountable for the practice of a profession to engage in the practice of that profession

  ▸ Also prohibits all others from legally doing protected practice

► Credentialing

  ▸ Process used to protect the public by ensuring a minimum level of professional competence

► Certification

  ▸ Is a credential that provides title protection

  ▸ Determines scope of practice (i.e., who NPs can see and what NPs can treat)

  ▸ Is the process by which a professional organization or association certifies that an individual licensed to practice as a professional has met certain predetermined standards specified by that profession for specialty practice

  ▸ Assures the public that an individual has mastery of a body of knowledge

- Assures that the individual has acquired the skills necessary to function in a particular specialty
- The American Nurses Credentialing Center (ANCC), which is a subsidiary of the American Nurses Association, is the only certifying body for advanced practice psychiatric nursing.
  - ▷ Certification offered as a Psychiatric Mental Health Nurse Practitioner (ANCC, 2013)

▶ Scope of practice
- Defines NP roles and actions
- Identifies competencies assumed to be held by all NPs who function in a particular role
- Has broad variations from state to state
- Advanced practice PMHNP standards are identified in *Scope and Standards of Psychiatric–Mental Health Clinical Nursing Practice* (ANA, 2007).

▶ Standards of practice
- Gives authoritative statements regarding the quality and type of practice that should be provided
- Provides a way to judge the nature of care provided
- Reflects the expectation for the care that should be provided to patients with various illnesses
- Reflects professional agreement focused on the minimum levels of acceptable performance
- Can be used to legally describe the standard of care that must be met by a provider
- May be precise protocols that must be followed or more general guidelines that recommend actions

Professional Role Responsibilities

▶ Confidentiality
- The patient's right to assume that information given to the healthcare provider will not be disclosed
- Protected under federal statute through the Medical Record Confidentiality Act of 1996 (S. 1360)
- Pertains to verbal and written patient information
- Requires that the provider discuss confidentiality issues with patients, establish consent, and clarify any questions about disclosure of information
- Requires that provider obtain a signed medical authorization and consent form to release medical records and information when requested by the patient or when requested by another healthcare provider

- ► HIPAA
  - ▻ The first national comprehensive privacy protection act
  - ▻ Guarantees patients 4 *fundamental rights:* (1) To be educated about HIPAA privacy protection, (2) to have access to their own medical records, (3) to request amendment of their health information to which they object, and (4) to require their permission for disclosure of their personal information.
- ► The Health Information Technology for Economic and Clinical Health Act (HITECH) of 2009
  - ▻ Incentive payments for sharing specific electronic health record (EHR) data
  - ▻ Meaningful use incentives
  - ▻ Electronic health records can improve both individual and population-based outcomes (Friedman, Parrish, & Ross, 2013).
  - ▻ Electronic health records can improve quality, safety, efficiency, effeteness, and outcomes (HRSA, 2013).
    - ▷ E-prescribing
    - ▷ Computerized physician order sets
    - ▷ Tracking care and avoiding duplication of services
- ► Exceptions to guaranteed confidentiality
  - ▻ When appropriate, individuals or organizations determine that the need for information outweighs the principle of confidentiality
    - ▷ If a patient reveals an intent to harm self or others
    - ▷ To attorneys involved in litigation
    - ▷ When records are released to insurance companies
    - ▷ When answering court orders, subpoenas, or summons
    - ▷ When meeting state requirements for mandatory reporting of diseases or conditions
    - ▷ *Tarasoff* principle (1976): Duty to warn potential victim of imminent danger of homicidal patients
    - ▷ In cases of child abuse or elder abuse
- ► Informed consent
  - ▻ The communication process between the provider and the patient that results in the patient's acceptance or rejection of the proposed treatment
  - ▻ An explanation of relevant information that enables the patient to make an appropriate and informed decision
  - ▻ The right of all competent adults or emancipated minors
    - ▷ **Emancipated minors:** Persons under 18 years of age who are married, parents, or self-sufficiently living away from the family domicile

- Elements of the informed consent
    - Nature and purpose of proposed treatment or procedure
    - Risks or discomforts and benefits of treatment
    - Risks and benefits of not undergoing treatment
    - Alternative procedures or treatments
    - Diagnosis and prognosis
  - Provider must document in the medical record that informed consent has been obtained from the patient
  - PMHNP is responsible for ensuring that the patient is cognitively capable of giving informed consent

► Ethics
  - An important aspect of the NP role that deals with moral duties, obligations, and responsibilities
  - What is right? vs. What is wrong?
  - Ethical principles that provide foundation and direction for complex decisions:
    - *Justice:* Doing what is fair; fairness in all aspects of care
    - *Beneficence:* Promoting well-being and doing good
    - *Nonmalfeasance:* Doing no harm
    - *Fidelity:* Being true and loyal
    - *Autonomy:* Doing for self
    - *Veracity:* Telling the truth
    - *Respect:* Treating everyone with equal respect
  - NP ethical behavior is defined in an ANA policy statement on ethics (*Code of Ethics for Nurses*, 2005) that provides guidelines related to delivering care that preserves patient's dignity, autonomy, rights, and confidentiality.

► Important ethical principles in psychiatry
  - Patients must be involved in decision-making to the full extent of their capacity (mutual decision-making).
  - Patients have a right to treatment in the least restrictive setting.
  - Patients have a right to refuse treatment unless a legal process resulting in a mandatory court order for treatment has been obtained.

► Ethical dilemma
  - Occurs in a situation in which there are two or more justifiable alternatives
  - Occurs when the choice is made to promote good
  - Which option sacrifices the fewest high-priority values (a harm reduction approach)?

- ▶ Theoretical approaches to ethical decision-making
  - ▹ *Deontological Theory:* An action is judged as good or bad based on the act itself regardless of the consequences
  - ▹ *Teleological Theory:* An action is judged as good or bad based on the consequence or outcome
  - ▹ *Virtue Ethics:* Actions are chosen based on the moral virtues (e.g., honesty, courage, compassion, wisdom, gratitude, self-respect) or the character of the person making the decision.

Ethics of Disclosure by Providers

- ▶ Patients have a right to know what is happening during the course of their treatment.
- ▶ Providers have an ethical responsibility to disclose medical errors, accidents, injuries, and negative results to patients.
- ▶ As a result of the disclosure, a patient may have legal right to compensation for harm suffered due to medical misadventures (Sadock & Sadock, 2007).

Risk vs. Benefits of Disclosure of Disability Regarding Employment

- ▶ The Americans with Disabilities Act (ADA) works to prevent discrimination by employers with 15 or more employees against qualified individuals in hiring, firing, advancement, job training, compensation, and workplace conditions (Buppert, 2012).
- ▶ Federal legislation grants Americans who have disabilities, including mental illness, the opportunity for employment on an equal basis with the nondisabled
- ▶ Employers are required to make reasonable accommodations for qualified applicants or employees with a disability

Risk of Disclosure

- ▶ Employers may find ways to avoid hiring persons known to have a disability
- ▶ Coworkers may harass or discriminate against persons with psychiatric illnesses
- ▶ Assumption that persons with psychiatric illnesses may be less productive
- ▶ May limit an employee's chance for advancement in career
- ▶ Feedback for improvement may not be given to employee because others may attribute the employee's behavior to the psychiatric illness
- ▶ Labeling oneself as "disabled" may affect one's beliefs or self-image

Benefits of Disclosure

- ▶ Able to request reasonable accommodations
- ▶ Opportunity to have a job coach come to the work site and communicate directly with employer

- Employee can involve an employment service provider, employee assistance program, or other third party in the development of accommodations
- Easier for employee to come to work during an exacerbation of symptoms
- May help with the recovery process
- Allows coworkers to offer personal support
- May empower another employee to disclose

Legal Considerations

- Malpractice insurance
  - Provides financial protection against claims of malpractice
    - Coverage for negligent professional acts
    - Coverage for highly technical or professional skills required by health professionals, including NPs
  - Recommended universally for all NPs
  - Does not protect NPs from charges of practicing outside their legal scope of practice
  - Provides NPs their own legal representation to advocate for them even if their agency also carries malpractice liability insurance protection
- Four elements of negligence that must be established to prove malpractice:
  1. *Duty:* The NP had a duty to exercise reasonable care when undertaking and providing treatment to the patient.
  2. *Breach of duty:* The NP violated the applicable standard of care in treating the patient's condition.
  3. *Proximate cause:* There is a causal relationship between the breach in the standard of care and the patient's injuries.
  4. *Damages:* There are permanent and substantial damages to the patient as a result of the breach in the standard of care.

Competency

- A legal, not a medical, concept
- A determination that a patient can make reasonable judgments and decisions regarding treatment and other health concerns
- A person is considered competent until a court rules the person to be incompetent.
- If a person is deemed incompetent, a court-appointed guardian will make health-related decisions for that person.

Commitment

- Process of involuntarily forcing a person to receive evaluation or treatment
- Process may differ from state to state

▶ Basic criteria include

- Person has a diagnosed psychiatric disorder.

- Person is harmful to self or others as a consequence of the disorder.

- Person is unaware or unwilling to accept the nature and severity of the disorder.

- Treatment is likely to improve functioning.

▶ Involuntary Admission

- Admission to a hospital or other treatment facility that is against the person's wishes

- Patients maintain all civil liberties except the ability to come and go as they please

- Amount of time patients can be kept against their wishes varies by state

- Voluntary Admission

- Admission to a hospital or other treatment facility that is desired by the person

- Patient maintains all civil liberties

- Patient consents to potential confinement within the structure of a hospital setting

Scholarly Activities

▶ It is important to engage in scholarly activities as an NP:

- Publishing

- Lecturing and presenting

- Preceptorship

- Continuing education

Mentoring

▶ A process in which a more experienced NP agrees to guide and support a junior colleague in the role, competencies, and skills

▶ Relationship consists of mutual respect and an interactive process of learning

▶ Needs involvement by both the mentor and the mentee in the relationship

Patient Advocacy

▶ Stand up for patients' rights and empowering them to become their own advocates

▶ Reduce the stigma of mental illness

▶ Help patients receive available services

▶ Promote mental health by participating in a professional organization:

- American Nurses Association (ANA)

- American Psychiatric Nurses Association (APNA)

- International Society of Psychiatric Nurses (ISPN)

HEALTH POLICY

▶ Advanced practice nurses have a legal and ethical responsibility to be a patient advocate

    ▸ Participation in local, state, national, and international health policy activities (Buppert, 2012)

▶ Involvement: Testify at a public meeting, lobby, or work with the media to bring an awareness to an issue

    ▸ Phases of policy-making: Formulation, implementation, and evaluation (Abood, 2007)

Case Management

▶ A system of controlled oversight and authorization of services and benefits provided to patients

▶ Consists of coordinating care, ensuring quality outcomes, monitoring plan of care, and doing advocacy

▶ Has overall goal to promote quality cost-effective outcomes

Leadership

Nurses should be leaders and engage with health professionals to transform and redesign health care (Institute of Medicine, 2010).

▶ The nurse practitioner is educated to lead interdisciplinary treatment teams

    ▸ Act as full partners in health care

    ▸ Design, implement, evaluate, and advocate to redesign the U.S. healthcare system

    ▸ Translate research into practice

▶ Team Leadership Model

    ▸ Decision 1: Should the leader monitor the team or take action?

        ▹ Seek out information to understand the team

        ▹ Analyze information

        ▹ Interpret the information and decide how to act

    ▸ Decision 2: Should the leader intervene to meet the task or relational need?

        ▹ Performance functions

        ▹ Task functions

    ▸ Decision 3: Should the leader intervene internally or externally?

        ▹ Assess for conflicts between group members—action to maintain group performance

        ▹ Assess for unclear goals

        ▹ Assess for proper support (Northouse, 2007, pp. 209–234)

Reflective Practice

▶ Reflection uses a model or framework to systematically "make sense of experience" (Sherwood & Horton-Deutsch, 2012, p. 4).

▶ Process to tell a story about self and others to gain insight into practice

▶ Enhances critical thinking to problem-solve and enhance clinical reasoning and decision-making

▶ Link theory and practice

Critical Thinking

▶ Defined as the acquisition of knowledge with an attitude of deliberate inquiry

▶ Making clinical decisions based on evidence-based practice

  ▸ Decreases the difficulty of choosing from conflicting or multiple recommendations when diagnosing and treating patients.

▶ Develops self-awareness though a metacognitive process to gain new insights about self, and in relation to self and others

Health Promotion and Disease Prevention Education

▶ Preventative care and screening practices essential aspects of the PMHNP role

▶ Screening for physical health problems in the psychiatric patient

▶ Usually guided by Healthy People 2010 (U.S. Department of Health and Human Services, 2005), which identifies national health objectives, including behavioral health

▶ Mental health promotion and education includes

  ▸ Teaching about interventions and ways to cope with specific stressors

  ▸ Validating "normalcy" of feelings; ensuring patients that they are not "crazy"

  ▸ Helping patients recognize and identify their feelings or behaviors

  ▸ Helping patients identify resources in the community

PUBLIC HEALTH PRINCIPLES

▶ *Primary prevention*: Aimed at decreasing the incidence (number of new cases) of mental disorders

  ▸ Helping people avoid stressors or cope with them more adaptively

    ▹ *Example*: Stress management classes for graduate students, smoking prevention classes, Drug Abuse Resistance Education (DARE)

▶ *Secondary prevention*: Aimed at decreasing the prevalence (number of existing cases) of mental disorders

  ▸ Early case-finding

  ▸ Screening

- Prompt and effective treatment
  - ▷ *Example*: Telephone hotlines, crisis intervention, disaster responses
- ▶ *Tertiary prevention:* Aimed at decreasing the disability and severity of a mental disorder
  - Rehabilitative services
  - Avoidance or postponement of complications
    - ▷ *Example*: Day treatment programs; case management for physical, housing, or vocational needs; social skills training.

Risk Factors

- ▶ Predisposing characteristics that make it more likely that a person will develop a disorder
- ▶ *Biological risk factors:* History of mental illness in family, poor nutritional status, poor general health
- ▶ *Psychological risk factors:* Poor self-concept, external locus of control, poor ego defenses
- ▶ *Social risk factors:* Stressful occupation, low socioeconomic status, poor level of social integration

Preventative Factors

- ▶ Factors that prevent or protect the person from the disorder
- ▶ Coping mechanisms or resources that facilitate a healthy response to stress
- ▶ *Biological preventative factors:* Without a history of mental illness in the family, healthy nutritional status, good general health
- ▶ *Psychological preventative factors:* Good self-esteem or self-concept, internal locus of control, healthy ego defenses
- ▶ *Social preventative factors:* Low-stress occupation, higher socioeconomic status, higher level of education

Risk Assessment

- ▶ Continuous monitoring of patients for high-risk situations
- ▶ Assessing patients for nonhealthy behaviors

Risk Management

- ▶ Activities or systems designed to recognize and intervene to reduce the risk of injury to patients
- ▶ Appropriate interventions that are implemented to reduce nonhealthy behaviors in patients and high-risk situations
- ▶ Functions to recognize and intervene to reduce subsequent claims against healthcare providers

Advance Directives

▶ May vary from state to state whether legally binding

▶ *Living will:* Document giving specific instructions while patient is mentally competent that providers must follow if client becomes incompetent

  ▸ Designates preferences for care if patient becomes incompetent or terminally ill

▶ *Durable power of attorney for health care:* Also known as *healthcare proxy*

  ▸ Designated in writing, an agent to act on behalf of an person should he or she become unable to make healthcare decisions

  ▸ Not limited to terminal illness, and also covers other aspects of illness, such as making financial decisions during a person's illness

  ▸ Should be considered as an aspect of relapse planning for patients with chronic psychiatric disorders

Culturally Competent Care

▶ Treating patients from diverse cultures, viewing each as a unique individual, and noting a potential relationship between the patients' cultural experiences and their symptom presentation and perceptions

▶ Assumes that if the NP becomes more sensitive to cultural issues surrounding the patient's symptoms and treatment, more comprehensive health care can be provided

▶ *Culture:* The learned beliefs and behaviors or the socially inherited characteristics that are common among all members of a group; may be a racial, social, ethnic, or religious grouping

▶ *Culture-bound syndromes:* Specific behaviors related to a person's culture and not linked to a psychiatric disorder

  ▸ Be cognizant of inaccurately judging a patient's behavior as psychopathology when it is really related to his or her culture.

Cultural Influences and Determinents of Health

▶ *Family:* A group of adults and children who are usually related and whose adults participate in carrying out the essential functions of providing food, clothing, shelter, safety, and education of children

  ▸ Concept broadened beyond the traditional husband–wife–children pattern

  ▸ Family initially teaches the belief patterns, religion, culture, and mores of a society.

▶ *Ethnicity:* Self-identified race, tribe, or nation with which a person or group identifies and which greatly influences beliefs and behavior

▶ *Community:* A group of families often sharing the same race, tribe, or culture and who have beliefs or behavior not shared by others

► *Environment:* Includes both physical and psychosocial factors; the general circumstances of a person's life:

- Social contacts
- Housing surroundings
- Climate
- Altitude
- Temperature
- Air pollution
- Fluoride in water
- Water contamination
- Crime
- Poverty
- Transportation

CULTURAL COMPETENCY

Homelessness

Homelessness is an enormous problem affecting the United States and the world. It can have devastating effects on individuals' and families' emotional and physical health. Drugs, alcohol, violence, and behavioral problems are just a few major issues faced by people who are homeless. The practitioner must be aware of the challenges faced by this vulnerable population. Possessing appropriate communication skills and knowledge of available resources are invaluable.

► Homeless individual or homeless person

  ▻ Persons who do not have stable or consistent nighttime housing or who maintain permanent residence at shelters, hotels, transitional housing, or public places not appropriate for human beings to live in; persons intended to be institutionalized who are in institutions for transitory residence

  ▻ Men, women, and children make up the homeless population. The number of homeless families is on the rise.

   ▻ The majority of homeless families are headed by a single parent, usually a woman.

    ▻ Female-headed households are at high risk for becoming homeless if the head of household has limited education or employment skills, low-paying employment with little or no benefits, and limited access to affordable housing.

    ▻ Teen mothers are at high risk due to lack of education and incomes that older parents possess.

   ▻ Reasons for homelessness:

    ▻ Mental illness

    ▻ Addictive disorders

    ▻ Poverty

    ▻ Unemployment

    ▻ Inadequate public assistance

    ▻ Domestic violence

    ▻ Lifestyle choice

- Mental illness and addictive disorders in the homeless population:

  - Approximately 50% of homeless people have co-occurring substance use disorders and serious mental illness, including bipolar disorder, schizophrenia, and depression.

  - Schizophrenia accounts for 15% to 45% of the U.S. homeless population (Sadock & Sadock, 2007).

  - Symptoms are often active and untreated.

  - Untreated serious mental illness results in symptoms such as paranoia, hallucinations, mania, anxiety, and depression, making it difficult for persons to maintain employment, relationships, and other activities of daily living.

  - Homeless people experiencing these problems with co-occurring disorders are at a greater risk for violence, medication noncompliance, and treatment resistance.

Strategies for Reducing Homelessness

- Outreach: Introducing services to homeless persons with serious mental illness in various settings, building an empathetic, consistent, and caring relationship to provide treatment.

- Integrated care: Treatment combining mental health and medical care to improve overall functioning in the community; may also include access to dental care and pharmacy services

  - Co-location: One site providing mental health and primary care services

- Supporting services to people in housing: Effective in moving homeless persons with serious mental illness directly to independent housing with support and intensive attention

- Prevention: Beginning with discharge planning in inpatient settings, provide resources for mental health care, housing, transitioning service, and follow-up

Migrant and Seasonal Farm Workers

- Migrants: Workers who leave their permanent residences to take agricultural jobs in different locations

- Seasonal: Workers who travel from their permanent residences seasonally for agricultural employment

- Men, women, and children of all cultures

- Estimated between 3 and 5 million in the United States (Hansen, 2003)

  - Hard to get an accurate census due to families and workers moving a great deal

- Working conditions, problems with the process of acculturation, isolation, discrimination, and impaired access to health care play a role in a high prevalence of mental illness among migrant and seasonal farm workers

- Very high incidence of depression, anxiety, and substance abuse

- Physical and emotional abuse of women is harder to address because of frequent changes of location.

▶ Meeting the mental health needs of this vulnerable population can pose a challenge because of the ways specific cultures perceive mental illness. Displaying an empathic, understanding, and culturally sensitive attitude is imperative when promoting care to this population.

Sexual Orientation

Possessing a thorough understanding of sexuality is of great importance when communicating with patients of different sexual orientations. The practitioner must possess an open, supportive, sensitive, empathetic attitude toward the patient. Understanding the patient's viewpoint and what he or she is seeking will help facilitate an effective psychiatric evaluation. In addition, an awareness of the factors the patient may have faced because of his or her sexuality is crucial.

▶ *Sexual identity:* How people identify psychologically on a continuum between female and male and to whom they are sexually or affectionately attracted (Sadock & Sadock, 2007)

▶ *Gender identity:* A person's identity along a continuum between normative constructs of masculinity and femininity

   ▸ Influences of gender identity may consist of biological and social factors.

   ▸ Biological factors may include pre- and postnatal hormone levels and gene expression.

   ▸ Social factors may include gender messages from family, mass media, and cultural attitudes.

   ▸ *Gender identity disorder* (GID) is the formal diagnosis to describe persons who experience significant gender dysphoria (discontent with their biological sex). It is a psychiatric classification in the *DSM-IV*.

▶ Sexual orientation: The direction of sexual attraction. Preferred over "sexual preference" or "lifestyle," which imply choice, whereas "orientation" does not. Some prefer "sexual identity" because it allows people to determine their own identities. Sexual orientation does not always relate to gender identity.

   ▸ *Asexual:* Not attracted to either sex

   ▸ *Bisexual:* Attracted to people of both sexes

   ▸ *Heterosexual:* Attracted to people of the opposite sex

   ▸ *Homosexual:* Attracted to people of the same sex

   ▸ *Transgender:* Umbrella term describing people whose gender identity does not conform to gender norms associated with the sex they were assigned at birth; does not imply a particular sexual orientation

   ▸ *Transsexual:* People who identify as the opposite gender from the one they were assigned at birth; some change their bodies hormonally and surgically to conform to their gender identity

   ▸ *GLBTQ:* Gay, lesbian, bisexual, transgender, and queer

   ▸ Many patients seek treatment from a provider of the same orientation

► *Sexual behavior:* The manner in which humans experience and express their sexuality; includes attracting partners, sexual interactions, and social interactions between individuals (Sadock & Sadock, 2007)

Forensics and Corrections

It is estimated that 15% to 24% of U.S. prisoners have severe mental illness resulting in the need for mental health care. Unfortunately, lack of synchronized care among criminal justice, mental, and public health systems results in repeat incarcerations (Baillargeon, Binswanger, Penn, Williams, & Murray, 2009; Kushel, Hahn, Evans, Bangsberg, & Moss, 2005). It is essential to remain neutral, calm, objective, and be skilled in self-reflective techniques as well as acknowledging one's own emotional response and biases when providing care for imprisoned patients. Lyons (2009) recommends that the practitioner compartmentalize emotional responses and biases temporarily then debrief after the fact.

► *Forensic:* The application of scientific knowledge to legal problems and legal proceedings, for example, in forensic anthropology, forensic dentistry, forensic medicine (legal medicine), forensic pathology, and forensic science

► *Forensic science:* The application of a broad range of sciences to answer questions of interest to the legal system; a high-technology field using electron microscopes, lasers, ultraviolet and infrared light, advanced analytical chemical techniques, and computerized databanks to analyze and research evidence

► *Forensic nursing:* The practice of nursing when health and legal systems intersect; the forensic nurse provides direct services to individual patients; consultation services to nursing, medical, and legal agencies; and expert court testimony in areas dealing with trauma or investigations of questioned deaths, adequacy of services delivery, and specialized diagnoses of specific conditions as related to nursing

Forensic vs. Correctional

► *Forensic:* Nurse–patient relationship based on crime committed and investigational aspect of the interaction

► *Correctional:* Nurse–patient relationship based on offender's current mental health and medical conditions

► Locations: Emergency departments, prisons (high-, medium-, and low-security units), courts, and police stations (Lyons, 2009)

Forensic Knowledge Base

► Relies on evidence-based practice and treatment practices as well as past clinical experience

► Incorporates both criminal justice and mental health systems

► Possess theoretical and practical knowledge of the criminal justice and mental health systems:

  ▻ Function of the court

  ▻ Litigation procedures

- Workings of the criminal justice system

- Relevant case law and health litigation

- Understanding of mental health, distorted thinking patterns, and impaired cognition

- Competence: Safety, security, management, and assessment of risk; management of aggression and violence; therapeutic relationship; offending behavior knowledge; prison culture; documentation; medical knowledge; psychopharmacology; and crisis de-escalation (Lyons, 2009)

Forensic Risk Assessment vs. Risk Assessment

► Forensic risk assessment: Protect the public from persons with known mental disorders having dangerous, violent, and criminal histories

- Risk assessment: Psychiatric evaluation performed in emergency department after arrest and before person is confined to a correctional facility (Lyons, 2009)

RESEARCH

► *Research utilization:* Process of synthesizing, disseminating, and using research-generated knowledge to make a change in practices; a subset of the broader evidence-based practice

- *Evidence-based practice:* The integration of best research evidence with clinical expertise and patient values and needs. *PMHNPs need to know the effectiveness of evidence-based interventions and select the intervention to be meet the patient need* (Perese, 2012, p. 29).

► Research utilization and evidence-based practice are two models for reducing the gap between research findings and application to practice

► *Research utilization process*

- Critique research

- Synthesize the findings

- Apply the findings

- Measure the outcomes

- Hierarchy of evidence has been identified by effectiveness of interventions (Figure 2–1) and effectiveness of meaning (Figure 2–2).

FIGURE 2-1. HIERARCHY OF EVIDENCE EFFECTIVENESS OF INTERVENTIONS

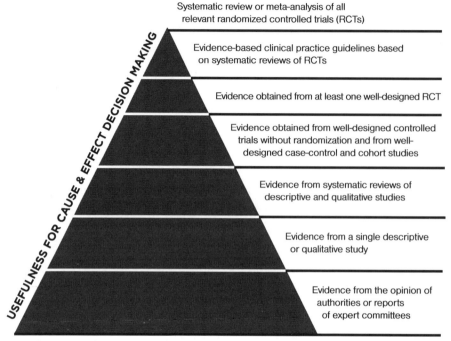

From "Transforming Health Care From the Inside Out: Advancing Evidence-Based Practice in the 21st Century" by E. Fineout-Overholt, B. M. Melnyk, & A. Schultz, 2005, *Journal of Professional Nursing, 21*(6), 335–344. Reprinted with permission.

FIGURE 2-2. EFFECTIVENESS OF MEANING

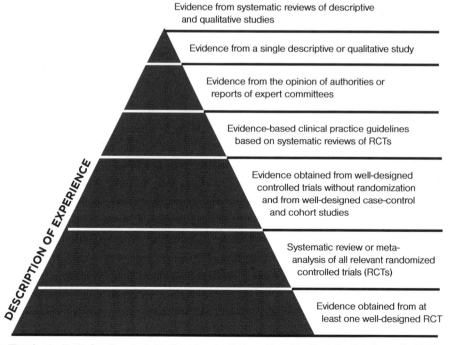

From "Transforming Health Care From the Inside Out: Advancing Evidence-Based Practice in the 21st Century" by E. Fineout-Overholt, B. M. Melnyk, & A. Schultz, 2005, *Journal of Professional Nursing, 21*(6), 335–344. Reprinted with permission.

- Develop a clinical question using the PICO method (Richardson, Wilson, Nishikawa, & Hayward, 1995).

  - P = patient, population of patients, problem

  - I = intervention

  - C = comparison (another treatment or therapy, placebo)

  - O = outcome

- Systematically search for relevant research evidence

- Critique the research evidence

- Make an evidence-based decision regarding implementation

- Implement the change, depending on the above decision

- Evaluate the change

Dissemination

- Presentations at local, regional and national conferences

- Publish in peer-reviewed journals

- Publish in professional newsletters (Melnyk, Fineout-Overholt, Stillwell, & Williamson, 2010).

Concepts in Interpreting Research Findings

- *Internal validity:* When the independent variable (the treatment) caused a change in the dependent variable (the outcome)

- *External validity:* When the sample is representative of the population and the results can be generalized

- *Descriptive statistics:* Used to describe the basic features of the data in the study; numerical values that summarize, organize, and describe observations; can be generated by either quantitative or qualitative studies

  - Examples include

    - *Mean:* Average of scores

    - *Standard deviation:* Indication of the possible deviations from the mean

    - *Variance:* How the values are dispersed around the mean; the larger the variance, the larger the dispersion of scores

- *Inferential statistics:* Numerical values that enable one to reach conclusions that extend beyond the immediate data alone; generated by quantitative research designs

  - Examples include

    - *t test:* Assesses whether the means of 2 groups are statistically different from each other

    - *Analysis of variance (ANOVA):* Tests the difference among 3 or more groups

▷ *Pearson's* r *correlation:* Tests the relationship between 2 variables

▷ *Probability:* Likelihood of an event occurring; lies between 0 and 1; an impossible event has a probability of 0, and a certain event has a probability of 1

▷ *p value:* Also known as *level of significance;* describes the probability of a particular result occurring by chance alone (if $p = .01$, there is a 1% probability of obtaining a result by chance alone)

► Ethical considerations in research

  ▸ *Institutional review boards (IRBs)* ensure that

    ▷ Risks to participants are minimized

    ▷ Participant selection is equitable

    ▷ Adverse events are reported and risks and benefits are reevaluated

    ▷ Informed consent is obtained and documented

    ▷ Data and safety monitoring plans are implemented when indicated

    ▷ Overall, the IRB protects the rights and welfare of human research participants and has the authority to approve, require modifications, or disapprove of any research activities

► All investigators and other persons involved in research studies must take and pass a test on protection of human participants—the *Belmont Report* (1979).

Quality Improvement

► Agency-specific projects that aim to improve systems, decrease cost, improve productivity

► Examine internal processes

► New knowledge is specific to an organization (Reinhardt & Ray, 2003)

Donabedian Model

► Structure

► Process

► Outcome

► May address the six dimensions of healthcare systems underpinnings of care: safe, effective, patient-centered, timely, efficient, and equitable (STEEP; IOM, 2001)

► Process of quality improvement can be PDSA cycle

  ▸ **Plan:** Plan the change

  ▸ **Do:** Carry out the plan

  ▸ **Study:** Examine the results

  ▸ **Act:** Decide what actions will improve the process

Healthcare Delivery Systems

► Health care is complex and fragmented; complexity science provides a framework to understand, design, and structure change

► Focus is on the interaction of the parts and relationships

► Nonlinear process (Matlow, Zimmerman, Thomson & Valente, 2006; Richardson, Cilliers & Lissack, 2001)

CASE STUDY

Karen Harris is a newly graduated PMHNP. She worked as a psychiatric nurse for 5 years before going to graduate school. She is considering a job at the local community mental health center. The director of the center has told her that her role would consist of seeing mainly adult patients with serious, chronic, and persistent mental illness.

On occasions when the psychiatrist is "busy," Ms. Harris is told she may be expected to see a few children in addition to adults. The director expects Ms. Harris to provide medication management to well-known patients and occasionally to assist in diagnostic evaluations of new patients or patients in crisis. He also expects that she will "from time to time" meet the emergent medical needs of patients who have limited access to primary care providers, including the routine, ongoing care of nonpsychiatric disorders such as diabetes, hypertension, and chronic pain. Ms. Harris has many issues to consider before deciding to take or not take the position:

► Would Ms. Harris be legally authorized to treat both children and adults?

► What regulation, rule, or standard should Ms. Harris consult to determine if she is legally allowed to treat both children and adults?

▸ What regulation, rule, or standard should Ms. Harris consult to determine if she is legally allowed to treat both physical and psychiatric disorders?

▸ What is the role of professional psychiatric nursing organizations in assisting Ms. Harris to determine the scope of practice that is appropriate for her as a new graduate?

Ms. Harris decides not to take that job and instead has been working for about a year as a PMHNP in a nurse-managed primary mental health clinic. One day she is asked to assess a patient who is clearly psychotic, experiencing hallucinations and delusions, and expressing verbal threats against many persons at another clinical practice in town who had "malpracticed me." The patient is adamant that he does not wish any treatment and that he is not ill. To care for this patient, Ms. Harris has many issues to consider:

► Is Ms. Harris able to treat the patient if he is not consenting to care?

► What legal standards must be met if she is to involuntarily treat this patient?

About 5 weeks later the above-mentioned patient returns to the clinic for follow-up care. He is clinically stable, on medication, and showing no active symptoms. He is interested in developing a relapse prevention plan and asks Ms. Harris to assist him in this process. Ms. Harris has many issues to consider:

▶ Is the inclusion of a durable power of attorney an appropriate strategy in relapse planning for this patient?

▶ What quality indicators should be considered in planning his care with the patient?

▶ What risk management and liability issues should Ms. Harris consider?

REFERENCES

Abood, S. (2007). Influencing health care in the legislative arena. *Online Journal of Issues in Nursing, 12*(1).

ACEN. (2013). *Influencing health care in the legislative arena.* Retrieved from http://www.nursingworld. org/MainMenuCategories/ANAMarketplace/ANAPeriodicals/OJIN/TableofContents/Volume122007/ No1Jan07/tpc32_216091.html

American Association of Critical-Care Nurses. (2013). *CCNE.* Retrieved from http://www.aacn.nche.edu/ ccne-accreditation/why-accreditation

American Nurses Association. (2000). *Medicare and "incidental to" payment: Coverage of nursing services in hospital outpatient clinics and emergency departments.* Washington, DC: American Nurses Association.

American Nurses Association. (2005). *Code of ethics for nurses.* Silver Spring, MD: Code of Ethics Project Task Force.

American Nurses Association. (2007). *Scope and standards of psychiatric mental health clinical nursing practice.* Silver Spring, MD: American Nurses Association.

American Psychiatric Association. (2000). *Diagnostic and statistical manual of mental disorders* (4th ed., text rev.). Washington, DC: American Psychiatric Association.

Brownson, R. C., & Petitti, D. (2006). *Applied epidemiology: Theory to practice* (2nd ed.). London: Oxford University Press.

Buppert, C. (2012). *Nurse practitioners business practice and legal guide* (4th ed.). Sudbury, MA: Jones & Bartlett Learning.

Burgess, A. W. (1998). *Advanced practice psychiatric nursing.* Stamford, CT: Appleton & Lange.

Cotroneo, M., Kurlowicz, L. H., Outlaw, F. H., Burgess, A. W., & Evans, L. K. (2001). Psychiatric mental health nursing at the interface: Revisioning education for the specialty. *Issues in Mental Health Nursing, 22,* 549–569.

Delaney, K., Chisholm, M., Clement, J., & Merwin, E. (1999). Trends in psychiatric mental health education. *Archives of Psychiatric Nursing, 13*(2), 67–73.

Donabedian, A. (1988). The quality of care. How can it be assessed? *JAMA, 260*(12), 1743-1748.

Edmunds, M. W., Horan, N. M., & Mayhew, M. S. (2000). *Adult nurse practitioner review manual.* Washington, DC: American Nurses Association.

Farnam, C., Zipple, A. M., Tyrell, W., & Chittiinanda, P. (1999). Health status risk factors of people with severe and persistent mental illness. *Journal of Psychosocial Nursing, 37,* 16–19.

Fineout-Overholt, E., Melnyk, B. M., & Schultz, A. (2005). Transforming health care from the inside out: Advancing evidence-based practice in the 21st century. *Journal of Professional Nursing, 21*(6), 335–344.

Ford, L. C. (1992). Advancing nursing practice: Future of the nurse practitioner. In L. H. Aiken & C. M. Fagin (Eds.), *Charting nursing's future: Agenda for the 1990s.* Philadelphia: J. B. Lippincott.

Friedman, D. J., Parrish, G., & Ross, D. A. (2013). Electronic health records and US public health: current realities and future promise. *American Journal of Public Health, 103*(9), 1560–1567.

Friedman, M. (2002). *Family nursing: Research, theory, and practice* (5th ed.). Stamford, CT: Appleton & Lange.

Harris, E., & Barraclough, B. (1999). Excess mortality of mental disorder. *British Journal of Psychiatry, 173,* 476–481.

Health Insurance Portability and Accountability Act (HIPAA). (1996). Public law 104-191.

Health Resources and Services Administration. (2013). *Health IT Adoption toolkit: Meaningful use.* Retrieved from http://www.hrsa.gov/healthit/toolbox/HealthITAdoptiontoolbox/index.html

Institute for the Future. (2000). *Health and health care 2010: The forecast, the challenge.* San Francisco: Jossey-Bass.

Institute of Medicine. (2001). *Crossing the quality chasm: A new health system for the 21st century.* Washington, DC: National Academic Press.

Institute of Medicine. (2010). *The future of nursing: Leading change, advancing health.* Retrieved from http://books.nap.edu/openbook/php?record_id=12956@page=R1.

Johnson, M., Maas, M., & Moorhead, S. (Eds.). (2003). *Nursing outcomes classification* (3rd ed). St. Louis, MO: Mosby.

Macnee, C., & McCabe, S. (2000). Micro stressors: The impact of hassles and uplifts. In V. H. Rice (Ed.), *Handbook of stress and coping: Implications for nursing research, theory, and practice* (pp. 125–142). Thousand Oaks, CA: Sage.

Matlow, A. G., Wright, J. G., & Zimmerman, B. (2006). How can the principles of complexity science be applied to improve the coordination of care for complex pediatric patients? *Quality and Safety in Health Care, 15,* 85–88.

McBride, A., & Austin, J. (1996). *Psychiatric mental health nursing: Integrating the behavioral and biological sciences.* Philadelphia: W. B. Saunders.

McCabe, S. (2000). Bringing psychiatric nursing into the twenty-first century. *Archives of Psychiatric Nursing, 14*(3), 109–116.

McCabe, S. (2002). The nature of psychiatric nursing: The intersection of paradigm, evolution, and history. *Archives of Psychiatric Nursing, 16*(2), 51–60.

McCabe, S., & Macnee, C. L. (2002). Weaving a new safety net of mental health care in rural America: A model of integrated practice. *Issues in Mental Health Nursing, 23,* 263–278.

McCloskey, J. C., & Bulechek, G. M. (Eds.). (2000). *Nursing interventions classification* (3rd ed.). St. Louis, MO: Mosby/Year Book.

Mellow, J. (1968). Nursing therapy. *American Journal of Nursing, 68,* 2365.

Melnyk, B. M., Fineout-Overholt, E., Stillwell, S. B., & Williamson, K. (2010). The seven steps of evidence-based practice. *American Journal of Nursing, 110*(1), 51–53.

Mirr Jansen, M., & Zwygart-Stauffacher, M. (2006). *Advanced practice nursing: Core concepts for professional role development* (3rd ed.). New York: Springer Publishing.

Nagle, M., & Krainovich-Miller, B. (2001). Shaping the advanced practice psychiatric nursing role: A futuristic model. *Issues in Mental Health Nursing, 22,* 461–482.

National Organization of Nurse Practitioner Faculties. (2003). *Psychiatric mental health nurse practitioner competencies.* Washington, DC: National Panel for Nurse Practitioner Faculties.

National Organization of Nurse Practitioner Faculties. (2006). *Domains and core competencies of nurse practitioner practice.* Washington, DC: National Panel for Nurse Practitioner Faculties.

Nettina, S. M., & Knudtson, M. (2001). *The family nurse practitioner review manual.* Washington, DC: American Nurses Credentialing Center.

North American Nursing Diagnosis Association. (2000). *Nursing diagnosis: Definitions and classifications 1999–2000*. Philadelphia: Author.

Northouse, P. G. (2007). *Leadership theory and practice* (4th ed). London: Sage Publications.

Peplau, H. (1952). *Interpersonal relations in nursing*. New York: GP Putnam's Sons.

Perese, E. F. (2012). *Psychiatric advanced practice nursing: A biopsychosoical foundation for practice*. Philadelphia: F. A. Davis.

Reinhardt, A. C., & Ray, L. N. (2003). Differentiating quality improvement from research. *Applied Nursing Research, 16*(1), 2–8.

Richardson, K. A., Cilliers, P., & Lissack, M. (2001). Complexity science: A "gray" science for the "stuff in between." *Emergence, 3*(2), 6–18.

Richardon, W. S., Wilson, M. C., Nishikawa, J., & Hayward, R. S. (1995). The well-built clinical question: A key to evidence based decisions. *ACP Journal Club, 123*(3), A12–A13.

Sadock, B., & Sadock, V. (2007). *Kaplan and Sadock's synopsis of psychiatry* (10th ed.). New York: Lippincott Williams & Wilkins.

Shea, C. A., Pelletier, L., Poster, E. C., Stuart, G. W., & Verhey, M. P. (1999). *Advanced practice nursing in psychiatric mental health care*. St. Louis, MO: Mosby.

Sherwood, G. D., & Horton-Deutsch, S. (2012). *Reflective practice transforming education and improving outcomes*. Indianapolis, IN: Sigma Theta Tau International.

Stuart, G. W., & Laraia, M. T. (2004). *Principles and practice of psychiatric nursing* (8th ed.). St. Louis, MO: Mosby.

Tarasoff v. The Regents at the University of California, Supreme Court of California. (1976).

U.S. Department of Health, Education, and Welfare. (1979). *The Belmont Report*. Washington, DC: Author.

U.S. Department of Health and Human Services. (2000). *Mental health: A report of the Surgeon General*. Washington, DC: Substance Abuse and Mental Health Service Administration, National Institute of Mental Health.

U.S. Department of Health and Human Services. (2005). *Healthy People 2010*. Washington, DC: Office of Disease Prevention and Health Promotion.

World Health Organization. (2007). *International classification of diseases* (9th rev.). Geneva: World Health Organization Assembly.

CHAPTER 3

THEORETICAL BASIS OF CARE

Although the psychiatric–mental health nurse practitioner (PMHNP) role is relatively new, psychiatric–mental health nursing has a long, well-established, and cherished tradition of advanced practice. As with all other specialty areas of nursing, advanced practice psychiatric nursing is theoretically grounded, and a wide array of theories form the basis of the PMHNP role. These theories help identify the foundational, core concepts of advanced-practice psychiatric nursing. The scope of practice for the PMHNP is based on an understanding of foundational core concepts and the theories (Marriner-Tomey & Alligood, 2005).

This chapter reviews the concepts of biopsychosocial theories that underpin PMHNP practice.

BIOPSYCHOSOCIAL FRAMEWORK OF CARE

RECOVERY

▶ Recovery is the single most important goal in the transformation of mental health care of the past 2 decades (Substance Abuse and Mental Health Services Administration [SAMHSA], 2006).

▶ In an effort to make recovery for person's with mental illness possible, there is a new emphasis on shared decision-making, peer support, and self-direction (SAMHSA, 2006).

▶ PMHNP interventions follow evidence-based practice guidelines, are always patient goal–directed, and take into account the patient's ethnicity and culture.

▶ PMHNPs help patients to recognize strengths, set attainable goals, and have hope for their future.

▶ A key part of the PMHNP's work is to utilize empirical evidence in educating their patients, patient families, and the community about psychiatric illness and effective management of their illness.

► The PMHNP oversees and guides the psychiatric–mental health nurse in designing evidence-based health information and educational programs that are geared to patient learning needs, ability, and readiness to learn.

► PMHNPs care for patients with co-occurring medical and psychiatric disorders.

► Principles of mental health recovery are integrated into all levels of mental health care (American Psychiatric Nurses Association, 2012).

CLASSIFICATION OF PSYCHIATRIC DISORDERS: *DSM-IV-TR, DSM-V*

DSM-IV-TR

► Prior to May of 2013, psychiatric disorders were classified using standard criteria of the *Diagnostic and Statistical Manual of Mental Disorders* (*DSM-IV-TR;* American Psychiatric Association, 2000).

► The *DSM-IV-TR* classifies mental illnesses on the basis of specific criteria that have been tested for reliability when used by mental health professionals.

► The *DSM-IV-TR* classification system uses a multiaxial approach (see Table 3–1) to diagnostic classifications that allows for holistic assessment.

► A patient is assessed in five general areas, and each area is individually coded as an axis.

► Each axis represents a specific assessment and, when taken together, the five axes represent the totality of a person's psychosocial–biological functioning, not merely the assessment of a single psychiatric disorder (see Table 3–1)

DSM-V

► The *DSM-V* classifies mental illnesses on the basis of specific criteria that have been tested for reliability when used by mental health professionals.

► Emphasizes dimensional assessments

► Aligns diagnosis with *The International Classification of Diseases* (ICD)

TABLE 3-1. *DSM-IV-TR* MULTIAXIAL CLASSIFICATION SCHEMA

DEFINITION	DISORDER EXAMPLE
▶ Clinical disorders; other conditions that may be the focus of clinical attention	▶ Mood disorders ▶ Anxiety disorders ▶ Psychotic disorders ▶ Disorders usually diagnosed in infancy, childhood, and adolescence
▶ Personality disorders ▶ Mental retardation ▶ Prominent maladaptive personality features ▶ Defense mechanisms	▶ Borderline personality disorder ▶ Antisocial personality disorder ▶ Image-distorting defense mechanisms
▶ General medical condition potentially relevant to the management of Axis I or II disorders	▶ Diseases of the nervous system ▶ Endocrine disorders ▶ Conditions originating in the perinatal period
▶ Psychosocial and environmental problems	▶ Problems with primary supports ▶ Problems related to social environment ▶ Housing problems ▶ Problems with access to health care
▶ Global assessment of functioning (GAF)	▶ Clinician's judgment of the client's overall functioning documented on a scale of 0–100, with the higher number indicating highest level of functioning. The highest and lowest GAF scored in the last 6 months (sometimes 1 year) is also documented.

THERAPEUTIC RELATIONSHIP

▶ Assumes the patient and nurse enter into a mutual, interactive, interpersonal relationship specifically to focus on the identified needs of the patient.

▶ Therapeutic relationships are focused on the patient's needs, and are goal-directed, theory-based, and open to supervision.

▶ Characteristics of a therapeutic relationship:

  ▹ Genuineness

  ▹ Acceptance

  ▹ Nonjudgmental attitude

  ▹ Authenticity

  ▹ Empathy

  ▹ Respect

  ▹ Professional boundaries

▶ The therapeutic relationship is seen as having specific and sequential phases (see Table 3–2).

▶ *Transference* and *countertransference* are key concepts in the nurse–patient relationship.

  ▹ *Transference:* Displacement of feelings for significant people in the patient's past onto the PMHNP in the present relationship

  ▹ *Countertransference:* Represents the nurse's emotional reaction to the patient based on her or his past experiences

TABLE 3-2. PHASES OF A THERAPEUTIC NURSE-PATIENT RELATIONSHIP

PHASE	NURSING ACTION	COMMON PATIENT BEHAVIOR
Introduction (Orientation)	▸ Creating a trusting environment ▸ Establishing professional boundaries ▸ Establishing the length of anticipated interaction ▸ Providing diagnostic evaluation ▸ Setting mutually agreed-upon treatment objectives	▸ Initial hesitancy by the patient to participate fully in assessment and treatment planning (approach avoidance)
Working (Identification and Exploitation)	▸ Clarifying patient expectations and mutually set goals ▸ Implementing treatment plan ▸ Monitoring health ▸ Undertaking preventative health care ▸ Measuring outcomes of care ▸ Evaluating outcomes of care ▸ Reprioritizing plan and objectives as indicated	▸ Transference—patient (countertransference—nurse) ▸ Patient resistance to care practices ▸ Patient resistance to change
Termination (Resolution)	▸ Reviewing patient's progress toward objectives ▸ Establishing long-term plan of care ▸ Focusing on self-management strategies ▸ Disengaging from relationship ▸ Referring patient to other services as needed	▸ Patient resistance to termination ▸ Regression ▸ Re-emergence of symptoms or problems

Adapted from *Psychiatric Nursing* (5th ed.) by N. Keltner, L. H. Schwecke, & C. E. Bostrom, 2006, St. Louis, MO: Mosby.

▸ Signs indicating the presence of countertransference in the PMHNP include:

- ▹ Intense emotional reactions, positive or negative, on first contact with patient

- ▹ Recurrent anxiety or uneasiness while dealing with the patient

- ▹ Uncharacteristic carelessness in interaction and follow-up with patient

- ▹ Difficulty empathizing

- ▹ Resistance to others treating or interacting with the patient

- ▹ Preoccupation or dreaming about the patient

- ▹ Frequently running overtime or cutting time short with patient

- ▹ Depression or other strong emotions during or after interaction with patient

- ▹ Feedback from others over involvement with patient

▸ The PMHNP is expected to monitor her or his reaction to patients to constantly assess for the presence of countertransference.

▸ If identified, countertransference is usually dealt with through the supervisory process and in talking to coworkers about the issues.

- ▹ Provided in peer–peer or peer–supervisor relationship

- ▹ Examines interpersonal dynamics inherent in the PMHNP's relationship with patients

DEVELOPMENTAL THEORIES

► Growth, change, and development are a part of the dynamic, constant life process of being human.

► Humans develop uniquely from simple to complex.

► The health states of individuals and families can be viewed over a continuum of development.

► Developmental stages and the milestones or tasks that accompany them give insight into age-appropriate behaviors, measure levels of comprehension for patient teaching, and provide a context within which to evaluate assessment data (see Table 3–3).

Example: The mental status finding of concrete thinking in a 9-year-old patient would be normal and expected; however, the same finding in a 29-year-old patient is nonnormative and suggestive of psychopathology (see Table 3–4 for typical age of onset for psychiatric disorders).

TABLE 3-3. ERIK ERIKSON'S (1902–1994) STAGES OF HUMAN DEVELOPMENT

DEVELOPMENTAL STAGE	AGE	DEVELOPMENTAL TASK	INDICATIONS OF DEVELOPMENTAL MASTERY	INDICATIONS OF DEVELOPMENTAL FAILURE
Infancy	0–1 year	Trust vs. mistrust	Ability to form meaningful relationships, hope about the future, trust in others	Poor relationships, lack of future hope, suspicious of others
Early childhood	1–3 years	Autonomy vs. shame and doubt	Self-control, self-esteem, willpower	Poor self-control, low self-esteem, self-doubt, lack of independence
Late childhood	3–6 years	Initiative vs. guilt	Self-directed behavior, goal formation, sense of purpose	Lack of self-initiated behavior, lack of goal orientation
School age	6–12 years	Industry vs. inferiority	Ability to work; sense of competency and achievement	Sense of inferiority; difficulty with working, learning
Adolescence	12–20 years	Identity vs. role confusion	Personal sense of identity	Identify confusion, poor self-identification in group settings
Early adulthood	20–35 years	Intimacy vs. isolation	Committed relationships, capacity to love	Emotional isolation, egocentrism
Middle adulthood	35–65 years	Generativity vs. self-absorption or stagnation	Ability to give time and talents to others, ability to care for others	Self-absorption, inability to grow and change as a person, inability to care for others
Late adulthood	> 65 years	Integrity vs. despair	Fulfillment and comfort with life, willingness to face death, insight and balanced perspective on life's events	Bitterness, sense of dissatisfaction with life, despair over impending death

Adapted from *Kaplan and Sadock's Synopsis of Psychiatry* (10th ed.) by B. Sadock, & V. Sadock, 2007, New York: Lippincott Williams & Wilkins.

TABLE 3–4. EXAMPLES OF TYPICAL AGE OF ONSET FOR COMMON PSYCHIATRIC DISORDERS

DISORDER	AGE OF ONSET
Mental retardation	Infancy—usually evident at birth
Attention-deficit hyperactivity disorder	4 to 6 years
Schizophrenia	18 to 25 years for men 25 to 35 years for women
Major depression	Late adolescence to young adulthood
Dementia	Most common after age 85

Adapted from *Kaplan and Sadock's Synopsis of Psychiatry* (10th ed.) by B. Sadock, & V. Sadock, 2007, New York: Lippincott Williams & Wilkins.

FOUNDATIONAL THEORIES SUPPORTING PMHNP ROLE

▶ Psychodynamic (Psychoanalytic) Theory (Sigmund Freud, 1856–1939)

- ► Focus is on concepts of intrapsychic conflict among the structures of the mind
- ► Initially designed to explain neurosis and conditions of high anxiety such as phobias and hysteria
- ► Theory later expanded to include normal and abnormal development and personality development.
- ► Basic tenets of psychodynamic theory
  - ▷ Psychoanalytic theory assumes that all behavior is purposeful and meaningful. All behavior has meaning.
  - ▷ *Principle of Psychic Determinism:* Even apparently meaningless, random, or accidental behavior is actually motivated by underlying unconscious mental content.

Example: A person forgets where he parked the car because he really does not wish to go wherever it was that he was headed.

- ► Most mental activity is unconscious—urges, feelings, and fantasies that would be unacceptable to the person's values if consciously experienced.
- ► Conscious behaviors and choices are affected by unconscious mental content.
- ► Past childhood experiences shape adult personality.
- ► Instincts, urges, or fantasies function as drives that motivate thoughts, feelings, and behaviors.
- ► Two types of normal drives: sexual drives (libido) and aggressive drives
- ► Drives affect behavior as a person attempts to deal with the associated feelings and seeks gratification through release of the tension that the drives produce.

- Normally, different actions and behaviors are used at different ages to discharge tension from drives and to therefore seek gratification.

- Psychosexual stages of development have been identified to show the age-related behaviors commonly used for discharging drives and obtaining gratification (see Table 3–5).

TABLE 3-5. FREUD'S PSYCHOSEXUAL STAGES OF DEVELOPMENT

STAGE	AGE	PRIMARY MEANS OF DISCHARGING DRIVES AND ACHIEVING GRATIFICATION	PSYCHIATRIC DISORDER LINKED TO FAILURE OF STAGE
Oral stage	0–18 months	Sucking, chewing, feeding, crying	Schizophrenia Substance abuse Paranoia
Anal stage	18 months– 3 years	Sphincter control, activities of expulsion and retention	Depressive disorders
Phallic stage	3–6 years	Exhibitionism, masturbation with focus on Oedipal conflict, castration anxiety, and female fear of lost maternal love	Sexual identity disorders
Latency stage	6 years– puberty	Peer relationships, learning, motor-skills development, socialization	Inability to form social relationships
Genital stage	Puberty forward	Integration and synthesis of behaviors from early stages, primary genital-based sexuality	Sexual perversion disorders

Adapted from *Kaplan and Sadock's Synopsis of Psychiatry* (10th ed.) by B. Sadock, & V. Sadock, 2007, New York: Lippincott Williams & Wilkins.

▶ Three primary psychic structures make up the mind and personality and are responsible for mental functioning:

- The Id

  ▷ Contains primary drives or instincts, urges (hunger, sex, or aggression), or fantasies

  ▷ Drives are largely unconscious, sexual or aggressive in content, and infantile in nature

  ▷ Operates on the pleasure principle; seeks immediate satisfaction

  ▷ Is present at birth and motivates early infantile actions

  ▷ The id says, "I want."

- The Ego

  ▷ Contains the concept of *external reality*

  ▷ Rational mind; responsible for logical and abstract thinking

  ▷ Functions in adaptation

  ▷ Mediates between the demands of drives and environmental realities

- ▷ Operates on the reality principle
- ▷ Begins to develop at birth as infant struggles to deal with environment
- ▷ Responsible for use of defense mechanisms
- ▷ The ego says, "I think, I evaluate."
- ▹ The Superego
  - ▷ Is the ego-ideal
  - ▷ Contains sense of conscience or right vs. wrong
  - ▷ Also contains aspirations, ideals, and moral values
  - ▷ Regulated by guilt and shame
  - ▷ Begins to fully develop around age 6 as a child comes into contact with external authority figures such as parents, schoolteachers, coaches, or religious figures
  - ▷ The superego says "I should or ought."
- ► Psychic structures commonly come into conflict over what to do to achieve gratification.
- ► Although the exact nature of conflict is often unconscious, conflict is experienced consciously as anxiety.
- ► The function of anxiety is to alert the conscious mind to the presence of conflict.
- ► Conflict is normally dealt with through the use of defense mechanisms (see Table 3–6), which:
  - ▹ Are a function of the ego
  - ▹ Are unconsciously called into action
  - ▹ Are used to reduce anxiety
  - ▹ Become part of the personality
  - ▹ Maintain a sense of safety
  - ▹ Promote self-esteem and a sense of well-being
  - ▹ May be used episodically or habitually
  - ▹ May be used constantly and become fixed, as seen in neurosis.

TABLE 3-6. DEFENSE MECHANISMS

DEFENSE MECHANISM	EXPLANATION
Denial	Avoidance of unpleasant realities by unconsciously ignoring their existence
Projection	Unconscious rejection of emotionally unacceptable personal attributes, beliefs, or actions by attributing them to other people, situations, or events
Regression	Return to more comfortable thoughts, behaviors, or feelings used in earlier stages of development in response to current conflict, stress, or threat
Repression	Unconscious exclusion of unwanted, disturbing emotions, thoughts, or impulses from conscious awareness
Reaction formation	Often called *overcompensation;* unacceptable feelings, thoughts, or behaviors are pushed from conscious awareness by displaying and acting on the opposite feeling, thought, or behavior
Rationalization	Justification of illogical, unreasonable ideas, feelings, or actions by developing an acceptable explanation that satisfies the person
Undoing	Behaviors that attempt to make up for or undo an unacceptable action, feeling, or impulse
Intellectualization	Attempts to master current stressor or conflict by expansion of knowledge, explanation, or understanding
Suppression	Conscious analog of repression; conscious denial of a disturbing situation, feeling, or event
Sublimation	Unconscious process of substitution of socially acceptable, constructive activity for strong unacceptable impulse
Altruism	Meeting the needs of others in order to discharge drives, conflicts, or stressors

Adapted from *Advanced Practice Nursing in Psychiatric Mental Health Care* by C. A. Shea, L. Pelletier, E. C. Poster, G. W. Stuart, & M. P. Verhey, 1999, St. Louis, MO: Mosby.

▶ Cognitive Theory (Jean Piaget, 1896–1980)

    ▸ Piaget believed that human development evolves through cognition, learning, and comprehending.

    ▸ He believed that factors such as native endowment and biological and environmental factors set the course for a child's development.

    ▸ He developed 4 stages of cognitive development:

        1. *Sensorimotor* (Birth–2 years): The critical achievement of this stage is *object permanence:* the ability to understand that objects have an existence independent of the child's involvement with them

        2. *Preoperational* (2–7 years): More extensive use of language and symbolism; magical thinking

        3. *Concrete Operations* (7–12 years): Child begins to use logic; develops concepts of reversibility and conservation

            ▷ *Reversibility:* The realization that one thing can turn into another and back again (e.g., water and ice)

▷ *Conservation:* Ability to recognize that although the shape of objects may change, it will still maintain characteristics that enable it to be recognized as that object (e.g., clay)

4. *Formal Operations* (12 years–adult): Ability to think abstractly; thinking operates in a formal, logical manner.

▶ Interpersonal Theory (Harry Stack Sullivan, 1892–1949)

» Behavior occurs because of interpersonal dynamics.

» Interpersonal relationships and experiences influence one's personality development, which is called the *self-system* (the total components of personality traits).

» Understanding behavior requires understanding the relationships in the person's life.

» Two drives for person's behavior: the *drive for satisfaction* (basic human drives such as sleep, sex, hunger) and the *drive for security* (conforming to social norms of a person's reference group).

» When the person's need for satisfaction and security is interfered with by the self-system, mental illness occurs.

» Humans experience anxiety and behavior is directed towards relieving the anxiety, which then results in *interpersonal security*.

» Sullivan also described *stages of interpersonal development* (see Table 3–7).

TABLE 3-7. SULLIVAN'S STAGES OF INTERPERSONAL DEVELOPMENT

STAGE	TIME PERIOD	DEVELOPMENTAL TASK
Infancy	Birth–18 months	Oral gratification; anxiety occurs for the first time
Childhood	18 months–6 years	Delayed gratification
Juvenile	6–9 years	Forming of peer relationships
Preadolescence	9–12 years	Same-sex relationships
Early adolescence	12–14 years	Opposite-sex relationships
Late adolescence	14–21 years	Self-identity developed

Adapted from *Kaplan and Sadock's Synopsis of Psychiatry* (10th ed.) by B. Sadock, & V. Sadock, 2007, New York: Lippincott Williams & Wilkins.

▶ Hierarchy of Needs Theory (Abraham Maslow, 1908–1970)

» Health model rather than illness model

» A hierarchical organization of needs

» Hypothesizes that certain needs are more important than others

» States that a person will attempt to meet more important needs first before satisfying other needs

- Hierarchy of needs:
  - Survival
    - Water
    - Air
    - Food
    - Sleep
  - Safety and security needs
    - Protection from harm: emotional and physical
  - Love and belonging
    - Affection, intimacy, and companionship
  - Self-esteem
    - Sense of worth
  - Self-actualization
    - Achieving one's potential
    - Being all that one can be

► Health Belief Model (Marshall Becker, 1940–1993)
  - Explains that healthy people do not always take advantage of screening or preventative programs because of certain variables:
    - Perception of susceptibility
    - Seriousness of illness
    - Perceived benefits of treatment
    - Perceived barriers to change
    - Expectations of efficacy

► Transtheoretical Model of Change
  - States that change such as in health behaviors occur in six predictable stages (Prochaska, Norcross, & DiClemente, 1992):
    - *Precontemplation:* The person has no intention to change.
    - *Contemplation:* The person is thinking about changing; is aware that there is a problem but not committed to changing.
    - *Preparation:* The person has made the decision to change; is ready for action.
    - *Action:* The person is engaging in specific, overt actions to change.
    - *Maintenance:* The person is engaging in behaviors to prevent relapse.

- Self-Efficacy/Social Learning Theory (Albert Bandura, born 1925)
  - Behavior is the result of cognitive and environmental factors.
  - People learn by observing others, relying on role-modeling.
  - *Self-efficacy* is the perception of one's ability to perform a certain task at a certain level of accomplishment.
  - Behavioral change and maintenance are a function of outcome expectations and efficacy expectations.

NURSING THEORIES

- Theory of Cultural Care (Madeline Leininger, born 1925)
  - Regardless of the culture, care is the unifying focus and the essence of nursing.
  - Health and well-being can be predicted through cultural care.
- Theory of Self Care (Dorothy Orem, 1914–2007)
  - *Self-care:* Activities that maintain life, health, and well-being
- Therapeutic Nurse–Patient Relationship Theory/Interpersonal Theory (Hildegard Peplau, 1909–1999)
  - First significant psychiatric nursing theory
  - Based in part on interpersonal theory (Sullivan)
  - Sees nursing as an interpersonal process in which all interventions occur within the context of the nurse–patient relationship.
  - States that the therapeutic nurse–patient relationship is central to nursing
  - Includes phases of the nurse–patient relationship (see Table 3–2):
    - Orientation phase
    - Working phase (identification, exploitation)
    - Termination phase (resolution)
  - Promotes concept that adaptive responses are the goal of nursing
  - States that behavior represents the person trying to adapt to internal or environmental forces
- Caring Theory (Jean Watson, born 1940)
  - Caring is an essential component of nursing.
  - "Carative factors" guide the core of nursing and should be implemented in health care.
  - Carative factors are those aspects of care which potentiate therapeutic healing and relationships.

CASE STUDY

Thomas is a 19-year-old college freshman. During the second week of classes, he presented to his college's student health services clinic seeking help for "shyness." As the PMHNP, you are responsible for assessment and care planning with this patient.

As you begin working with him, he gives a chief complaint of feeling uncomfortable around the new people he meets and of a desire to return home and drop out of school. There are several issues for you to consider as you continue to work with Thomas.

▶ Chronologically, what stage of development should Thomas be experiencing?

▶ What are the tasks of this stage?

▶ How would you assess the actual developmental issues that he is experiencing?

    ▹ What factors do you need to consider to determine whether he is experiencing normative or nonnormative behaviors?

    ▹ What characteristic do you as the PMHNP need to display to establish a therapeutic relationship with him?

Thomas reported that he has not been sleeping well, has experienced a decrease in appetite, and just wants to talk to someone about his problems in adjusting to school. In planning the follow-up care for Thomas, you have many issues to consider.

▶ What would be the goal of continued work with Thomas?

▶ If you were to start therapy with him, what kind of therapy would you consider?

▶ Would you consider him to have a mental illness?

REFERENCES

American Nurses Association. (2010). *Nursing: Scope and standards of practice* (2nd ed.). Silver Spring, MD: Nursebooks.org.

American Psychiatric Association. (2000). *Diagnostic and statistical manual of mental disorders* (4th ed., text rev.). Arlington, VA: American Psychiatric Publishing,

American Psychiatric Association. (2013). *Diagnostic and statistical manual of mental disorders* (5th ed.). Arlington, VA: American Psychiatric Publishing.

American Psychiatric Nurses Association. (2012). *Psychiatric mental health nursing: Scope and standards of practice (Draft).*

Burgess, A. W. (1998). *Advanced practice psychiatric nursing.* Stamford, CT: Appleton & Lange.

Erikson, E. H. (1963). *Childhood and society.* New York: Basic Books.

Haley, J. (1996). *Learning and teaching therapy.* New York: Guilford Press.

Keltner, N., Schwecke, L. H., & Bostrom, C. E. (2006). *Psychiatric nursing* (5th ed.). St. Louis, MO: Mosby.

Kerr, M., & Bowen, M. (1989). *Family evaluation: An approach based on Bowen theory.* New York: W. W. Norton.

Freud, S. (1934). *The ego and the id.* New York: W. W. Norton.

Freud, S. (1936). *The problem of anxiety.* New York: Basic Books.

Marsh, D. (1998). *Serious mental illness and the family: The practitioner's guide.* New York: John Wiley.

Minuchin, S., & Fishman, H. (1981). *Family therapy techniques.* Cambridge, MA: Harvard University Press.

Mohr, W. (2000). Partnering with families. *Journal of Psychosocial Nursing, 38,* 15–19.

National Institute of Mental Health (NIMH). (1990). *Decade of the brain.* Washington, DC: Author.

Peplau, H. (1952). *Interpersonal relations in nursing.* New York: Putnam.

Prochaska, J., & DiClemente, C. (1984). *The transtheoretical approach: Crossing traditional boundaries therapy.* Homewood, IL: Dow Jones Irwin.

Prochaska, J., Norcross, J., & DiClemente, C. (1992). In search of how people change: Applications to addictive behaviors. *American Psychologist, 47*(9), 1102–1112.

Sadock, B., & Sadock, V. (2007). *Kaplan and Sadock's synopsis of psychiatry* (10th ed.). New York: Lippincott Williams & Wilkins.

Shea, C. A., Pelletier, L., Poster, E. C., Stuart, G. W., & Verhey, M. P. (1999). *Advanced practice nursing in psychiatric mental health care.* St. Louis, MO: Mosby.

Sherman, C. (2000). Assessment is good opportunity to change family dynamics. *Clinical Psychiatric News, 3,* 25–29.

Stuart, G. W., & Laraia, M. (2004). *Principles and practice of psychiatric nursing.* St. Louis, MO: Mosby.

The Substance Abuse and Mental Health Services Administration. (2005). *Transforming mental health care in America. The Federal Action Agenda: First steps.* DHHS Pub. No. SMA-05-4060. Rockville, MD: Author.

Sullivan, H. S. (1953). *Interpersonal theory of psychiatry.* New York: Basic Books.

Yalom, I. (2005). *The theory and practice of group psychotherapy* (5th ed.). New York: Basic Books.

CHAPTER 4

NEUROANATOMY, NEUROPHYSIOLOGY, AND BEHAVIOR

A tremendous expansion of knowledge about the brain has occurred in the past two decades. As more has been learned about the brain and its complex functioning, assessment and treatment for psychiatric disorders have been altered dramatically. Increasingly, the links among genetics, altered brain anatomy and physiology, and the symptoms of psychiatric disorders have been identified (Sadock & Sadock, 2007).

This growing knowledge base will continue to alter the treatment of psychiatric disorders. As new knowledge is disseminated, it is helping diminish the stigma long associated with psychiatric illness.

This chapter reviews the basics of neuroanatomy and physiology that provide the scientific rational for many of the psychiatric–mental health nurse practitioner (PMHNP) care practices, including psychopharmacological interventions described elsewhere in this review book. PMHNPs need a solid grounding in neurobiology. Increasingly, the roles of the PMHNP require the application of this knowledge to clinical practice.

THE NERVOUS SYSTEM

- ▶ All human thoughts, feelings, and actions are seated in and start with actions of the nervous system.
- ▶ Necessary for the PMHNP's role functioning is an understanding of the following basic neuroanatomy and physiology:
  - » Neurodeficits that underlie psychiatric disorders
  - » Actions of and patient responses to psychopharmacological treatment agents.
- ▶ The nervous system's primary function is to transfer and exchange information.

The Neuron ("Nerve Cells")

▶ The basic cellular unit of the nervous system

▶ The microprocessor of the brain responsible for conducting impulses from one part of the body to another

▶ Components of the neuron:

  ▹ *Cell body*: Also known as *soma;* made up of the nucleus and cytoplasm within cell

  ▹ membrane

  ▹ *Stem or axon*: Transmits signals *away* from the neuron's cell body to connect with other neurons and cells

  ▹ *Dendrites*: Collect incoming signals from other neurons and send the signal *toward* the neuron's cell body.

Nervous System

▶ Composed of two separate, interconnected divisions:

  ▹ Central nervous system (CNS)

    ▹ Composed of the spinal cord and the brain

  ▹ Peripheral nervous system (PNS)

    ▹ Composed of the peripheral nerves that connect the CNS to receptors, muscles, and glands

    ▹ Includes the cranial nerves just outside the brainstem

    ▹ Composed of the somatic nervous system and the autonomic nervous system:

      ▹ *Somatic nervous system*: Conveys information from the CNS to skeletal muscles; responsible for voluntary movement

      ▹ *Autonomic nervous system:* Regulates internal body functions to maintain homeostasis; conveys information from the CNS to smooth muscle, cardiac muscle, and glands; responsible for involuntary movement; divided into the sympathetic nervous system and the parasympathetic nervous system:

        ▹ *Sympathetic nervous system:* The excitatory division; prepares the body for stress (fight or flight); stimulates or increases activity of organs

        ▹ *Parasympathetic nervous system:* Maintains or restores energy; inhibits or decreases activity of organs.

NEUROANATOMY AND THE BRAIN

▶ Brain tissue is categorized as either white matter or gray matter.

  ▹ *White matter* is the myelinated axons of neurons.

  ▹ *Gray matter* is composed of nerve cell bodies and dendrites; is the working area of the brain; and contains the synapses or area of neuronal connection.

▶ *Outermost surface of the brain:* Structured to contain grooves and dips of corrugated wrinkles within the brain tissue to provide anatomical landmarks or reference points.

  ▹ Functions to increase brain's surface area

   ▷ Increases working area and cell communication area

  ▹ Grooves and dips named by size and depth

   ▷ *Sulci:* Small, shallow grooves

   ▷ *Fissures:* Deeper grooves extending into the brain

  ▹ *Gyri* are the raised tissue areas.

▶ Distinct anatomical areas of brain

  ▹ The brain is subdivided into the cerebrum and the brainstem.

Cerebrum

▶ Largest part of the brain, which is divided into two halves, the right and left cerebral hemispheres

  ▹ *Left hemisphere:* Dominant in most people; controls most right-sided body functions

  ▹ *Right hemisphere:* Controls most left-sided body functions

  ▹ Normal functioning requires effective coordination of two hemispheres

  ▹ Both hemispheres connected by a large bundle of white matter, the *corpus callosum,* an area of sensorimotor information exchange between the two hemispheres

  ▹ Each hemisphere is divided into four major lobes, which work in an interactive and integrated manner, and each with a distinct function.

   ▷ *Frontal lobe:* Largest and most developed lobe

    ▹ Functions include

     ▷ *Motor function:* Responsible for controlling voluntary motor activity of specific muscles

     ▷ *Premotor area:* Coordinates movement of multiple muscles

     ▷ *Association cortex:* Allows for multimodal sensory input to trigger memory and lead to decision-making

     ▷ *Seat of executive functions:* Working memory, reasoning, planning, prioritizing, sequencing behavior, insight, flexibility, judgment, impulse control, behavioral cueing, intelligence, abstraction

     ▷ *Language (Broca's area):* Expressive speech

     ▷ *Personality variables:* The most focal area for personality development

     ▷ Problems in the frontal lobe can lead to personality, emotional, and intellectual changes.

▷ *Temporal lobe*

  ▸ Functions include:

    ▷ Language (Wernicke's area): Receptive speech or language comprehension

      ▸ Primary auditory area

    ▷ Memory

    ▷ Emotion

    ▷ Integration of vision with sensory information

  ▸ Problems in the temporal lobe can lead to visual or auditory hallucinations, aphasia, and amnesia.

▷ *Occipital lobe*

  ▸ Functions include:

    ▷ Primary visual cortex

    ▷ Integration area: Integrates vision with other sensory information

  ▸ Problems in the occipital lobe can lead to visual field defects, blindness, and visual hallucinations.

▷ *Parietal lobe*

  ▸ Functions include:

    ▷ Primary sensory area

    ▷ Taste

    ▷ Reading and writing

  ▸ Problems in the parietal lobe can lead to sensory–perceptual disturbances and agnosia.

► Cerebrum includes important areas of brain, including cerebral cortex, limbic system, thalamus, hypothalamus, and basal ganglia.

  ▸ Cerebral cortex

    ▷ Controls wide array of behaviors

    ▷ Controls the *contralateral* (opposite) side of the body: The right hemisphere controls the left side of the body, and the left hemisphere controls the right side of the body.

    ▷ Sensory information is relayed from thalamus and then processed and integrated in the cortex.

    ▷ Responsible for much of the behavior that makes us human: speech, cognition, judgment, perception, and motor function

  ▸ Limbic system

    ▷ Essential system for the regulation and modulation of emotions and memory

    ▷ Composed of the hypothalamus, thalamus, hippocampus, and amygdala

- *Hypothalamus:* Plays key roles in various regulatory functions such as appetite, sensations of hunger and thirst, water balance, circadian rhythms, body temperature, libido, and hormonal regulation

- *Thalamus:* Sensory relay station except for smell; modulates flow of sensory information to prevent overwhelming the cortex; regulates emotions, memory, and related affective behaviors

- *Hippocampus:* Regulates memory and converts short-term memory into long-term memory

- *Amygdala:* Responsible for mediating mood, fear, emotion, and aggression; also responsible for connecting sensory smell information with emotions.

- Basal Ganglia: Also known as the *corpus striatum*

  - Serves as a complex feedback system to modulate and stabilize somatic motor activity (information conveyed from the CNS to skeletal muscles)

  - Plays a role in movement initiation; complex motor functions with association connections

  - Functions in learning and automatic actions such as walking or driving a car

  - Contains extrapyramidal motor system or nerve track

  - Functions in involuntary motor activities (e.g., muscle tone, posture, coordination of muscle movement and common reflexes)

  - Many psychotropic medications can affect the extrapyramidal motor nerve track, causing involuntary movement side effects.

  - Contains both the caudate and the putamen

  - Problems in the basal ganglia can lead to bradykinesia, hyperkinesias, and dystonia.

▶ Brainstem

- Includes the midbrain, pons, cerebellum, medulla, cerebellum, and reticular formation

- Is made up of cells that produce neurotransmitters

- *Midbrain:* Houses the ventral tegmental area and the substantia nigra (areas of dopamine synthesis)

- *Pons:* Houses the locus ceruleus (area of norepinephrine synthesis)

- *Medulla:* Together with the pons, contain autonomic control centers that regulate internal body functions

- *Cerebellum:* Responsible for maintaining equilibrium; acts as a gross movement control center (e.g., control movement, balance, posture)

  - Each hemisphere of cerebellum has *ipsilateral* control (same side of body).

  - Problems with the cerebellum can lead to ataxia (uncoordinated and inaccurate movements).

  - Rhomberg test is important for detecting deficiencies in cerebellar functioning.

- *Reticular formation system*: The primitive brain
  - ▷ Receives input from cortex; an integration area for input from postsensory pathways
  - ▷ Innervates thalamus, hypothalamus, and cortex
  - ▷ Regulation functions include
    - ▸ Involuntary movement
    - ▸ Reflex
    - ▸ Muscle tone
    - ▸ Vital sign control
    - ▸ Blood pressure
    - ▸ Respiratory rate
    - ▸ Is critical to consciousness and ability to mentally focus, to be alert and pay attention to environmental stimuli

NEUROPHYSIOLOGY AND THE BRAIN

▶ Two classes of cells are in the nervous system: glia and neurons.
  - ▸ *Glia*: Structures that form the myelin sheath around axons and provide protection and support
  - ▸ *Neurons*: Nerve cells responsible for conducting impulses from one part of the body to another

▶ Components of a neuron include
  - ▸ *Cell body*: Also known as *soma*; made up of the nucleus and cytoplasm within the cell membrane
  - ▸ *Dendrites*: Receive information to conduct impulse *toward* the cell body
  - ▸ *Axon*: Sends or conducts information *away* from cell body

▶ *Synapse or synaptic cleft*: The connection site and area of communication between neurons where neurotransmitters are released
  - ▸ The synapse converts an electrical signal (action potential) from the presynaptic neuron into a chemical signal (neuron transmitter) that is transferred to the postsynaptic neuron.
  - ▸ Neurotransmitters are released at the synaptic cleft as the result of an electrical activity (action potential).

Two phases of an action potential include
  - ▷ *Depolarization:* The initial phase of the action potential; an excitatory response; influx of sodium and calcium ions into the cell
  - ▷ *Repolarization*: The restoration phase; an inhibitory response; potassium leaves cell or chloride enters cell.

- Problems in either the structure or chemistry of the synapse interrupts normal flow of impulses and stimuli, which then contributes to symptoms commonly seen in psychiatric disorders.

▶ *Neurotransmitters*: Chemicals synthesized from dietary substrates that communicate information from one cell to another.

  ▷ The neurotransmitter will be released from the presynaptic neuron, cross the synapse, and then bind to a specific finite receptor on the postsynaptic neuron.

  ▷ Specific criteria must be met for a molecule to be classified as a neurotransmitter (see Table 4–1).

TABLE 4–1. CLASSIFICATION NOMENCLATURE FOR NEUROTRANSMITTERS

Criteria	1. Neurotransmitter must be present in the nerve terminal.
	2. Stimulation of neuron must cause release of neurotransmitter in sufficient quantities to cause an action to occur at postsynaptic membrane.
	3. Effects of exogenous transmitter on postsynaptic membrane must be similar to those caused by stimulation of presynaptic neuron.
	4. A mechanism for inactivation or metabolism of the neurotransmitter must exist in the area of the synapse.
	5. Exogenous drugs should alter the dose–response curve of the neurotransmitter in a manner similar to the naturally occurring synaptic potential.

Adapted from *Kaplan and Sadock's Synopsis of Psychiatry* (10th ed.) by B. Sadock, & V. Sadock, 2007, New York: Lippincott Williams & Wilkins.

▶ *Categories of neurotransmitters*: Monoamines, amino acids, cholinergics, peptides

  ▶ **Monoamines:** "Biogenic amines"; dopamine, norepinephrine, epinephrine, serotonin

    ▷ *Dopamine*: Known as a *catecholamine*; produced in the substantia nigra and the ventral tegmental area; precursor is tyrosine; removed from the synaptic cleft by monoamine oxidase (MAO) enzymatic action

    ▷ *Four dopaminergic pathways*: Mesocortical, mesolimbic, nigrostriatal, tuberoinfundibular (see Chapter 9).

    ▷ *Norepinephrine*: Also known as a *catecholamine*; produced in the locus ceruleus of the pons; precursor is tyrosine; removed from the synaptic cleft and returned to storage via an active reuptake process; major neurotransmitter implicated in mood, anxiety, and concentration disorders

    ▷ *Epinephrine*: Also known as a catecholamine; produced by the adrenal glands; epinephrine system referred to as the adrenergic system.

    ▷ *Serotonin*: Known as an *indole*; produced in the raphe nuclei of the brainstem; precursor is tryptophan; removed from the synaptic cleft and returned to storage via an active reuptake process; major neurotransmitter implicated in mood and anxiety disorders

▶ **Amino Acids:** Glutamate, γ-aminobutyric acid (GABA), glycine, aspartate

   ▹ *Glutamate:* Universal excitatory neurotransmitter; major neurotransmitter involved in process of kindling, which is implicated in seizure disorders and possibly bipolar disorder; imbalance implicated in mood disorders and schizophrenia

   ▹ *Aspartate:* Another excitatory neurotransmitter that works with glutamate

   ▹ *GABA:* Universal inhibitory neurotransmitter; site of action of benzodiazepines, alcohol, barbiturates, and other CNS depressants.

   ▹ *Glycine:* Another inhibitory neurotransmitter that works with GABA.

   ▹ *Cholinergics:* Acetylcholine

   ▹ *Acetylcholine:* Synthesized by the basal nucleus of Meynert; precursors are acetylcoenzyme A and choline.

▶ **Neuropeptides:** Nonopioid type (substance P, somatostatin); opioid type (endorphins, enkephalins, dynorphins)

   ▹ Modulate pain; decreased amount of neuropeptides is thought to cause substance abuse

   ▹ See Table 4–2 for identification of neurotransmitters' role in symptom expression in common psychiatric disorders.

TABLE 4–2. COMMON PSYCHIATRIC DISORDERS AND NEUROTRANSMITTERS IMPLICATED IN THE COMPLEX PATHOPHYSIOLOGY OF COMMON PSYCHIATRIC DISORDERS

NEUROTRANSMITTER	SUSPECTED IMBALANCE	PSYCHIATRIC PRESENTATION
Acetylcholine	▶ Decrease ▶ Decrease ▶ Increase	▶ Alzheimer's disease ▶ Impaired memory ▶ Parkinsonian symptoms
Dopamine	▶ Increase ▶ Decrease ▶ Decrease ▶ Decrease	▶ Schizophrenia/psychosis ▶ Substance abuse ▶ Anhedonia ▶ Parkinson's
Norepinephrine	▶ Decrease ▶ Increase	▶ Depression ▶ Anxiety
Serotonin	▶ Decrease ▶ Decrease ▶ Decrease	▶ Depression ▶ Obsessive–compulsive disorder, anxiety disorders ▶ Schizophrenia
γ-aminobutyric acid (GABA)	▶ Decrease	▶ Anxiety disorders
Glutamate	Increase Decrease	▶ Bipolar affective disorder ▶ Psychosis from ischemic neurotoxicity/ excessive pruning ▶ Memory and learning difficulty or; negative symptoms of schizophrenia
Opioid neuropeptides	Decrease	Substance abuse

Adapted from *Anatomy and Physiology* (6th ed.), by G. Thibodeau, & K. Patton, 2006, St. Louis, MO: Mosby.

NEUROANATOMY, NEUROPHYSIOLOGY, AND BEHAVIOR 63

▶ Recovery and degradation of neurotransmitters

  ▹ After the neurotransmitter reaches the postsynaptic neuron, it may then diffuse off its receptor to be destroyed by enzymes or to be transported back to the presynaptic neuron for reuse.

  ▹ *Enzymatic destruction* occurs either in the cytosol or in the synapse. The neurotransmitter can be destroyed by the enzymes monoamine oxidase (MAO) in the cytosol or catechol-O-methyl transferase (COMT) intracellularly or in the synapse.

  ▹ *Reuptake pumps* can remove the neurotransmitter from acting in the synapse. The neurotransmitter will be reloaded into the presynaptic neuron and will be recycled.

▶ Function of neurotransmitters (see Table 4–3)

TABLE 4-3. COMPARISON OF COMMON CNS NEUROTRANSMITTERS

NEURO-TRANSMITTER	RECEPTORS	GENERAL FUNCTION	SYMPTOMS OF DEFICIT	SYMPTOMS OF EXCESS
Dopamine	D_1-like D_2-like	▶ Thinking ▶ Decision-making ▶ Reward-seeking behavior ▶ Fine muscle action ▶ Integrated cognition	Mild: ▶ Poor impulse control ▶ Poor spatiality ▶ Lack of abstractive thought Severe: ▶ Parkinson's ▶ Endocrine alterations ▶ Movement disorders	Mild: ▶ Improved creativity ▶ Improved ability for abstract thinking ▶ Improved executive functioning ▶ Improved spatiality Severe: ▶ Disorganized thinking ▶ Loose association ▶ Tics ▶ Stereotypic behavior
Norepinephrine	α1 α2	▶ Alertness ▶ Focused attention ▶ Orientation ▶ Primes "fight–flight" ▶ Learning ▶ Memory	▶ Dullness ▶ Low energy ▶ Depressive affect	▶ Anxiety ▶ Hyperalertness ▶ Increased startle ▶ Paranoia ▶ Decreased appetite

CONTINUED ▶

TABLE 4-3. COMPARISON OF COMMON CNS NEUROTRANSMITTERS CONTINUED ▶

NEURO-TRANSMITTER	RECEPTORS	GENERAL FUNCTION	SYMPTOMS OF DEFICIT	SYMPTOMS OF EXCESS
Serotonin	▶ 5HT1a ▶ 5HT1d ▶ 5HT2 ▶ 5HT2a ▶ 5HT3 ▶ 5HT4	▶ Regulation of sleep ▶ Pain perceptions ▶ Mood states ▶ Temperature ▶ Regulation of aggression ▶ Libido ▶ Precursor for melatonin	▶ Irritability ▶ Hostility ▶ Depression ▶ Sleep dysregulation ▶ Loss of appetite ▶ Loss of libido	▶ Sedation ▶ Serotonin syndrome: Restlessness, agitation, myoclonus, blood pressure, pulse and temperature abnormalities ▶ Hallucinations (rare)
Acetylcholine	▶ Nicotinic ▶ Muscarinic	▶ Attention ▶ Memory ▶ Thirst ▶ Mood regulation ▶ REM sleep ▶ Sexual behavior ▶ Muscle tone	▶ Lack of inhibition ▶ Decreased memory ▶ Euphoria ▶ Antisocial action ▶ Speech decrease ▶ Dry mouth, blurred vision, constipation	▶ Over-inhibition ▶ Anxiety ▶ Depression ▶ Somatic complaints ▶ Self-consciousness ▶ Drooling ▶ Extrapyramidal movements
GABA	▶ GABAa ▶ GABAb	▶ Reduces arousal ▶ Reduces aggression ▶ Reduces anxiety ▶ Reduces excitation	▶ Irritability ▶ Hostility ▶ Tension and worry ▶ Anxiety ▶ Seizure activity	▶ Reduced cellular excitability ▶ Sedation ▶ Impaired memory
Glutamate	▶ AMPA ▶ MNDA	▶ Memory ▶ Sustained automatic functions	▶ Poor memory ▶ Low energy ▶ Distractible	▶ Kindling ▶ Seizures ▶ Anxiety or panic
Peptides: Opiod type	μ mu Ќ kappa ε epsilon δ delta σ sigma	▶ Modulate emotions ▶ Reward-center function ▶ Consolidation of memory ▶ Modulate reactions to stress	▶ Hypersensitivity to pain and stress ▶ Decreased pleasure sensation ▶ Dysphoria	▶ Insensitivity to pain ▶ Catatonic-like movement disturbance ▶ Auditory hallucinations ▶ Decreased memory

Adapted from *Kaplan and Sadock's Synopsis of Psychiatry* (10th ed.) by B. Sadock, & V. Sadock, 2007, New York: Lippincott Williams & Wilkins.

NEUROIMAGING ASSESSMENT AND DIAGNOSTIC PROCEDURES

▶ Techniques that permit observation of the brain can be divided into three categories: structural imaging, functional imaging, and structural and functional imaging.

▶ *Structural imaging*: Provides evidence of size and shape of anatomical structures

▶ Common structural imaging tests include

    ▻ *Computed tomography (CT)*: Provides a three-dimensional view of the brain structures; differentiates structures based on density; provides suggestive evidence of brain-based problems but no specific testing for psychiatric disorders

        ▹ *Advantages:* Widely available, relatively inexpensive

        ▹ *Disadvantages:* Lack of sensitivity, cannot differentiate white matter from gray matter, and cannot view structures close to the bone tissue; underestimation of brain atrophy; inability to image sagittal and coronal views

    ▻ *Magnetic resonance imaging (MRI)*: Provides a series of two-dimensional images that represent the brain

        ▹ *Advantages:* Can view brain structures close to the skull and can separate white matter from gray matter; readily available; resolution of brain tissue superior to CT scanning

        ▹ *Disadvantages:* Expensive; many contraindications to its use (e.g., patients with pacemakers, patients on ventilators, patients with any metallic implants such as orthopedic screws or plates); patients with claustrophobia often are unable to complete study because of design of machinery (an enclosed tubelike structure with a confining environment)

▶ *Functional imaging:* Technique that measures function of areas of the brain and bases the resulting assessment on blood flow to the brain; may use radioactive pharmaceuticals to cross the blood-brain barrier; mainly used for research purposes.

▶ Common functional imaging tests include

    ▻ *EEG and evoked potentials testing:* Least expensive tests that convey information on electrical functioning of the CNS

        ▹ *Magnetoencephalography (MEG):* Similar to the EEG but detects different electrical activities; often used in a complementary fashion with EEG testing

        ▹ *Single photon emission computed tomography (SPECT):* Provides information on the cerebral blood flow; limited availability; expensive but less than positron emission tomography

        ▹ *Positron emission tomography (PET):* Provides images of the brain when positron-emitting radionuclei interact with electrons; expensive procedure that requires extensive resources and support team

▶ *Structural and Functional Imaging:* The newest imaging; attempts to examine structure in conjunction with function; currently mainly used for research purposes

▶ Available tests include

  ▸ Functional MRI (fMRI)

  ▸ 3-dimensional event-related functional MRI (3fEMRI)

  ▸ Fluorine magnetic spectroscopy

  ▸ Dopamine D_2 receptor binding

GENOMICS

Family History, Family Tree, Pedigree

▶ Tool in determining likelihood of genetic disorder in family, inheritance patterns, and risk of recurrence in family members

▶ Surgeon General recommended that families know their family history (U.S. Department of Health & Human Services, n.d.)

▶ Pedigree symbols in drawing a family tree indicate male, female, marriage, divorce, adoption, twins, pregnancy, consanguinity (relatives having children), conditions

▶ Family history starts with current family and moves back to grandparents

▶ Autosomal dominant conditions may be present in more than one generation and in up to 50% of offspring when one parent is affected (e.g., Marfan syndrome)

▶ Recessive conditions appear only in one generation, affecting individuals who have two copies of a faulty gene, one from each (unaffected) parent (e.g., hemochromatosis, cystic fibrosis)

▶ X-linked disorders are caused by faulty genes on an X chromosome (e.g., fragile X syndrome, color blindness)

▶ Risk assessment is based on inheritance patterns and may be by percentage of risk

Genetic Counseling

▶ Genetic counseling is a communication process used whenever there is genetic risk and often involves offering a test that could provide information about the genetic status of the person and possible implications for the family.

▶ A genetic counselor is someone whose primary role is to offer information and support to persons concerned about an illness that may have a genetic basis.

▶ A referral to a genetic counselor may be needed when anticipating a pregnancy and being concerned for the health of the fetus.

Genetic Terms

▶ *Chromosomes* are structures of DNA (deoxyribonucleic acid) in nucleus of cells; there are normally 46 total (23 pairs).

▶ DNA is made up of two twisted, paired strands, composed of sugars linked by 4 nucleotide bases—adenine (A), thymine (T), cytosine (C), and guanine (G)—specifying the amino acids that make proteins. A is always paired with T and G is always paired with C.

▶ *Genes* are a sequence of DNA that cause human characteristics to be passed to the next generation; genes direct the production of proteins.

▶ Messenger RNA (mRNA) codes for an amino acid.

▶ The Human Genome Project mapped the entire nucleotide sequence of the human genome in 2003. The genome is a complete set of DNA.

▶ A *phenotype* is the observable characteristic of a specific trait and is connected to the genetic contributions to that trait (e.g., fast metabolizer of CYP4502D6 medications).

▶ Gene therapy involves replacing a faulty copy of a gene with a healthy copy of the same gene.

▶ Personalized medicine is health care based on genetic variability.

Studies of Population Genetics

▶ Family studies investigate the occurrence of disorders in first-degree relatives (parents, siblings, and offspring) and second-degree relatives (grandparents, cousins, aunts, and uncles).

▶ Twin studies survey the concordance rate (presence) of a disorder in monozygotic (identical) and dizygotic (fraternal) twins.

▶ Adoption studies investigate the risk of a disorder developing in children raised in a different environment from the biological parent with a specific disorder.

▶ Strong genetic contributions have been found for most psychiatric disorders, with a range of 40% to 90% heritability for some disorders (e.g., attention-deficit hyperactivity disorder, bipolar disorder).

▶ Genes are risk factors that make a person vulnerable to developing the illness when combined with certain environmental risk factors that increase susceptibility of developing the disorder.

▶ Environmental risk factors include prenatal insults, stress, infections, poor nutrition, exposure to toxins, catastrophic loss, and physical and sexual abuse.

▶ Most diseases are multifactorial, caused by both environmental and genetic factors; single-gene disorders are rare.

Gene Expression and Disease

► Single nucleotide polymorphisms (SNP) detect single base changes in DNA sequence.

► Reduced penetrance of a gene decreases chances of disease in person at genetic risk.

► Variable expression of a gene for a disorder occurs at the cellular level.

Pharmacogenomics

► Genes account for differences in the way enzymes metabolize drugs.

► Medications may act differently based on how genes affect metabolism.

► Genetic testing or profiling helps identify the presence of gene variants that may help determine dosing of medication (e.g., CYP450 test of CYP4502D6 and CYP4502C19 genes).

► Testing for presence of HLA-B*1502 allele, an inherited variant of HLA-B gene, is required by the FDA in people of Asian descent prior to being prescribed the anticonvulsant carbamazepine due to risk of Stevens-Johnson syndrome and toxic epidermal necrolysis (TEN) .

CASE STUDY

Ms. Franklin is a 24-year-old sales clerk. She has a strong family history of mental illness and is worried that she may experience some problems in her life because of her family history. She presents to her local primary care provider complaining of the following symptoms:

► Hyperalertness

► Increased startle response

► Concern that people are staring at her and watching what she eats

► Decreased appetite

► Difficulty falling asleep

Ms. Franklin is trying to determine if these experiences are the beginning of a mental illness. She wants to have a brain scan done to determine the answer. She also is getting married soon and wants to know what the risk is that her future children will experience mental illness, as she believes it runs in her family. In working with Ms. Franklin, the PMHNP must consider many issues.

► Are the symptoms described by Ms. Franklin consistent with a psychiatric disorder?

► Do psychiatric disorders run in families, as Ms. Franklin believes?

► Do the symptoms as described by Ms. Franklin link with any known neuroanatomical or neurophysiologic deficit?

► Is a brain scan warranted for Ms. Franklin?

► Can the risk of Ms. Franklin's children developing psychiatric disorders be determined?

REFERENCES

Alexander, E., Chen, K., Pietrini, P. Rapoport, S. I., & Reiman, E. M. (2002). Longitudinal PET evaluation of cerebral metabolic decline in dementia: A potential outcome measure in Alzheimer's disease treatment studies. *American Journal of Psychiatry, 159,* 238–245.

Amen, D. G. (1998). Brain SPECT imaging in psychiatry. *Primary Psychiatry, 5,* 83–87.

American Nurses Association. (2000). *Scope and standards of psychiatric mental health practice.* Washington, DC: American Nurses Association.

Carlson, N. R. (2006). *Physiology of behavior* (9th ed.). Boston: Allyn & Bacon.

Doyle, A. E., Roe, C. M., & Faraone, S. V. (2001). The genetics of attention deficit hyperactivity disorder. *Primary Psychiatry, 8*(9), 65–71.

Dubin, M. W. (2002). *How the brain works.* Williston, VT: Blackwell Science.

Goff, D., & Coyle, J. (2001). The emerging role of glutamate in the pathophysiology and treatment of schizophrenia. *American Journal of Psychiatry, 158,* 1367–1377.

Gribbin, J. (2002). *How the brain works: A beginner's guide to the mind and consciousness.* New York: Dorling Kindersley.

Gross-Isseroff, R., Bigeon, A., Voet, H., & Weizman, A. (1998). The suicide brain: A review of postmortem receptor transporter binding studies. *Neuroscience Biobehavioral Review, 22,* 653.

Gur, R. (2002). Functional imaging is fulfilling some promises. *American Journal of Psychiatry, 159,* 693–694.

Keltner, N. L., Folks, D. G., Palmer, C. A., & Powers, R. E. (1998). *Psychobiological foundations of psychiatric care.* St. Louis, MO: Mosby.

McCabe, S. (2001a). The biological foundations of psychiatric nursing. In M. A. Boyd (Ed.), *Psychiatric nursing* (2nd ed., pp. 94–126). Philadelphia: Lippincott Williams & Wilkins.

McCabe, S. (2001b). Psychopharmacology and other biological treatments. In M. A. Boyd (Ed.), *Psychiatric nursing* (2nd ed., pp. 128–175). Philadelphia: Lippincott Williams & Wilkins.

McLeod, T. M., Lopez-Figueroa, A., & Lopez-Figueroa, M. O. (2001). Nitric oxide, stress, and depression. *Psychopharmacology Bulletin, 35,* 24–41.

Mohr, W. K., & Mohr, B. (2001). Brain, behavior, connections, and implications: Psychodynamics no more. *Archives of Psychiatric Nursing, 15,* 171–181.

Mujica-Parodi, L. R., Corcoran, C., Greenberg, T., Saceim, H. A., & Malaspina, D. (2002). Are cognitive symptoms of schizophrenia mediated by abnormalities in emotional arousal? *CNS Spectrums, 7*(1), 58–69.

Raemaekers, M., Johannus, M. J., Cahn, W., Van der Geest, J. N., van der Linden, J. A., Kahn, R. S., et al. (1999). Neuronal substrate of the saccadic inhibition deficit in schizophrenia investigated with 3-dimensional event-related functional MRI. *Archives of General Psychiatry, 59,* 313–320.

Raine, T., Lencz, T., Bihrle, S., LaCasse, L., & Colletti, P. (2000). Reduced gray matter volume and reduced autonomic activity in antisocial personality disorder. *Archives of General Psychiatry, 57,* 119–129.

Sadock, B., & Sadock, V. (2007). *Kaplan and Sadock's synopsis of psychiatry* (10th ed.). New York: Lippincott Williams & Wilkins.

Schindler, K. M., Pato, M. T., Torre, C. D., Valente, J., Azevedo, M. H., Coelho, I., et al. (2001). Candidate genes for schizophrenia: Further evaluation of KCNN3. *Primary Psychiatry, 8*(9), 51–53.

Shihabuddin, L. S., Ray, J., & Gage, F. H. (1999). Stem cell technology for basic science and clinical applications. *Archives of Neurology, 6,* 29–32.

Stahl, S. M. (2000). *Essential psychopharmacology: Neuroscientific basis and practical applications* (2nd ed.). New York: Cambridge University Press.

Stuart, G. W., & Laraia, M. T. (2004). *Principles and practice of psychiatric nursing* (8th ed.). St. Louis, MO: Mosby.

Thibodeau, G., & Patton, K. (2006). *Anatomy and physiology* (6th ed.). St. Louis, MO: Mosby.

U.S. Department of Health & Human Services. (n.d.). *Surgeon General's Family Health History Initiative.* Retrieved from http://www.hhs.gov/familyhistory

Young, G. B., & Pigott, S. E. (1999). Neurobiologic basis of consciousness. *Archives of Neurology, 56,* 153–157.

CHAPTER 5

ASSESSMENT OF ACUTE AND CHRONIC DISEASE STATES

This chapter reviews the role of psychiatric–mental health nurse practitioners (PMHNPs) in assessment. It reviews the process of history-taking, physical exam, mental status exam, differential diagnosis, and the appropriate use of diagnostic and laboratory testing in providing competent nursing care for patients and families experiencing psychiatric disorders. The chapter specifically highlights the PMHNP role in assessing and diagnosing common psychiatric disorders.

STATISTICS FOR PSYCHIATRIC DISORDERS

General Incidence and Demographics

▶ Epidemiology: The study of the distribution, incidence, prevalence, and duration of disease

▶ Incidence rate: The number of new cases occurring over a specified time (usually 1 year)

▶ Prevalence rate: The number of existing cases of a disorder at a specified time

  ▸ One in 4 adults will be diagnosed with a psychiatric disorder within their lifetime.

  ▸ An estimated 26.2% of Americans ages 18 and older have a diagnosable psychiatric disorder in a given year. On the basis of census data (National Institute of Mental Health, 2006), this figure translates to 57.7 million Americans with a psychiatric disorder in any given year.

  ▸ Mental illness is the leading cause of disability in the United States and Canada.

  ▸ Psychiatric disorders have common, frequently occurring comorbidities; that is, people often have more than one psychiatric disorder at a given time. Also, people often have a psychiatric disorder and another common health disorder at a given time.

- Four of the 10 leading causes of disability in Americans are psychiatric disorders: major depression, bipolar disorder, schizophrenia, and anxiety disorders.

ASSESSMENT OF PSYCHIATRIC DISORDERS

General Considerations

▶ Interviewing is the primary form of assessment and data collection.

▶ The psychiatric assessment process is a structured, organized, and systematic process that includes multiple components: patient history, physical examination, mental status examination, and diagnostic and laboratory tests.

Fundamentals of Interviewing

▶ Psychiatric interviewing requires many skills on the part of the PMHNP:

- Openness

- Respect for the patient and family

- Appropriate use of therapeutic communication

- Ability to form rapport with the patient

- Subjective and objective data collection skills using all senses

- Critical thinking to identify the needs of the patient.

▶ The psychiatric assessment process is a focused, goal-directed, interactional process between the PMHNP and the patient and family.

▶ Primary goals of the assessment process:

- Gather intentional specific data

- Identify the health needs of the patient

- Plan for care

- Evaluate outcomes of care

- Evaluate ongoing health needs of the patient.

▶ Assessment requires the PMHNP to form an *effective relationship with the patient* by

- Learning about the patient's interest and motivation for care

- Having open and respectful engagement with the patient using a nonjudgmental approach

- Exploring current emotional status

- Validating assumptions about emotional status of patient

- Displaying empathy

- Instilling hope that patient's concern can be addressed

- Developing a sense of partnership with patient and family.

ASSESSMENT OF ACUTE AND CHRONIC DISEASE STATES **73**

▶ The *initial assessment* of the patient focuses on the process of differential diagnostic assessment.

▶ *Subsequent assessments* with the patient focus on monitoring client outcomes, on general health status, and on modifying care practices based on clinical outcomes.

THERAPEUTIC COMMUNICATION CONSIDERATIONS

▶ Therapeutic communication techniques (see Table 5–1) need to be used in all interactions with the patient and family.

▶ Active listening

  ▸ Paying attention to nonverbal communication (such as loss of eye contact, shift in body posture, increase in fidgeting or restlessness, clenched fists, bouncing legs)

  ▸ Maintaining an open and engaging posture (positioning oneself at patient's eye level, being relaxed and unhurried, leaning slightly forward)

  ▸ Maintaining eye contact that is matched to client's comfort level and cultural background.

▶ Facilitative communication techniques

  ▸ Intended to foster greater disclosure by patient

  ▸ Allow patient to pace conversation

  ▸ Avoid interrupting the patient unnecessarily

  ▸ Avoid nonstop questions directed at patient

  ▸ Use open-ended questioning initially

  ▸ Avoid much self-disclosure by the PMHNP

  ▸ Use encouraging vocalizations such as "go on" or "tell me more"

  ▸ Request clarification when needed

  ▸ Summarize key points to ensure congruency of understanding

  ▸ Follow up with directive and closed questions for confirmatory data assessment.

▶ Paraphrasing: Repeating the patient's thoughts or feelings with similar words

▶ Confrontation: Pointing out to a patient something that he or she is not paying attention to, is missing, or is denying

▶ Silence: May be constructive; may allow patients to contemplate, to cry, or just sit in an accepting and supportive environment

TABLE 5-1. THERAPEUTIC COMMUNICATION TECHNIQUES

TECHNIQUE	EXAMPLE
Broad opening	▶ "How are things for you?" ▶ "What brings you here today?" ▶ "What's happened since we last saw each other?"
Accepting	▶ "I can imagine that it has been very difficult for you" (nodding).
Summarizing	▶ "So what you are most concerned about is …. " ▶ "So let me see if I understand …."
Reflection	▶ Patient: "I keep worrying about what will happen next." PMHNP: "You're worried about the future."
Focusing	▶ "Could we talk about the suicidal thoughts a little more?" ▶ "Tell me more about when this all started."
Validating	▶ "It sounds like you are saying …." ▶ "So I am hearing you say …."
Exploring	▶ "How does the depression affect your husband?" ▶ "Tell me what was happening in your life when the voices started."
Clarifying	▶ "Could you explain to me how that mattered?" ▶ "I'm not sure I understand. Could you tell me how that happened?"
Sequencing	▶ "Which came first …." ▶ "Was that before or after you were in the hospital?"
Recognizing	▶ "I notice that you are looking very sad today." ▶ "I see that you still have some trouble with tremors in you hands."
Theming	▶ "We have talked for a while now, and I've noticed that we are mainly talking about your feeling unsupported by your family."

▶ Always compare patient's current symptoms with his or her premorbid symptoms.

▶ Ask how the client was functioning 6 months ago.

Other Assessment and Planning Considerations

▶ Milieu considerations

  ▷ The interview location should be conducive to data collection (a comfortable, private, and quiet, low-sensory-stimulus area), which will decrease anxiety and promote a sense of safety and security for the patient.

  ▷ The milieu also needs to be public enough to access needed equipment, supplies, or assistance as needed.

► Cultural considerations

    ► *Culture*: The pattern of behavior of a group (racial, social, ethnic, religious grouping) that includes the thoughts, customs, beliefs, values, or communication pattern of that particular group

    ► *Cultural competence*: Viewing the patient as a unique individual and providing care that is sensitive to issues related to culture, race, gender, and sexual orientation

        ▷ Reduce health disparities and improve access to care (NIH, 2013)

    ► Demonstrating respectfulness of diversity

    ► *Types of diversity*: Age, gender, sexual orientation, race, ethnicity, language, disability, religion, social class, education, occupation

    ► Being aware of the need to modify the interview to match cultural differences (e.g., regarding behavioral etiquette, inappropriate or taboo topics, gender differences, differences in affective expressions)

    ► Accommodating the interview style to cultural needs (e.g., with regard to language, family structure, health beliefs, health practices)

    ► Online cultural assessment is available through the National Center for Cultural Competence at Georgetown University at www11.georgetown.edu/research/gucchd/nccc/

► Focal areas for assessment of cultural issues

    ► Family roles: Who is the primary caretaker? Who makes most of the decisions?

    ► Family customs

    ► Religious beliefs

    ► Beliefs about death and dying

    ► Dietary preferences

    ► Meaning of nonverbal gestures

    ► Physical space.

► It is important to be aware of the various cultural perspectives of mental health.

► Keep in mind that cultural factors may affect the expression of mental disorders: Be aware of incorrectly judging a person's behavior as psychopathology, when it is in fact culturally related.

► *Culturally bound syndromes:* Those specific behaviors related to a person's culture and not linked to a psychiatric disorder

► *Acculturation:* The process by which the person acquires the culture of the society that he or she inhabits

► When intervening in psychiatric situations that are affected by cultural influences

  ► Listen with empathy

  ► Explain your perceptions of the client's problem

  ► Acknowledge similarities and differences in perceptions between the two cultures

  ► Recommend treatment

  ► Negotiate treatment

► Age considerations

  ► Assessment in children

    ▷ Modify language use according to age of child.

    ▷ Exhibit nurturing behavior.

    ▷ Use play and fantasy in the interview process.

    ▷ Allow more time for the assessment.

    ▷ Use a direct and clear questioning style for adolescents.

  ► Assessment in older adults

    ▷ Allow more time for the assessment.

    ▷ Allow the patient to pace the conversation.

    ▷ Allow time for rapport-building before asking sensitive questions.

    ▷ Allow time for the patient to reminisce and share past history.

► Collateral sources of data

  ► Sometimes comparing what the patient says with what other family members, friends, peers, or significant others say about situations or previous treatment can be helpful.

  ► Using collateral sources of data can be useful with persons with

    ▷ Impaired insight

    ▷ Cognitive deficits

    ▷ Substance abuse problems

    ▷ Unstable behavior

    ▷ All patients, especially children, adolescents, and older adults

ASSESSMENT OF SPIRITUAL NEEDS

► Patient definition of spirituality vs. religion

  ▸ Assess beliefs, practices, and traditions

► HOPE Questions (Anandarahah & Hight, 2001, p. 86)

  ▸ **H:** Sources of hope, meaning, comfort, strength, peace, love connection

  ▸ **O:** Organized religion

  ▸ **P:** Personal spirituality and practices

  ▸ **E:** Effects on medical care and end of life

NATURE OF SYMPTOM PRESENTATION OF PSYCHIATRIC DISORDERS

► Generally, psychiatric symptoms are nonspecific. Ensure that the assessment has been broad and holistic. Identify *clusters* and *patterns* emerging in assessment data rather than looking for discrete signs or symptoms.

► Symptoms of psychiatric disorders often are best observed in the behavioral manifestation of the patient and may not initially be recognized by the patient or family as a symptom. It often is helpful to specifically ask the patient if a particular sign or symptom has been present. Use nonmedical words, avoid jargon, and be aware of the regional or cultural vocabulary used to describe common psychiatric symptoms.

► Many symptoms of common psychiatric disorders have a *somatic component*.

  ▸ The patient initially may be reluctant to view a symptom as an indication of a psychiatric disorder.

  ▸ Sensitivity is needed in forming questions.

  ▸ The stigmatizing nature of psychiatric disorders often will initially limit patient disclosure.

► The presence of certain active symptoms in the patient may increase the difficulty of obtaining assessment data. The following assessment techniques may be used when certain symptoms are present:

  ▸ Anger

    ▷ Take time to establish rapport.

    ▷ Extend courtesy and respect.

    ▷ Use humor to defuse the situation.

    ▷ Get quickly to the patient's agenda and expectations for assessment.

    ▷ Be clear and honest about the goal of assessment and how the data will be used.

    ▷ Use limit-setting when needed.

- Psychosis
  - Frequently reestablish reality for the patient.
  - Use clear and concise language.
  - Avoid word choices that the patient can interpret in concrete ways.
  - Avoid unnecessary physical touch.
- Suspiciousness
  - Explain carefully to the patient any physical touch that is necessary before initiating it with him or her.
  - Be clear and honest about the goals of assessment and how the data will be used.
  - Acknowledge the patient's suspiciousness.
- Controlling features
  - Provide the patient with information about what is happening and will happen.
  - Focus initially on intellectual aspects to match the patient's control needs.
  - Allow the patient to control aspects of interview as appropriate.
- Dependent features
  - Set limits as needed.
  - Allow time for and show patience during interview process.
  - Express an interest in dealing with the patient.
  - Maintain professional boundaries.
- Anxiety
  - Attend to milieu considerations.
  - Notice that the patient may have a decreased ability to process information.
  - Repeat questions as needed.
  - Refocus the patient as needed.

COMPONENTS OF THE PMHNP ASSESSMENT PROCESS

- History
  - Elements of a psychiatric history:
    - Identifying demographic information: age, gender, marital status, race, referral source
    - Chief complaint:
      - The patient's presenting problem
      - The patient's explanation, regardless of how bizarre or irrelevant it is, should be recorded verbatim and placed in quotation marks.

- History of present illness (HPI):
  - Provides a comprehensive and chronological picture of events leading up to the current moment in the patient's life
  - The most helpful part in making a diagnosis and the most important aspect of the history
  - Requires ascertaining information about the presenting problem:
    - *Palliative*: What makes it better?
    - *Provocative*: What makes it worse?
    - *Quality*: How and where does the presence of the complaint affect the patient's quality of life?
    - *Radiation*: Is the problem radiating to other areas of the patient's life, such as work?
    - *Severity*: How much does the patient's complaint affect day-to-day life? On a scale of 0 to 10, with 0 least severe and 10 most severe, rate the severity of the problem.
    - *Timing*: Is this a new complaint? How long has it been a problem? Is there any particular time of day the complaint occurs?
  - Acronym to use when collecting HPI: *OLDCARTS*
    - **O**nset
    - **L**ocation
    - **D**uration
    - **C**haracter
    - **A**lleviating and **A**ggravating factors
    - **R**adiation
    - **T**emporal pattern (time of day)
    - **S**everity
  - Goals for the HPI
    - Develop rapport
    - Record at least one-half of the mental status exam (MSE)
    - Keep track of cues for further exploration of facts or feelings
    - Develop and devise a preliminary diagnosis
  - Past psychiatric history
    - Important to determine the course and severity of the disorder
    - Entails past mental disorders, any remissions or exacerbations, family psychiatric history, past treatments and response, past suicidal or homicidal ideations or attempts

- Past medical history
  - Important to distinguish between organic and psychiatric disorders
  - Gives a chronological history of medical problems
- Social history
  - Home situation
  - Family constellation, marital history, children, dependents
  - Work and school situation
  - Social network, relationship with others
  - Typical pattern of activity
  - Spirituality
  - Recent stressors
  - Legal history
  - Substance use history and current use
- Family history (family of origin and nuclear family)
  - Structure
  - Health history, cause of death of relatives if deceased, psychiatric disorders and treatment
  - Family risk factors
  - Conflicting and supportive relationships, cutoffs
  - Family strengths
- Developmental history
  - Maternal history of pregnancy
  - Adverse perinatal events
  - History of delivery
- Important aspects to include in developmental and social history for child or adolescent:
  - Relevant birth and infancy history (e.g., temperament, motor development)
  - Cognitive development (e.g., school performance, milestones)
  - Emotional development (e.g., self-esteem, self-efficacy, sense of right and wrong)
  - Losses, including divorce
  - Abuse, including neglect
  - Sexual activity, birth control, and pregnancies
  - Childhood illnesses
  - Childhood psychiatric disorders, learning disabilities

- Secondary sexual characteristics (e.g., onset of puberty, onset of menses)
- Parental pressures
- Sense of personal identity

- Key principles of child development
  - Development proceeds along a predictable pathway marked by milestones.
  - Children mature and develop at different rates.
  - Development may be affected by many factors such as abuse or poverty.

- Clues to developmental and behavioral problems in children
  - Enuresis and encopresis
  - Night terrors
  - Thumb-sucking
  - Frequent tantrums
  - Excessive isolation
  - Fire setting
  - Cruelty to animals
  - Frequent school truancy

- Functional assessment
  - Looks at the degree to which the patient's abilities and performance match the demands of his or her life
  - Determines the impact of the illness on the overall functioning
  - Is used to differentiate depression from dementia in older adults
  - Is used to track patient improvement or decline from his or her baseline
  - Includes activities of daily living (ADLs) and instrumental activities of daily living (IADLs)
    - *ADLs*: Basic self-care skills, such as eating, bathing, dressing, and toileting
    - *IADLs*: Activities needed for independent functioning, such as shopping, cooking, taking medications, driving, housekeeping

- History-taking during crisis
  - Determine as the first priority the status of the emergency and assess danger to the patient and others.
  - Always be alert for risk of impending violence.
  - Attend to the safety of the physical surroundings.
  - Focus on the presenting complaint or problem and obtain a supplemental history from others if necessary.
  - Assess drug or alcohol use, mental status, current medications, and past effective coping skills.

▷ Be straightforward, calm, honest, and nonthreatening.

▶ Physical exam

- Reasons to be familiar with the physical exam in psychiatry:

  ▷ To be able to detect underlying medical problems

  ▷ To be familiar with a screening neurological exam and to be able to rule out neurological problems that may manifest as symptoms of a psychiatric problem

  ▷ To be able to differentiate normal and abnormal signs and symptoms

  ▷ To know when to refer

- Done by the PMHNP in the context of his or her primary psychiatric care role

- Goals are identifying presence of psychiatric disorders, identifying general health status, and screening for other nonpsychiatric disorders

- Focuses on physical assessment required to accomplish differential diagnoses to determine patient health needs

- Specifically focuses on assessing for disorders or conditions that explain patientpresentation

  ▷ Psychiatric disorders

  ▷ Nonpsychiatric disorders

- Not intended to replace the role of primary healthcare provider for the patient

  ▷ PMHNP should assist patient to establish primary care provider.

- Avoids highly personal or intrusive procedures that may make the formation of a therapeutic alliance more difficult (e.g., Pap exam, male genital exam, rectal exam, breast exam), but it is important to be familiar with these exams and be able to differentiate normal from abnormal

- Requires the PMHNP to have depth of knowledge regarding the common health disorders that can mimic symptoms of a psychiatric disorder

  ▷ Differential diagnostic considerations

- Requires the PMHNP to have depth of knowledge regarding the common psychiatric disorders that can mimic or produce symptoms of other disorders

  ▷ Differential diagnostic considerations

  ▷ Comorbid condition and clinical management issues

- Generally, if patient health issues are determined to be nonpsychiatric, patient is referred to primary care providers other than the PMHNP

- Because of the brain-based nature of psychiatric disorders, the PMHNP role requires the ability to perform an in-depth neurological exam.

▶ Neurological exam

- Reflexes (biceps, triceps, brachioradialis, patellar, Achilles, plantar)

  ▷ Grade reflexes and note symmetry between right and left sides.

ASSESSMENT OF ACUTE AND CHRONIC DISEASE STATES   83

▷ Check primitive reflexes in infants (head lag, flexion, rooting, grasping, Moro, glabellar, Babinski).

▷ A positive Babinski (fanning of toes and dorsiflexion of the great toe) is normal in infants up to age 2 years.

▸ Cranial nerves

  ▷ *Olfactory* —1st (On)

    ▸ Test sense of smell and ensure patency of the nasal passages.

    ▸ Have the patient close eyes and test each nostril separately while other is occluded, asking the patient to identify familiar odors.

  ▷ *Optic* —2nd (Old)

    ▸ Test vision using Snellen chart or other suitable chart depending on the patient's acuity and ability to cooperate.

    ▸ Examine the inner aspect of the eyes with the ophthalmoscope.

    ▸ Test peripheral vision using the confrontation test.

  ▷ *Oculomotor* —3rd (Olympus')

    ▸ This is the motor nerve to the five extrinsic eye muscles. Test together with cranial nerve 4 (trochlear) and cranial nerve 6 (abducens; see below).

    ▸ Test the extraocular movements (EOMs).

    ▸ Check the equality of pupils, their reaction to light, and their ability to accommodate.

    ▸ Test the corneal light reflex (when shining a light at the bridge of the nose, the light should appear symmetrically in both eyes).

  ▷ *Trochlear* —4th (Towering)

    ▸ Use the same process as cranial nerve 3 (oculomotor) and cranial nerve 6 (abducens).

  ▷ *Trigeminal* —5th (Motor Division; Top)

    ▸ Palpate the masseter muscles with the fingertips while the patient clenches his or her teeth.

    ▸ Look for disparity in tension between the two muscles, which can indicate paralysis on the weak side.

    ▸ Look for tremor of the lips, involuntary chewing movements, and spasm of the masticatory muscles.

  ▷ *Trigeminal*—5th (Sensory Division)

    ▸ Test tactile perception of the facial skin by touching with a wisp of cotton.

    ▸ Test corneal reflex with wisp of cotton.

    ▸ Test superficial pain of the skin and mucosa with pinpricks.

    ▸ Test the sense of touch in the oral mucosa.

▷ *Abducens*—6th (A)

  ▸ Use the same process as for cranial nerves 3 (oculomotor) and 4 (trochlear).

▷ *Facial*—7th (Motor Division; Finn)

  ▸ Inspect the face in repose for evidence of flaccid paralysis.

  ▸ Test by asking the patient to elevate eyebrows, wrinkle forehead, close eyes, frown, smile, and puff cheeks.

▷ *Facial*—7th (Sensory Division)

  ▸ Test taste for sugar, vinegar, and salt.

▷ *Acoustic*—8th (And)

  ▸ Check hearing with the audiometer or by the whisper test.

  ▸ Check for hearing loss using the Weber and the Rinne tests.

▷ *Glossopharyngeal*—9th (German)

  ▸ Test together with cranial nerve 10 (vagus; see below).

▷ *Vagus*—10th (Viewed)

  ▸ Test for elevation of the uvula by having the patient open his or her mouth and say "ah."

  ▸ Test the gag reflex by touching the back of throat with a tongue blade.

▷ *Accessory spinal*—11th (Some)

  ▸ Test the strength of the sternocleidomastoid and trapezius muscles against resistance of your hands.

▷ *Hypoglossal*—12th (Hops)

  ▸ Look for tremors and other involuntary movement when the patient protrudes his or her tongue.

► Coordination and fine motor skills

  ▸ Equilibrium: Check by administering the Romberg test: have the patient stand up straight with feet together, arms by sides, and eyes closed. Only slight swaying would be normal, and the patient will be able to sustain this pose for approximately 5 seconds. More than slight swaying suggests cerebellar ataxia or vestibular dysfunction.

  ▸ Diadochokinesia: Ability to perform rapid alternating movements (such as patting knees alternating palm and back of hands, touching thumb to each finger); the patient should be able to smoothly execute these movements and maintain the rhythm.

  ▸ Dyssynergia: Finger-to-nose test, heel-to-knee test

  ▸ Handwriting

  ▸ Gait: Observe patient walking.

► Sensory functions

  ▹ Pain: Check sensation to pain with safety pinprick, and compare on each side of body.

  ▹ Temperature: Check temperature if sensation to pain is abnormal.

  ▹ Superficial touch: Test with wisp of cotton.

  ▹ Two-point discrimination: Apply pins to skin simultaneously; ask the patient if he or she feels one or two pinpricks.

  ▹ Stereognosis: Tests the ability to distinguish forms by placing objects in the patient's hands while his or her eyes are closed.

  ▹ Graphesthesia: Tests the ability to identify figures, letters, or words by tracing the figure on the skin of the palm of the hand.

► Motor functions

  ▹ Muscle mass: Measure muscle mass to check for atrophy or hypertrophy.

  ▹ Muscle tone: Tension is present when the muscle is resting.

  ▹ Muscle strength: Check muscular strength against resistance.

  ▹ Be aware of abnormal muscle movements.

► Neurological soft signs

  ▹ Dysdiadochokinesia: Inability to perform rapid alternating movements; result of a lesion to the posterior lobe of the cerebellum.

  ▹ Astereognosis: Inability to discriminate between objects based on touch alone; result of a lesion in the parietal lobe.

  ▹ Choreiform movements

  ▹ Tics

  ▹ Agraphesthesia: Inability to recognize letters or numbers "drawn" on the client's hand with a pointed object.

  ▹ Facial grimacing

  ▹ Impaired fine-motor skills

  ▹ Abnormal blinking

  ▹ Abnormal motor tone.

► Be alert for extrapyramidal symptoms (as in Parkinsonism, dystonia, akathisia) in the patient taking antipsychotics.

► Vital signs

  ▹ Measure height, weight, blood pressure (on children ages 2 or older), pulse, respirations, temperature, and (during the first 2 years) head circumference.

  ▹ Use growth charts for infants and children.

    ▷ Greater than 85th percentile for body mass index (BMI) places a child at increased risk for being overweight.

- Use BMI charts
  - Normal: 20 to 25
  - Overweight: 26 to 29
  - Obese: 30 to 35
- High BMI is a risk factor for diabetes, heart disease, stroke, hypertension, osteoarthritis, and some forms of cancer.

▶ Be alert for high BMI if the client also is being prescribed psychotropic meds with a propensity for weight gain, especially atypical antipsychotics.

- If a patient is presenting with elevated temperature and also is taking psychotropic meds such as carbamazeptine (Tegretol) or clozapine (Clozaril), be alert for agranulocytosis.

▶ Head, skin, nails

- Note the color and integrity of the skin and whether lesions are present.
- Note if the skin is well hydrated, dry, or scaly.
- Assess skin turgor.
- Palpate the skin's temperature.
- Note any unusual moles or other lesions.
- Look at hair texture and distribution.
- Determine the quality of the nails, noting splitting, clubbing, or onychomycosis.
- Check capillary refill.
- Examine head, scalp, sutures, and fontanelles (if infant).
- Check cranial nerve 7 (facial nerve) for symmetry (have client smile, frown, wrinkle forehead, puff cheeks).

▶ Be alert for Stevens-Johnson syndrome (life-threatening rash) especially if the patient is taking carbamazepine or lamotrigine (Lamictal).

- Cancerous moles can be detected by using the acronym ABCDE—*a*ssymetry, *b*order irregularity, *c*olor variation, *d*iameter greater than 6 millimeters, and *e*levation.

▶ Eyes

- Check visual acuity using the Snellen chart (tests cranial nerve 2–optic nerve).
- Test peripheral vision using the confrontation test (tests cranial nerve 2–optic nerve).
- Note the symmetry of eyes and the appearance of orbits, eyelids, and brows.
- Inspect the sclera.
- Assess corneal sensation with wisp of cotton (tests cranial nerves 5 and 7).
- Assess papillary reaction to light and accommodation (tests cranial nerves 3, 4, and 6).

- Assess the six cardinal fields of gaze (extraocular movements; tests cranial nerves 3, 4, and 6).

- Assess corneal light reflex. Light reflections should appear symmetrically in both pupils (tests cranial nerves 3, 4, and 6).

- Examine the inner aspect of the eyes with the ophthalmoscope (tests cranial nerve 2).

▶ Be aware that many psychotropics can cause blurry vision (an anticholinergic side effect).

- Quetiapine (Seroquel) may cause cataracts.

▶ Ears

- Check for configuration, position, and alignment of auricles.

- Test auditory acuity (cranial nerve 8) with the whisper test or audiometer.

- Inspect external auditory canals with otoscope for redness, swelling, or excess cerumen.

- Tympanic membrane should be translucent pearly gray without retractions or bulges.

▶ Nose and sinuses

- Note the appearance of the external nose and whether it is smooth, intact, symmetric, midline, has discharge, or is flaring

- Assess nasal patency.

- Assess sense of smell.

- Inspect internal nasal cavity for patency and septal deviation.

- Palpate maxillary and frontal sinuses.

▶ Neck

- Palpate the lymph nodes (preauricular, postauricular, tonsillar, submandibular, submental, anticervical) for swelling or masses.

- Palpate thyroid (usually not palpable except in very thin people).

- Palpate or auscultate carotid pulse and note any bruits.

▶ Back

- Inspect skin and respiratory pattern on posterior chest.

- Palpate cervical, thoracic, lumbar, and sacral spine.

- Palpate thoracic expansion.

- Percuss posterior chest for tympany.

- Auscultate posterior chest for vesicular or bronchovesicular sounds and note any adventitious breath sounds.

► Thorax and lungs

  ▸ Assess respiratory rate and depth, regularity, and ease of respirations.

  ▸ Note anterior–posterior (AP) diameter, which should be less than the transverse diameter.

  ▸ Percuss anterior chest for resonance and note the quality and symmetry of percussion notes.

  ▸ Auscultate anterior chest for lung sounds; normal breath sounds include vesicular over peripheral lung, bronchovesicular over first and second intercostal spaces at the sternal border, and bronchial over the trachea.

► Breasts

  ▸ Inspect breasts in different positions: with client arms relaxed and by side, with arms elevated above head, and with hands on hips. Look for dimpling, retractions, and orange-peel appearance.

  ▸ Palpate breasts for lumps, including Tail of Spence.

  ▸ Palpate axillary and epitrochlear lymph nodes.

  ▸ Palpate supraclavicular lymph nodes (also known as sentinel or Virchow nodes).

► Be aware that typical antipsychotics as well as atypical antipsychotics may cause galactorrhea.

► Heart

  ▸ Inspect, palpate, and auscultate the carotid pulse.

  ▸ Palpate peripheral pulses and check for symmetry (carotid, brachial, radial, femoral, popliteal, pedal, and posterior tibial).

  ▸ Assess heart rate, rhythm, amplitude, and contour.

  ▸ Assess anatomic location of the apical pulse.

  ▸ Palpate precordium for pulsations, thrills, heaves, and lifts.

  ▸ Auscultate heart sounds with bell and diaphragm and note characteristics of the first and second heart sounds.

  ▸ Assess for jugular venous distention (JVD).

► Be alert for possible electrocardiogram (ECG) changes if the patient is taking tricyclic antidepressants or antipsychotics.

► Be aware that lithium and anorexia nervosa can cause peripheral edema.

► Abdomen

  ▸ Inspect the contour of the abdomen and for scars, abdominal aortic pulsations, and the umbilical cord in the newborn.

  ▸ Auscultate for bowel sounds and the abdominal aorta for bruits.

  ▸ Percuss the abdomen, and note areas of tympany and dullness. It is normal to hear tympany over the small and large intestines and dullness over organs and a distended bladder.

ASSESSMENT OF ACUTE AND CHRONIC DISEASE STATES   89

- Percuss the size of liver and spleen.

- Palpate the abdomen for masses and tenderness. Also palpate the liver and spleen, which are not normally palpable (sometimes the liver can be palpable in thin patients).

▶ Musculoskeletal

- Assess patient's posture for alignment of extremities and spine and for symmetry of body parts.

- Test muscle strength of upper and lower extremities.

- Note symmetry of muscle mass, tone, and strength.

- Assess active range of motion in neck and upper and lower extremities, and note any presence of pain with movement.

- Palpate muscles and joints to elicit pain, deformities, crepitus, and passive range of motion.

- Check for hip dysplasia in infants.

- Check for scoliosis in children and adolescents.

▶ Common indicators of physical child abuse

- History of unexplained multiple fractures

- Burns, hand, or bite marks

- Injuries at various stages of healing

- Evidence of neglect

- Bruising on padded parts of body

MENTAL STATUS EXAMINATION (MSE)

▶ The MSE is the examiner's observations of the patient at the time of the interview.

▶ The MSE is part of the overall process of the psychiatric assessment. It does not stand alone but is used in conjunction with the history, physical exam, and diagnostic and laboratory findings.

▶ Performing the MSE is a key role function of the PMHNP; the MSE should be performed on every patient at every visit.

▶ The MSE a systematic method of evaluating a patient's behavioral, emotional, and cognitive functioning.

- Goals

  ▷ Establish a baseline of a patient's emotional and cognitive functioning

  ▷ Identify a patient's behavioral–psychiatric needs

  ▷ Monitor a patient's functioning and symptom levels over time

  ▷ Function as a screening tool for at-risk patients

  ▷ Readily identify clients experiencing psychotic symptoms (secondary goal).

▶ Structure

▪ Appearance

▷ Assess the patient's overall appearance related to age or culture.

▷ Assess the patient's hygiene and grooming.

▷ Assess the patient's appropriateness of clothing to age, weather, or occasion.

▷ Assess the patient's posture and mannerisms.

▪ Behavior

▷ Describe the patient's general behavior.

▷ Assess the patient's motor behavior.

▷ Describe the patient's attitude—cooperative, confrontative, or evasive.

▪ Mood

▷ Sustained emotional state of the person; internal feelings that influence behavior.

▷ Mood is recorded as the subjective state of emotions as described by the patient.

▪ Affect

▷ Variation of emotional expression in facial expression, body language, nonverbal communication, and voice intonation.

▷ Recorded as the objectively observed state of emotions as determined by the PMHNP

▪ Thought processes (see Table 5–2)

▷ How the patient is thinking: stream of thought; continuity and logic in thought.

▷ Ability to correctly identify abnormalities is essential to effective differential diagnosing of patient needs.

▷ Note problems with word-finding and thought-blocking.

▶ Keep in mind that thought processes can be assessed during the interview before completing the MSE.

▪ Thought content (see Table 5–3)

▷ What the patient is thinking about: ideas, obsessions, and preoccupations

▷ Ability to correctly identify abnormalities is essential to effective differential diagnosing of patient needs.

TABLE 5-2. COMMON FINDINGS OF THOUGHT DISORDER

FINDING	DESCRIPTION
Flight of ideas	► Speech pattern characterized by accelerated speech and rapid shifts in topic ► Often disorganized and difficult to follow, but syntax and vocabulary remain intact
Loose association (derailment)	► Shift in thinking in which ideas move from one apparently unrelated topic to another ► Person remains unaware of the juxtaposed topics
Poverty of content	► Vague, repetitive, and abstractive form of speech that contains many words but little information
Neologisms	► Word inventions or unusual application of current words that, while having personal significance to the person, have no apparent meaning for the listener
Circumstantiality	► Inclusion of unnecessary detail and parenthetical information into the conversation
Tangentiality	► Shifts in topics that often start as related shifts but progressively move farther and farther away from the original topic
Clanging	► Form of loose association in which topics change on the basis of sounds of words rather than meaning of words
Word salad	► Form of very disorganized speech in which syntax is lost and word use is random and idiosyncratic
Perseveration	► Persistent repetition of words or phrases
Confabulation	► Fabrication of facts and details to fill gaps in memory
Blocking	► Sudden stoppage of speech attributed to losing thought or forgetting what was being talked about
Echolalia	► Echoing of words or phrases just spoken by another

TABLE 5-3. ABNORMALITIES OF THOUGHT CONTENT

ABNORMALITY	DESCRIPTION
Hallucination	False sensory perception without stimuli present; can be tactile, olfactory, gustatory, auditory, or visual; can be pervasive or episodic
Delusion	False belief firmly maintained despite evidence to the contrary
Illusion	False perception of a real external stimulus
Homicidal ideation	Thoughts of wishes or intentions to kill someone else
Suicidal ideation	Thoughts of wishes or desires to kill oneself
Hopelessness	A belief that things will not improve and that nothing can be done
Helplessness	A belief that one will not be able to change the course of events, affect a situation, or alter the outcome of things
Anhedonia	Inability to derive pleasure from ordinarily pleasurable activities
Somatic preoccupation	Preoccupation with bodily functions, process, and sensations that may not be based in any realistic alteration in body functioning
Depersonalization	Feeling self far away, disconnected
Derealization	Sense that one's environment has changed and is different than the way it had been before

► Types of delusions

   ► *Religious*: Having an unrealistic or special relationship with God

   ► *Grandiose*: Believing in one's special powers or mission

   ► *Persecution*: Believing that others are conspiring against the person or have malevolent intentions toward him or her

   ► *Of reference*: Other people's thoughts, words, or actions refer to the person (such as thought insertion, thought withdrawal, thought broadcasting, thought control)

      ▷ Thought insertion: Delusion that thoughts are being placed into a person's mind by another person or force

      ▷ Thought withdrawal: Delusion that thoughts are being removed by another person or force

      ▷ Thought broadcasting: Delusion that others can hear a person's thoughts or a person's thoughts are being broadcast over the air

      ▷ Thought control: Delusion that a person's thoughts are being controlled by another person or force

   ► *Somatic*: False beliefs involving functioning of the body

STRUCTURED (TESTED) DATA SET OF THE MSE

▶ Data collected through use of standardized questions; in general, a well-established way to assess for impairment in tested area of functioning

▶ Narrower range of possible findings

▶ Requires a degree of patient cooperation to complete

▶ Includes the following:

   » *Orientation*: Person, time, and place

   » *Attention*: Attentive or distractible

   » *Concentration*

      ▷ Digit-span testing

      ▷ Serial-number testing

      ▷ Backward-spelling testing

   » Memory

      ▷ Long-term testing

      ▷ President testing

      ▷ Event testing

      ▷ Short-term testing

      ▷ Three-object testing

      ▷ Immediate recall testing

      ▷ Number-string testing

   » *Abstraction* (used only if patient is aged 12 or older)

      ▷ Proverb testing

      ▷ Similarity testing

   » *Insight*: Patient's recognition of need for treatment; can be impaired in delirium, dementia, psychosis, frontal-lobe syndrome, substance abuse or dependence

   » *Judgment*: Is patient making realistic decisions based on his or her age, knowledge, assets, and liabilities?

      ▷ Personal welfare testing

      ▷ Social welfare testing

      ▷ Delirium and dementia will show a clouded or wandering sensorium.

      ▷ When testing cognition, depressed patients will usually say, "I don't know," and patients with dementia will usually confabulate.

MINI-MENTAL STATUS EXAM (MMSE)

- The MMSE is a brief instrument designed to assess a patient's cognitive functioning, which can assist in diagnosing an organic component to his or her symptoms.
- Education and intelligence can skew the results.

▶ Orientation
- Time: Year, season, month, date, day
- Place: Name of this place, floor, city, county, state

▶ Registration (memory)
- Repeat three objects, such as *apple, table,* and *penny,* immediately after the PMHNP and have patient recall the same three objects in 5 minutes

▶ Attention and calculation
- Subtract serial 7s from 100
- Spell "world" backward

▶ Recall
- Recall the three objects previously named

▶ Naming
- Show patient items such as a watch and a pencil and have him or her name them

▶ Repeat
- Repeat the words "No ifs, ands, or buts"

▶ Three-stage verbal command
- "Take this paper in your right hand."
- "Fold it in half."
- "Put it on the floor."

▶ Written command
- Print on blank paper the sentence "Close your eyes," and have the patient follow the directions.

▶ Write a sentence
- Have patient write a sentence with a subject, verb, and logical progression of thought.

▶ Intersecting pentagons
- Copy intersecting pentagons on a piece of paper.

▶ MMSE scoring
- 25 to 30: Normal
- 21 to 24: Mild cognitive impairment

- 16 to 20: Moderate cognitive impairment

- Less than 15: Severe cognitive impairment

- Below 24: Possible indicator of dementia

MONTREAL COGNITIVE ASSESSMENT (MoCA) AND SHORT PORTABLE MENTAL STATUS QUESTIONNAIRE (SPMSQ)

▶ In public domain

▶ Translated to many languages

▶ Score: 0–30

- A score of 26 or higher is considered in normal range

Diagnostic and Laboratory Testing

▶ Assessment of diagnostic and laboratory testing is an essential element of the PMHNP role. It is important for the PMHNP to know when to order such tests, how to interpret the findings, and how to appropriately alter care based on the findings.

▶ *Reasons to assess diagnostic and laboratory testing in psychiatry:*

- To assist in the establishment of a diagnosis; as knowledge of underlying pathophysiology grows, diagnostic and laboratory testing use will grow as well

- Used to rule out other disorders such as medical causes of psychiatric symptoms; helpful in differential diagnostic assessment

- Used to determine whether a patient's symptoms are better explained by a nonpsychiatric disorder or by factors such as drug use or abuse

  ▷ For routine ongoing monitoring such as general health screening, monitoring drug levels of certain psychiatric meds, and assessment and monitoring for complications of psychiatric disorders or adverse effects of drugs.

▶ Thyroid function tests

- Function of thyroid gland is to take iodine from the circulating blood, combine it with the amino acid tyrosine, and convert it to the thyroid hormones T3 and T4.

- It also stores T3 and T4 until they are released into the bloodstream under the influence of thyroid-stimulating hormone (TSH) released from the pituitary gland.

- Only a small amount of T3 and T4 are bound to protein.

- The free portion of the thyroid hormones is the true determinant of thyroid status.

▶ Free thyroxine T4 (FT4: normal values 0.8 to 2.8 ng/dL)

  ▸ FT4 composes a small portion of the total thyroxine, is available to the tissues, and is the metabolically active form of this hormone.

  ▸ FT4 test is commonly done to determine thyroid status, to rule out hypo- and hyperthyroidism, and to evaluate thyroid therapy.

    ▷ Increased levels:

      ▸ Graves' disease

      ▸ Thyrotoxicosis due to T4

      ▸ Acute thyroiditis

    ▷ Decreased levels:

      ▸ Primary hypothyroidism

      ▸ Secondary hypothyroidism (pituitary insufficiency)

      ▸ Tertiary hypothyroidism (hypothalamic failure)

      ▸ Thyrotoxicosis due to T3

      ▸ Renal failure

      ▸ Cushing's syndrome

      ▸ Cirrhosis

      ▸ Hashimoto's thyroiditis

    ▷ Interfering factors:

      ▸ Values can be increased during treatment with heparin, aspirin, and propranolol.

      ▸ Values can be decreased during treatment with furosemide (Lasix) or methadone.

▶ Thyroid-stimulating hormone (TSH; normal values 0.4–0.5 mU/L)

  ▸ Stimulation of the thyroid gland by TSH causes release and distribution of stored thyroid hormones.

    ▷ When T4 and T3 are high, TSH secretion decreases.

    ▷ When T4 and T3 are low, TSH secretion increases.

  ▸ In primary hypothyroidism, TSH levels rise because of low levels of thyroid hormone.

    ▷ If the pituitary gland fails, TSH is not secreted and blood levels of TSH fall.

  ▸ TSH testing is commonly performed to establish the diagnosis of primary hypothyroidism.

    ▷ Increased levels:

      ▸ Primary hypothyroidism

      ▸ Thyroiditis

    ▷ Decreased levels:

      ▸ Hyperthyroidism

      ▸ Secondary and tertiary hypothyroidism

> ▷ Interfering factors:
>
> > ▻ Values can be decreased during treatment with T3, acetylsalicylic acid, corticosteroids, and heparin.
> >
> > ▻ Values can be increased during drug therapy with lithium.

▶ Systemic effects of hypothyroidism (decreased T4, increased TSH)

> ▻ Mimics symptoms of unipolar mood disorders
>
> > ▷ Confusion
> >
> > ▷ Decreased libido
> >
> > ▷ Impotence
> >
> > ▷ Decreased appetite
> >
> > ▷ Memory loss
> >
> > ▷ Lethargy
> >
> > ▷ Constipation
> >
> > ▷ Headaches
> >
> > ▷ Slow or clumsy movements
> >
> > ▷ Syncope
> >
> > ▷ Weight gain
> >
> > ▷ Fluid retention
> >
> > ▷ Muscle aching and stiffness
> >
> > ▷ Slowed reflexes
> >
> > ▷ Somatic discomfort including aching and joint stiffness
> >
> > ▷ Slowed speech and thinking
> >
> > ▷ Sensory disturbances, including hearing
> >
> > ▷ Cerebellar ataxia
> >
> > ▷ Loss of amplitude in ECG

▶ Systemic effects of hyperthyroidism (increased T4, decreased TSH)

> ▻ May mimic symptoms of bipolar affective disorders
>
> > ▷ Motor restlessness
> >
> > ▷ Emotional lability
> >
> > ▷ Short attention span
> >
> > ▷ Compulsive movement
> >
> > ▷ Fatigue
> >
> > ▷ Tremor
> >
> > ▷ Insomnia

- Impotence

- Weight loss

- Increase in appetite

- Abdominal pain

- Excessive sweating

- Flushing

- Elevated upper eyelid leading to decreased blinking, staring, fine tremor of eyelid

- Tachycardia

- Dysrhythmias

► Electrolytes

- Carried out as a part of routine screening in acute and critical illness or where there is a known or suspected disorder associated with fluid, electrolyte, or acid–base balance.

► Calcium (Ca; normal values 8.8–10.5 mg/dL)

- Abnormal values:

- < 7.0 mg/dL—associated with tetany

- > 11.0 mg/dL—associated with hyperparathyroidism

- > 13.5 mg/dL—associated with hypercalcemic coma and metastatic cancer.

- Most Ca (99%) is located in bone and the remainder is in the plasma and body cells.

- Of the Ca in the plasma, 50% is bound to plasma proteins and 40% is in the free or ionized form. The remaining fraction circulates in the blood.

- Ca is the major cation for the structure of bones and teeth.

- Functions:

- Enzymatic cofactor for blood clotting

- Required for hormone secretion

- Required for function of cell receptors

- Required for plasma membrane stability and permeability

- Required for transmission of nerve impulses and the contraction of muscles

- Ca balance is mediated by interactions among three hormones: parathyroid hormone, vitamin D, and calcitonin.

- Acting together, these substances determine the amount of dietary Ca absorbed and the renal reabsorption and excretion of Ca by the kidney.

- Increased levels:

- Acidosis

- Hyperparathyroidism

- Cancers (for example, of bone, leukemia, myeloma)

- Drugs (such as thiazide diuretics, hormones, vitamin D, Ca)
- Vitamin D intoxication
- Addison's disease
- Hyperthyroidism
▷ Decreased levels:
  - Alkalosis
  - Hypoparathyroidism
  - Renal failure
  - Pancreatitis
  - Inadequate dietary intake of calcium, vitamin D
  - Drugs, including barbiturates, anticonvulsants, acetazolamide, adrenocorticosteroids
▷ Interfering factors:
  - Values are higher in children because of growth and active bone formation.
  - Values can be increased by excessive ingestion of milk or during treatment with lithium, thiazide diuretics, alkaline antacids, or vitamin D.
  - Values can be decreased during treatment with anticonvulsants, aspirin, calcitonin, corticosteroids, heparin, laxatives, diuretics, albuterol, and oral contraceptives.

► Systemic effects of hypocalcemia (Ca < 8.5 mg/dL):
- Increase in neuromuscular excitability
- Confusion
- Paraesthesias around the mouth and in the digits
- Muscle spasms in the hands and feet
- Hyperreflexia
- Convulsions
- Tetany
- Continuous, severe muscle spasm
- ECG changes: prolonged QT interval
- Intestinal cramping
- Hyperactive bowel sounds

► Systemic effects of hypercalemia (Ca > 12.0 mg/dL):
- Fatigue
- Weakness
- Lethargy

- Anorexia
- Nausea
- Constipation
- Behavioral changes
- Impaired renal function
- ECG changes: shortened QT interval, depressed T-waves
- Bradycardia
- Heart block

► Sodium (Na; normal values 135–148 mEq/L)

- Na accounts for 90% of the extracellular fluid cations and is the most powerful cation in the extracellular fluid.
- It regulates osmolality (interstitial and intravascular fluid volume).
- It works with potassium and calcium to maintain neuromuscular irritability for conduction of nerve impulses.
- It regulates acid–base balance.
- It participates in cellular chemical reactions and membrane transport.
- It regulates renal retention and excretion of water.
- It maintains systemic blood pressure.
  - Increased levels:
    - Hypovolemia
    - Dehydration
    - Diabetes insipidus
    - Excessive salt ingestion
    - Gastroenteritis
    - Drugs such as adrenocorticosteroids, methyldopa, hydralazine, or cough medication
  - Decreased levels:
    - Addison's disease
    - Renal disorder
    - GI fluid loss from vomiting, diarrhea, nasogastric suction, ileus
    - Diuresis
    - Drugs such as lithium, vasopressin, or diuretics

► Systemic effects of hyponatremia (Na < 135 mEq/L):

  ▸ Lethargy

  ▸ Headache

  ▸ Confusion

  ▸ Apprehension

  ▸ Seizures

  ▸ Coma

  ▸ Hypotension

  ▸ Tachycardia

  ▸ Decreased urine output

  ▸ Weight gain

  ▸ Edema

  ▸ Ascites

  ▸ Jugular vein distention

► Systemic effects of hypernatremia (Na >147 mEq/L):

  ▸ Convulsions

  ▸ Pulmonary edema

  ▸ Thirst

  ▸ Fever

  ▸ Dry mucous membranes

  ▸ Hypotension

  ▸ Tachycardia

  ▸ Low jugular venous pressure

  ▸ Restlessness

► Magnesium (Mg: normal values 1.3–2.1 mEq/L)

  ▸ Mg is a major intracellular cation; 40%–60% is stored in bone and muscle, with 30% in cells.

  ▸ A small amount is in the serum, where one-third is bound to plasma proteins and the rest is in ionized form.

  ▸ Regulation of Mg metabolism is primarily by the kidney.

  ▸ Low serum levels cause renal conservation of Mg.

  ▸ Mg is a cofactor in intracellular enzymatic reactions.

  ▸ Mg is a cause of neuromuscular excitability.

    ▷ Increased levels:

- Addison's disease
- Adrenalectomy
- Renal failure
- Diabetic ketoacidosis
- Dehydration
- Hypothyroidism
- Hyperthyroidism

▷ Decreased levels:

- Hyperaldosteronism
- Hypokalemia
- Diabetic ketoacidosis
- Malnutrition
- Alcoholism
- Acute pancreatitis
- GI loss from vomiting, diarrhea, nasogastric suction, and fistula
- Malabsorption syndrome
- Pregnancy-induced hypertension

▷ Interfering factors:

- Hemolysis of a sample leads to falsely elevated levels.
- Numerous drugs can alter levels.
- Values can be increased by drugs such as antacids, laxatives containing Mg, salicylates, and lithium.
- Values can be decreased by drugs such as thiazide diuretics, calcium gluconate, insulin, amphotericin B, neomycin, aldosterone, and ethanol.

▶ Systemic effects of hypomagnesemia (Mg < 1.5 mEq/L):

- Depression
- Confusion
- Irritability
- Increased reflexes
- Muscle weakness
- Ataxia
- Nystagmus
- Tetany
- Convulsions

► Systemic effects of hypermagnesemia (Mg >2.5 mEq/L):

  ▹ Nausea and vomiting

  ▹ Muscle weakness

  ▹ Hypotension

  ▹ Bradycardia

  ▹ Respiratory depression

  ▹ Depressed skeletal muscle contraction and nerve function

► Chloride (normal values 98–106 mEq/L)

  ▹ Chloride is the major anion in the extracellular fluid.

  ▹ It provides electroneutrality in relation to sodium (see above).

  ▹ Transport of chloride is passive and follows the active transport of sodium so that increases or decreases in chloride are proportional to changes in sodium.

    ▷ Increased levels:

      ▹ Acidosis

      ▹ Hyperkalemia, hypernatremia

      ▹ Dehydration

      ▹ Renal failure

      ▹ Cushing's syndrome

      ▹ Hyperventilation

      ▹ Anemia

    ▷ Decreased levels:

      ▹ Alkalosis

      ▹ Hypokalemia

      ▹ Hyponatremia

      ▹ GI loss from vomiting, diarrhea, nasogastric suction, and fistula

      ▹ Diuresis

      ▹ Overhydration

      ▹ Addison's disease

      ▹ Burns

    ▷ Interfering factors:

      ▹ Elevated serum triglyceride levels and myeloma proteins may lead to falsely decreased levels.

      ▹ Values can be increased by potassium chloride, acetazolamide, methyldopa, diazoxide, and guanethidine.

- Values can be decreased by ethacrynic acid, furosemide, thiazide diuretics, and bicarbonate.
  - No specific symptoms are associated with chloride increase or decrease.
- Potassium (K+ ; normal values 3.5–5.1 mEq/L)
  - K+ is the major intracellular electrolyte.
  - Total body K+ is about 4,000 mEq, with most of it located in the cells.
  - Intracellular concentration of K+ is 150 to 160 mEq/L; extracellular concentration is 3.5 to 4.5 mEq/L.
  - As the predominant intracellular ion, K+ regulates intracellular fluid osmolality and provides the balance for intracellular electrical neutrality.
  - K+ is required for glycogen deposition in liver and skeletal muscle cells.
  - K+ maintains resting membrane potential and assists in transmission and conduction of nerve impulses, maintenance of normal cardiac rhythms, and skeletal and smooth muscle contraction.
  - K+ balance is regulated by the kidney, aldosterone levels, insulin secretion, and changes in pH.
    - Increased levels:
      - Acidosis
      - Insulin deficiency
      - Addison's disease
      - Acute renal failure
      - Hypoaldosteronism
      - Infection
      - Dehydration
    - Decreased levels:
      - Alkalosis
      - Excessive insulin
      - GI loss
      - Laxative abuse
      - Burns
      - Trauma
      - Surgery
      - Cushing's syndrome
      - Hyperaldosteronism
      - Thyrotoxicosis

- Anorexia nervosa
- Diet deficient in meat and vegetables
- Interfering factors:
  - False elevations can occur with vigorous pumping of the hand during venipuncture, hemolysis of the sample, or high platelet counts during clotting.
  - False decreases are seen in anticoagulated samples left at room temperature.
  - Values can be decreased by drugs such as furosemide, ethacrynic acid, thiazide diuretics, insulin, aspirin, prednisone, cortisone, gentamycin, lithium, and laxatives.
  - Values can be increased by drugs such as amphotericin B, tetracycline, heparin, epinephrine, potassium-sparing diuretics, and isoniazid.
  - Chronic marijuana use can elevate K+ level.

► Systemic effects of hyperkalemia (K+ > 5.5m Eq/L):
  - Muscle weakness
  - Paralysis
  - Tingling of lips and fingers
  - Restlessness
  - Intestinal cramping
  - Diarrhea
  - ECG changes: narrow and taller T-waves
    - Mild hyperkalemia: shortened QT interval
    - Severe hyperkalemia: depressed ST segment, prolonged PR interval, widened QRS complex leading to cardiac arrest

► Systemic effects of hypokalemia (K+ < 3.5 mEq/L):
  - Impaired carbohydrate metabolism
  - Impaired renal function
  - Polyuria
  - Polydipsia
  - Skeletal muscle weakness
  - Smooth muscle atony
  - Cardiac dysrhythmias
  - Paralysis and respiratory arrest

▶ Liver function tests

    ▸ Used to monitor liver disease or damage caused by hepatotoxic drugs, as confirmed by elevated levels

▶ Alanine aminotransferase (ALT; normal values 5–35 U/L)

    ▸ Formerly known as glutamic–pyruvic transaminase (SGPT), ALT is an enzyme produced by the liver that acts as a catalyst in the transamination reaction necessary for amino acid production.

    ▸ ALT is found in liver cells in high concentrations and in moderate amounts in body fluids, heart, kidneys, and skeletal muscles.

    ▸ When liver damage occurs, serum levels of ALT rise to as much as 50 times normal.

        ▷ Pronounced elevated levels (> 300 U/L):

            ▸ Liver disease or damage, such as hepatic cancer, hepatitis, or infectious mononucleosis

        ▷ Moderately elevated levels (100–300 U/L):

            ▸ Biliary tract obstruction

            ▸ Recent cerebrovascular accident

            ▸ Muscle injury from intramuscular injections, trauma, infection, and seizures

            ▸ Muscular dystrophy

            ▸ Acute pancreatitis

            ▸ Intestinal injury

            ▸ Myocardial infarction

            ▸ Congestive heart failure

            ▸ Renal failure

            ▸ Severe burns

        ▷ Interfering factors:

            ▸ Uremia and hemodialysis can cause falsely decreased levels.

            ▸ Values can be increased with acetaminophen, allopurinol, aspirin, ampicillin, carbamazepine, cephalosporins, codeine, digitalis, indomethacin, heparin, isoniazid, methotrexate, methyldopa, oral contraceptives, phenothiazines, propranolol, tetracycline, and verapamil.

▶ Aspartate amino transferase (AST; normal values 5–40 U/L)

    ▸ Previously known as serum glutamate oxaloacetate transaminase (SGOT), AST measures the level of the enzyme that catalyzes the reversible transfer of an amino group between the amino acid, aspartate, and alphaketoglutamic acid.

- AST exists in large amounts in both liver and myocardial cells and in smaller but significant amounts in skeletal muscles, kidneys, the pancreas, and the brain.

- Serum AST rises when there is cellular damage to the tissues in which the enzyme is found.

  - Pronounced elevation (> 5× normal):

    - Acute hepatocellular damage

    - Myocardial infarction

    - Shock

    - Acute pancreatitis

    - Infectious mononucleosis

  - Moderate elevation (3–5× normal):

    - Biliary tract obstruction

    - Cardiac arrhythmias

    - Congestive heart failure

    - Liver tumors

    - Chronic hepatitis

    - Muscular dystrophy

    - Dermatomyositis

  - Slight elevation (2–3× normal):

    - Pericarditis

    - Cirrhosis, fatty liver

    - Pulmonary infarction

    - Delirium tremens

    - Cerebrovascular accident

    - Hemolytic anemia

  - Interfering factors:

    - Numerous drugs may elevate levels, including antihypertensives, cholinergic agents, anticoagulants, digitalis, erythromycin, isoniazid, methyldopa, oral contraceptives, opiates, salicylates, hepatotoxic medications, and verapamil.

    - Exercise can cause increased levels.

► Gamma glutamyl transpeptidase (GGT; normal values 10–38 IU/L)

- GGT is an isoenzyme of alkaline phosphatase and assists with the transfer of amino acids and peptides across cellular membranes.

- Hepatobiliary tissues and renal tubular and pancreatic epithelium contain large amounts of GGT.

- Other sources of GGT include the prostate gland, brain, and heart.

- GGT is used to evaluate and monitor a patient with known or suspected alcohol abuse, because levels rise even after ingestion of small amounts of alcohol.

- Also used to evaluate elevated alkaline phosphatase of uncertain etiology.

- Pronounced early increases in GGT are found in in hepatic disease.

- Modest elevation in GGT occurs in cirrhosis and in pancreatic or renal disease.

  - Elevated GGT:
    - Hepatobiliary tract disorders
    - Hepatocellular carcinoma
    - Hepatocellular degeneration such as cirrhosis
    - Hepatitis
    - Pancreatic or renal cell damage or neoplasm
    - Congestive heart failure
    - Acute myocardial infarction (after 4–10 days)
    - Hyperlipoproteinemia
    - Diabetes mellitus with hypertension
    - Seizure disorder
    - Significant alcohol ingestion
  - Interfering factors:
    - Alcohol, barbiturates, and phenytoin can elevate GGT levels.
    - Late pregnancy, oral contraceptives, and clofibrate can lower GGT levels.

Disease Prevention Activities

Immunizations are critical to preventing disease, according to the U.S. Centers for Disease Control and Prevention (CDC). Immunizations protect individual children and adults from developing potentially serious diseases while also protecting the community by reducing the spread of infectious disease.

- ▶ Schedules for children and adults are available on the CDC website at www.cdc.gov/vaccines/schedules/index.html.

- ▶ Seasonal influenza vaccination (as live attenuated influenza vaccine or inactivated type)

  - Vaccinate all children ages 6 months to 18 years; all persons aged 50+ years; persons ages 19 through 49 years who live in nursing homes, long-term care, or assisted living facilities or who have chronic health conditions (asthma, diabetes mellitus, renal or hepatic dysfunction; immunocompromising conditions caused by HIV or medication; cognitive, neurologic, or neuromuscular disorders; and pregnancy); and all persons who wish to decrease their risk for influenza.

- ‣ Vaccinate all healthcare personnel and caregivers of children younger than 5 years.

- ‣ Use live vaccine or inactivated vaccine for healthy nonpregnant adults younger than 50 years of age with no high-risk medical conditions. All others should receive the inactivated vaccine only.

▶ HPV vaccination for girls is recommended at age 11 or 12 years with catch-up vaccination at ages 13 through 26 years to prevent genital human papillomavirus infection, which can cause cervical cancer and genital warts.

- ‣ HPV4 may be administered to males age 9 through 26 years to prevent genital warts.

▶ Measles, mumps, rubella (MMR; live vaccine)

- ‣ Not for pregnant women; people with cancer, weakened immune systems, or HIV/AIDS with T-cell counts below 200; or people currently being treated with high-dose steroids or who have received a blood transfusion within the previous 2 weeks.

▶ Diphtheria, tetanus, acellular pertussis

- ‣ Td (tetanus, diphtheria) vaccine should be given every 10 years beginning at age 11 years, with Tdap (tetanus, diphtheria, acellular pertussis) substituted once for Td but no less than 5 years after the last DTaP dose was given. DTaP should not be given to anyone 7 years of age or older.

▶ Shingles (also known as *herpes zoster*) vaccine

- ‣ Recommended for anyone age of 60 or older who has had chickenpox.

- ‣ Do not give shingles vaccine to people with weakened immune systems or HIV/AIDS with T-cell counts below 200, or to patients being treated with high-dose steroids.

- ‣ Shingles is an inflammatory condition in which a virus produces painful vesicular eruptions along the distribution of the nerves from one or more dorsal root ganglia (National Institutes of Health, 2010).

▶ Varicella (chickenpox) vaccine

- ‣ Not for pregnant women, people with weakened immune systems, HIV/AIDS with T-cell counts below 200, or cancer; not for people being treated with high-dose steroids or who received a blood transfusion within the previous 2 weeks.

Anticipatory guidance is a framework for implementation of prevention strategies.

▶ Based on the premise that information can be provided to people to help them cope more effectively with events that occur along the lifespan. Within the framework of anticipatory guidance, the practitioner seeks to determine the specific informational needs of the patient in a systematic, standard way.

▶ Pediatrics: Soliciting information from parents about their concerns in parenting and providing information specific to their concerns. Teaching parents about health hazards and strategies to prevent harm, such as car seat safety, water safety, wearing helmets, and so forth.

- *Bright Futures* (www.brightfutures.org/) is a national health promotion initiative (launched by the Health Resources and Services Administration in partnership with other agencies) dedicated to the principle that every child deserves to be healthy and that optimal health involves a trusting relationship among the health professional, the child, the family, and the community as partners in health practice. Expansion of the model includes screening, care management, and education about mental health problems and disorders in developmental context.

- In specific healthcare situations, anticipatory guidance can be used to assist people in meeting healthcare challenges across the life span. Some examples include

  - Coping with terminal illness or death and dying (anticipatory grief)

  - Coping with disease progression, such as with Alzheimer's dementia, in a loved one

  - Coping with change and limitations resulting from spinal cord injuries

  - Can be implemented in each "well check" to identify information needs pertinent to the patient's current life situation. Some examples:

    - Responsible alcohol use for the adolescent going off to college

    - Domestic violence

    - Life after the loss of a loved one (through divorce or death)

    - Planning for retirement

GENDER-BASED MEDICAL TESTING AND SCREENING RECOMMENDATIONS FOR THE GENERAL PUBLIC

Tanner Stages

Defines physical measurements of development in children, adolescents, and adults. The development of primary and secondary sex characteristics (breasts, genitalia, and pubic hair) are assessed by stages to describe the onset and progression of puberty in both males and females. Because of natural variability, males and females pass through the stages at different rates based on timing of puberty.

Boys: Development of External Genitalia

- Stage 1: Prepubertal

- Stage 2: Enlargement of scrotum and testes; scrotum skin reddens and changes in texture

- Stage 3: Enlargement of penis (length at first); further growth of testes

- Stage 4: Increase in size of penis with growth in breadth and development of glans; testes and scrotum larger, scrotum skin darker

- Stage 5: Adult genitalia (Jarvis, 2000)

ASSESSMENT OF ACUTE AND CHRONIC DISEASE STATES   111

Girls: Breast Development

▶ Stage 1: Prepubertal

▶ Stage 2: Breast bud stage with elevation of breast and papilla; enlargement of areola

▶ Stage 3: Further enlargement of breast and areola; no separation of their contour

▶ Stage 4: Areola and papilla from a secondary mound above level of breast

▶ Stage 5: Mature stage: projection of papilla only, related to recession of areola (Jarvis, 2000)

Boys and Girls: Pubic Hair

▶ Stage 1: Prepubertal (can see velus hair similar to adominal wall)

▶ Stage 2: Sparse growth of long, slightly pigmented hair, straight or curled, at base of penis or along labia

▶ Stage 3: Darker, coarser and more curled hair, spreading sparsely over junctions of pubes

▶ Stage 4: Hair adult type, but covering smaller area than in adult, no spread to medial surface of thighs

▶ Stage 5: Adult type and quantity, with horizontal distribution (Jarvis, 2000).

Women

▶ Ages 18 through 39

  ▹ Monthly: Skin and oral self-exams

  ▹ Yearly: Blood pressure; blood tests and urinalysis; physical exam; Pap smear (beginning at age 21 or within 3 years of sexual activity, whichever comes first), pelvic exam, sexually transmitted infection (STI) detection

▶ Ages 40 through 49

  ▹ Monthly: Skin and oral self-exams

  ▹ Yearly: Blood pressure; blood tests and urinalysis; physical exam; Pap smear (every 2 or 3 years after 3 consecutive negative smears), pelvic exam, STI detection; electrocardiogram (ECG) every 4 years

▶ Ages 50+

  ▹ Monthly: Skin and oral self-exams

  ▹ Yearly: Blood pressure; blood tests (complete blood count, metabolic panel, thyroid-stimulating hormone) and urinalysis; physical exam; Pap smear (65 and older not recommended if person had proper recent normal Pap smear and is not at high risk for cervical cancer), pelvic exam, STI detection; mammography every 2 years; routine bone density screening starting at age 65 and older (beginning at 60 if increased risk for osteoporotic fractures)

  ▹ Every 4 years: ECG

  ▹ Every 5 years through age 75, flexible sigmoidoscopy or double-contrast barium enema or CT colonography (if any of these tests are positive, a colonoscopy should be done), *or* colonoscopy every 10 years

  ▹ Consult provider: Hearing, vision

► Additional colorectal cancer screening for high-risk women

   ▪ The American Cancer Society recommends that some people be screened using a different schedule because of their personal or family history.

Men

► Ages 18 through 39

   ▪ Monthly: Self-exams (testicles, skin, and oral)

   ▪ Yearly: Blood pressure; blood tests (complete blood count, metabolic panel, thyroid-stimulating hormone) and urinalysis; physical exam

► Ages 40 through 49

   ▪ Monthly: Testicles, skin, and oral self-exams

   ▪ Yearly: Blood pressure; blood tests (complete blood count, metabolic panel, thyroid-stimulating hormone) and urinalysis; physical exam; ECG every 4 years

► Ages 50+

   ▪ Monthly: Testicles, skin, and oral self-exams

   ▪ Yearly: Blood pressure; blood tests (complete blood count, metabolic panel, thyroid-stimulating hormone) and urinalysis; physical exam; ECG every 3 years

   ▪ 5 years through age 75: Flexible sigmoidoscopy or double-contrast barium enema or CT colonography (if any of these tests are positive, a colonoscopy should be done), *or* colonoscopy every 10 years

   ▪ Consult provider: Testosterone blood test; hearing and vision screening

DEVELOPING AND PRIORITIZING A DIFFERENTIAL DIAGNOSIS LIST

Differential diagnosis: A systematic method for diagnosing a disorder that lacks unique symptoms, signs, or characteristics. Through this process, the practitioner settles upon a final and correct diagnosis.

► Establishment of a differential diagnosis allows the clinician to

   ▪ Identify disorder-specific questions to be included during the interview

   ▪ Establish a list of appropriate and cost-effective diagnostic tests

   ▪ Logically and systematically eliminate inaccurate diagnoses

   ▪ Prioritize diagnoses from imminently dangerous to chronic or nonacute.

▶ Steps

    ▹ Establish a therapeutic, collaborative relationship with patient

    ▹ Elicit the patient's chief complaint

    ▹ Validate symptoms through the interview process, screening tools, and collateral resources

▶ Rule out the influence of medications, toxins, or substances on central nervous system functioning

    ▹ Through interview, screening tools, physical examination, and diagnostic testing

    ▹ Establish the timing of symptoms and substance use

    ▹ Determine whether the substance used, amount, and duration are consistent with the psychiatric symptoms

    ▹ When substances are present, determine whether a causal relationship exists:

        ▷ Direct effect: Are the presenting symptoms a direct result of substance use?

        ▷ Consequence: Is substance use the result of having a psychiatric illness?

        ▷ Simultaneous: Did substance use and presenting symptoms occur together?

        ▷ Independent: Are symptoms and substance use independent?

        ▷ Alternatives: Are there other or better explanations for the symptoms?

▶ When substance use is suspected of being the primary Axis I diagnosis, *DSM-IV* criteria guide diagnostic decision-making. Competing diagnoses are eliminated before a final diagnosis is made. Rule out a general medical condition as the basis of symptoms.

    ▹ Through interview, screening tools, physical examination, and diagnostic testing

    ▹ When a medical condition is present, determine whether a causal relationship exists

    ▹ Congruence: Are the onset, pattern, and course of the medical condition mirrored in that of the psychiatric illness?

        ▷ Direct effect: Are the psychiatric symptoms a direct result of a medical condition?

        ▷ Psychological: Does the medical condition cause the psychiatric symptoms through psychological means?

        ▷ Treatment effect: Are psychiatric symptoms related to the treatment of the medical condition?

        ▷ Coincidental: Do the psychiatric symptoms and medical condition occur together but remain unrelated?

    ▹ When a medical condition is suspected of being the primary Axis I disorder, *DSM-IV* criteria guide diagnostic decision-making. Competing diagnoses are eliminated before a final diagnosis is made.

- Settle on the primary or principal disorder on Axis I.
  - Use *DSM-IV* criteria to determine the disorder that best accounts for the patient's symptoms
- If symptom severity or duration does not meet *DSM-IV* criteria, decide if the stressor is likely to have caused the symptoms.
  - Adjustment disorder: Symptoms represent a maladaptive response to a specific stressor.
  - Not otherwise specified: Does not meet criteria for particular disorder and the symptoms are not caused by a specific stressor.
- Determine whether the symptoms are causing a level of distress or impairment in social, occupational, or other areas of functioning (American Psychological Association, 2000).
- Multiple Axis I disorders are common and often necessary to describe the patient's symptoms. The principal diagnosis is listed first (First, Frances, & Pinus, 2002).

HEALTH BEHAVIOR GUIDELINES

Exercise

Exercise benefits both physical and mental health. Inactivity has a direct link to obesity, a major health problem in this country. In results of recent studies, exercise has demonstrated effects comparable to antidepressant therapy in the treatment of depression.

- Key factor in staying healthy: Strengthens bones, heart, and lungs, tones muscles, improves vitality, relieves depression, and helps to improve sleep. It is particularly beneficial to persons with comorbid medical conditions such as diabetes, obesity, and hypertension.
- Mind–body connection: Improves cognition and enhances mood
- Neurobiological explanation: Promotes increased concentrations of serotonin, norepinephrine, and endorphins
- Integrative psychiatry includes strategies to improve lifestyle practices (diet, exercise, smoking cessation, drug and alcohol use) and reduce stress to prevent illness
- Patient teaching regarding exercise:
  - Check with provider before starting an exercise program.
  - Begin exercising gradually. Don't expect results overnight. If you are consistent, you will see improvement within 3 months.
  - Work hard enough to sweat, but not so hard that you cannot carry on a conversation.
  - Plan an exercise routine that lasts 20 to 30 minutes, and perform the workout at least 3 to 5 days a week. Warming up before exercise helps avoid injury.

- Include both aerobic and strengthening activities in exercise program.

- Exercise programs need to be modified for children, pregnant women, the older adults, patients who are obese or disabled, and heart attack survivors as well as modified for high altitudes and extreme hot or cold conditions.

- Monitor the intensity of exercise by measuring heart rate. The target heart rate during physical activity should be 60% to 90% of the maximum heart rate. Use the following formula to calculate target heart rate:

  - 220 (beats per minute) minus age = maximum heart rate

  - Maximum heart rate multiplied by the intensity level = target heart rate

  - Physical activity at 60% to 70% of the maximum heart rate is considered moderate-intensity exercise.

▶ CDC recommends **60 minutes (1 hour) or more of physical activity each day for children and adolescents.**

▶ CDC recommends 150 minutes of moderate-intensity aerobic activity (such as brisk walking) every week **and** muscle-strengthening activities 2 or more days a week for adults, including healthy older adults (www.cdc.gov/physicalactivity/everyone/ guidelines/adults.html#Musclestrengthening; U.S. Department of Health and Human Services, 2008; Centers for Disease Control and Prevention, 2010).

Access to Care Model

Access to care is a patient-centered care model based on the principle that healthcare services should be coordinated and directed by a single physician or other provider. In this model, patients can access services from multiple entry points. Services can be located in the same facility, or an integrated care network of providers in different locations can be accessed when needed.

Patient-Centered Care Model (PCC)

▶ Welcoming environment: Provide a physical space and an initial personal interaction that is welcoming and familiar, not intimidating.

▶ Respect for patients' values and expressed needs: Obtain information about the patient's care preferences and priorities; inform and involve the patient and family or caregivers in decision-making; tailor care to the individual; promote a mutually respectful, consistent patient–provider relationship.

▶ Patient empowerment or "activation": Educate and encourage the patient to expand his or her role in decision-making, health-related behaviors, and self-management.

▶ Sociocultural competence: Understand and consider culture, economic and educational status, health literacy level, family patterns and situation, and traditions (including alternative and folk remedies); communicate in language and at a level that the patient understands.

▶ Coordination and integration of care: Assess the patient's need for formal and informal services that may have an impact on health or treatment; provide team-based care, care management, and referrals as needed; advocate for the patient and family; and ensure smooth transitions between different providers and phases of care.

▶ Comfort and support: Emphasize physical comfort, privacy, emotional support, and involvement of family and friends.

▶ Access and navigation skills: Provide what the patient can consider a "medical home"; keep waiting times to a minimum; provide convenient service hours; promote access and patient flow; help patient attain skills to better navigate the healthcare system.

▶ Community outreach: Make demonstrable, proactive efforts to understand and reach out to the local community (Silow-Carroll, Alteras, & Stepnick, 2006).

THERAPEUTIC COMMUNICATION PRINCIPLES

Conflict of Interest

A conflict of interest (COI) is a situation in which a person's financial, professional, or personal situation may affect or appear to affect the person's judgment in his or her professional responsibilities, including healthcare decisions, research, and other matters, with the potential for personal or professional gain or advantage—or, conversely, loss or disadvantage—of any kind and the possibility of potential harm to patients.

▶ Disclosure of potential conflicts of interests should be done at least annually and whenever new significant financial interests are acquired.

▶ Disclosure is required to be reported to employers, boards, professional agencies, and wherever there is potential for a COI.

▶ Action should be carried out to resolve the potential or actual conflicts of interest and reduce bias.

▶ Healthcare agencies and educational and research institutions have policies to require the disclosure of any potential conflict of interest and to define the limits allowed in any relationship with external organizations and companies.

▶ A conflict of interest form indicating any financial or other relationship with the products being discussed must be completed prior to any professional presentation. In addition, if any off-label uses of medications or medical devices will be discussed, this information must also be disclosed.

▶ Types of conflict of interest

   ▸ Relationships with pharmaceutical, medical supply, or insurance companies

   ▸ Money, gifts in kind

   ▸ Referrals

   ▸ Fee splitting

Self-Awareness

▶ Requires reflection on one's personal beliefs, thoughts, emotions, motives, biases, and limitations and being aware of how they influence your behavior toward others.

▶ Helpful to have a trusted person who can give open, honest feedback to self-examination

▶ Personal experiences influence communication patterns and responses to patients

▶ Social biases, feelings, and beliefs projected onto the patient may affect the nurse–patient relationship

▶ Being nonjudgmental and objective cultivates trust in the relationship

▶ Clinical supervision by colleague provides ongoing feedback for therapeutic development of the helper, including supporting change as needed

▶ If personal values and beliefs make it difficult to be therapeutic with a particular patient, refer the patient to another provider.

Self-Disclosure

▶ Revealing personal information to the patient changes the focus away from the patient.

▶ When asked personal questions, self-disclosure can be limited by redirecting, giving a vague answer, or reminding patient that you will not share your personal information.

▶ Self-disclosure may be therapeutic only when it is purposeful and has an identified therapeutic outcome, such as role-modeling.

ASSESSMENT TOOLS

Screening Tools

▶ Purpose

　▷ Identification of risks associated with a particular disease

　▷ Part of a diagnostic workup; screening tools may be a small part of a diagnostic evaluation

　▷ Identification of key factors the clinician should include in the clinical evaluation or assessment

　▷ Early detection of disease

Diagnostic Tools

▶ Purpose

　▷ Detection of disease

　▷ Assessment of disease severity

　▷ Establish and assess efficacy of treatment regimens

► Terms

- *Validity:* The extent to which a particular screening tool actually identifies the disorder for which it is used

- *Reliability:* The extent to which a particular screening tool consistently identifies the disorder for which it is used

- *Sensitivity:* The proportion of actual positives that are correctly identified as such. A tool with high sensitivity is important when the cost of failing to detect the disorder is high. Example: failing to identify a high potential for suicide.

- *Specificity:* The proportion of true negatives that are correctly identified. A tool with high specificity is important when the cost of a false positive is high. Example: labeling a person as alcohol-dependent when he or she is not.

- *Gold-standard test:* A test or tool with a sufficiently high sensitivity and specificity to be considered definitive or the best available

► Types

- *Screening tools:* Brief, easily administered and scored scales that, when positive, suggest the need for additional evaluation. Examples include the CAGE and CRAFFT screening tools for substance use.

- *Assessment tools:* Used to evaluate and assess the presence of specific symptoms and their severity. Examples include the Abnormal Involuntary Movement Scale (AIMS) used to monitor adverse treatment effects and the Global Assessment of Functioning (GAF). When used repeatedly, assessment tools provide valuable information on treatment efficacy and disease management.

- *Treatment-directed tools:* These scales assist in the rational utilization of specific treatments. For example, the Clinical Institute Withdrawal Assessment of Alcohol Scale (CIWA) monitors alcohol withdrawal symptoms and is often linked to specific treatment protocols, such as administration of benzodiazepines to promote safe detoxification.

► Tool audience

- Self-report

  ▷ Advantages: The screening tool is completed at the person's convenience; allows time for self-reflection

  ▷ Problems: Exaggeration or underreporting of symptoms; deliberate misrepresentation for secondary gain; comorbid conditions that have symptoms similar or identical to those being assessed can invalidate the results

- Collateral: Family member, teacher, friends

  ▷ Advantages: Offers additional assessment depth, especially when the person being screened its too young, too ill, or unable or unwilling to participate

  ▷ Problems: Perspectives of others may not be more accurate or insightful that those of the person; responses may represent bias or prejudices not germane to the person; adult patients typically must consent

- Clinician

  - Advantages: The tool is administered in the appropriate setting and manner; process offers an additional opportunity to assess the person

  - Problems: Can be time-consuming; may not have been validated in specific population or comorbid condition

▶ Comments

  - Scales used by researchers are often not appropriate for clinical use due to the number of questions, time required to complete the questionnaire, difficulty with scoring, and lack of evidence supporting clinical application.

  - Not all scales are congruent with *DSM-IV* criteria.

  - Time frames for reporting of symptoms vary from test to test. Some ask for symptoms in the last week, others in the last month.

  - Scales used by clinicians and patients are typically not diagnostic. They are one component of a comprehensive clinical evaluation.

120 PSYCHIATRIC–MENTAL HEALTH NURSE PRACTITIONER REVIEW MANUAL, 3RD EDITION

TABLE 5–4. SELECTED ASSESSMENT TOOLS

ASSESSMENT TOOLS	CHARACTERISTICS	COMMENTS
ADVERSE TREATMENT EFFECTS		
AIMS* **Abnormal Involuntary Movement Scale** (STABLE National Coordinating Counsel, 2008)	▸ Assessment of symptoms associated with tardive dyskinesia in patients receiving antipsychotic medications ▸ A 12-item tool with two items related to current dental health and 10 items referring to atypical movements in seven body areas. First, the individual describes any unusual movements and rates the impact on daily activities. The clinician then asks the patient to perform a series of movements; the presence of any atypical movements is rated, according to severity, and contributes to the overall score. ▸ Rating: 0 [no abnormal movement] to 4 [severe abnormal movement] ▸ Scoring: Dyskinesia is present if movements were 2 [mildly abnormal] in at least two body areas or 3 [moderately abnormal] in one area. A score > 2 warrants a diagnosis of tardive dyskinesia. The clinician should discontinue or reduce the dose of the antipsychotic medication.	▸ Clinician-administered ▸ Age 8 and older; both genders; validated in diverse cultures; used in multiple psychiatric illnesses and with a variety of antipsychotic medications ▸ Recommended that serial testing be done every 3 to 6 months for all patients receiving antipsychotics ▸ Although interrater reliability has been found to be > 90%, erroneous scores may occur, especially with clinicians lacking experience with the tool ▸ http://www. testandcalc.com/etc/ tests/bprs.asp
BARS* **Barnes Akathisia Rating Scale** (Barnes, 2003; Hamilton, 1959)	▸ Assessment of objective and subjective symptoms associated with akathisia in patients receiving antipsychotic medications or SSRIs ▸ A four-item scale assessing the presence and severity of drug-induced akathisia; includes both objective items (observed restlessness) and subjective items (patient's awareness of restlessness and related distress), and a clinical evaluation for symptoms of akathisia ▸ The Global Clinical Assessment of Akathisia uses a 6-point scale ranging from 0 through 5. ▸ Score of 0 [absent]; 1 [questionable]; 2 [mild akathisia a];, 3 [moderate akathisia]; 4 [marked akathisia]; or 5 [severe akathisia]	▸ Clinician-administered ▸ Age 8 and older; both genders; validated in diverse cultures; used in multiple psychiatric illnesses and with a variety of antipsychotic medications ▸ Most widely used scale to measure akathisia ▸ http://www. outcometracker.org/ library/BAS.pdf

* indicates public domain

CONTINUED ▸

ASSESSMENT OF ACUTE AND CHRONIC DISEASE STATES   121

TABLE 5–4. CONTINUED ▶

ASSESSMENT TOOLS	CHARACTERISTICS	COMMENTS
ADHD		
CRS-R Connors Rating Scales – Revised **ADHD Parent and Teacher Scales** (Massachusetts General Hospital, 2010)	▶ Long form contains parent scale (80 questions) and teacher scale (59 questions) ▶ Subset scales for Oppositional Behaviors, Cognitive Problems, Hyperactivity, ADHD Index, Anxious–Shy, Perfectionism, Social Problems, *DSM-IV* Symptom Subscales, and Connors' Global Index ▶ Short form has parent scale (27 items) and teacher scale (28 items) ▶ Interpretable scores range from a low T-score of 61 [mildly atypical] to above 70 [markedly atypical]	▶ Self-, parent-, or teacher-reported, or clinician-administered ▶ Ages 3–17; both genders ▶ One component of a complete work-up ▶ Further information can be obtained from http://portal. wpspublish.com/ portal/page?_ pageid=53,235050&_ dad=portal&_ schema=PORTAL
Vanderbilt ADHD* Parent and Teacher (Massachusetts General Hospital, 2010)	▶ Consists of parent (55 items) and teacher (43 items) scales ▶ Initial assessment tool that rates both symptoms and impairment in academic and behavioral performance	▶ Children ages 6–12 ▶ Parent and teacher report ▶ Copies can be obtained from http://www2. massgeneral.org/ schoolpsychiatry/ screeningtools_table. asp
ASRS-1* Adult ADHD Self-Report Scale Kessler, Adams, Ames, Demlar et al. (2005)	▶ A two-part screening tool for adult ADHD ▶ Part A: Six questions reflecting common ADHD symptoms ▶ Rating: For questions 1–3: 1 point for any positive response (sometimes, often, or very often). For questions 4–6: 1 point for a positive response (often or very often). ▶ Scoring: The presence of at least four symptoms is strongly indicative of adult ADHD and warrants further attention ▶ Part B: 12 questions that explore the type and frequency of symptoms ▶ Scoring: There is no scoring for this section of the tool; it is used to clarify and quantify additional, less sensitive, symptoms	▶ Self-reported or clinician-administered ▶ Age 16 and older; both genders. ▶ Questions meet *DSM-IV* criteria for diagnosis

* indicates public domain

CONTINUED ▶

TABLE 5–4. SELECTED ASSESSMENT TOOLS CONTINUED ▶

ASSESSMENT TOOLS	CHARACTERISTICS	COMMENTS
ALCOHOL AND DRUG USE		
AUDIT-C* Alcohol Use Disorders Identification Test – Consumption (Bradley, Bush, & Epler, 2003; Bush, Kivlahan, McDonell, Fihn, & Bradley, 1998; Halverson & Chan, 2004; National Institute on Alcohol Abuse and Alcoholism, 2005; STABLE National Coordinating Counsel, 2008)	▶ Documents the use and frequency of alcohol or drug intake during the last year; eight questions regarding the frequency and quantity on a single occasion ▶ Rating: 0 [never] to 4 [four or more times per week]. Two questions cover the impact of substance use; rated 0 [no], 2 [yes, but not in the last year], or 4 [yes, in the last year] ▶ Scoring: Females with a score > 3 are considered positive ▶ Males with a score > 4 are considered positive ▶ A score of 8 or higher, for either gender, indicates hazardous drinking	▶ Self-reported or clinician-administered ▶ Age 13 and older; both genders; validated in diverse cultures and in a variety of comorbid conditions ▶ Heavy or hazardous drinking: ▷ Males: > 4: sensitivity 95%; specificity 60% ▷ Females: > 3: sensitivity 66%; specificity 94% ▷ Active *DSM-IV* alcohol abuse or dependence: ▷ Males: > 4: sensitivity 90%; specificity 45% ▷ Females: > 3: sensitivity 80%; specificity 87%
CAGE-AID* (acronym of four questions used in screening) (Brown & Rounds, 1995; Halverson & Chan, 2004; National Institute on Alcohol Abuse and Alcoholism, 2005; STABLE National Coordinating Counsel, 2008)	▶ Identification of problem drinking or drug use by asking: have you tried to **C**ut down; do people **A**nnoy you about it; do you feel **G**uilty about it; do you need an **E**ye-opener; and Altered to Include Drugs ▶ Rating: Four questions rated as 0 [no] or 1 [yes] ▶ Scoring: One point for each "yes" answer. Two or more points indicate clinically significant substance use and *may* indicate dependence	▶ Self-reported or clinician-administered ▶ Age 13 and older; both genders; validated in diverse cultures and a variety of comorbid conditions ▶ Can screen for alcohol and substance used simultaneously ▶ One positive response: sensitivity 79%; specificity 77% ▶ Two or more positive responses: sensitivity 93%; specificity 76% ▶ May be less sensitive in women and some minorities
CRAFFT* (acronym of six questions used in screening) (Knight, Sherritt, Shrier, Harris, & Chang, 2002; Massachusetts Department of Public Heath Bureau of Substance Abuse Services, 2009)	▶ Six-item instrument used to screen for alcohol and other drug use in adolescents ▶ By asking: have you ridden in a **C**ar driven by someone high or intoxicated; do you use to **R**elax; do you use when **A**lone; do you **F**orget when using; do **F**amily or **F**riends tell you to stop; have you ever gotten into **T**rouble when using ▶ Rating: Six questions, rated 0 [no] or 1 [yes] ▶ Scoring: Two or more points suggest alcohol or drug abuse	▶ Self-reported or clinician-administered ▶ Age 14–18 ▶ Sensitivity: 80%; specificity: 86% ▶ http://www.mass.gov/ eohhs/docs/dph/ substance-abuse/sbirt/ crafft-provider-guide.rtf

* indicates public domain

CONTINUED ▶

ASSESSMENT OF ACUTE AND CHRONIC DISEASE STATES 123

TABLE 5-4. CONTINUED ▶

ASSESSMENT TOOLS	CHARACTERISTICS	COMMENTS
ANXIETY		
SOCIAL ANXIETY		
BAI **Beck Anxiety Inventory** (Halverson & Chan, 2004; Leyfer, Ruberg, & Woodruff-Borden, 2005)	▶ Measures presence and impact of 21 symptoms commonly associated with anxiety ▶ Does not assess worry, difficulty concentrating, irritability, or sleep problems ▶ Rating: 0 [not at all bothersome] to 3 [very bothersome] ▶ Scoring: 0–21 [very low anxiety]; 22–35 [moderate anxiety]; 36+ [serious anxiety]	▶ Self-reported or clinician-administered ▶ Age 17 and older; both genders; validated in diverse cultures ▶ Is best in detecting panic disorder: sensitivity 97%; specificity 81% ▶ GAD: sensitivity 98%; specificity 84% ▶ Phobia: sensitivity 81%; specificity 44% ▶ Any anxiety disorder: sensitivity 84%; specificity 67%
HAM-A* **Hamilton Anxiety Scale** (Hamilton, 1959)	▶ Based on 14 domains of anxiety: anxious mood, fears, sleep disturbance, somatic complaints, tension, and observed behavior at interview ▶ Rating: Severity of symptomatology 0 [not present] to 4 [severe] ▶ Scoring: 14–17 [mild anxiety]; 18–24 [moderate anxiety]; 25–30 [severe anxiety]	Clinician-administered ▶ Most commonly used anxiety rating scale ▶ Best used in the evaluation of symptom severity and treatment efficacy over time
LSAS–CA* **Liebowitz Social Anxiety Scale–Child/ Adolescent Version** (Masia-Warner, Storch, Pincus, Klein, Heimberg, & Liebowitz, 2003)	▶ The questionnaire includes 24 items. Each item consists of a given situation, the rate of anxiety (0 to 3 = none, mild, moderate, severe) and the rate of avoidance (0 to 3 = never, occasionally, often, usually) ▶ Assessment by investigation of 12 social interactions and 12- performance situations ▶ Rating: Four-point fear rating from 0 [none] to 3 [severe]; avoidance behavior rated 0 [never] to 3 [usually] ▶ Scoring: 55–65 (moderate social phobia); 65–80 (marked social phobia); 80–95 (severe social phobia); > 95 (very severe social phobia)	Clinician-administered and -evaluated ▶ Age 7 and older; both genders; validated in diverse cultures ▶ Frequently used in pharmacologic studies and the evaluation of cognitive behavioral therapy ▶ http://healthnet. umassmed.edu/ mhealth/LiebowitzSocial AnxietyScale.pdf

* indicates public domain

CONTINUED ▶

TABLE 5–4. SELECTED ASSESSMENT TOOLS CONTINUED ▶

ASSESSMENT TOOLS	CHARACTERISTICS	COMMENTS
COGNITIVE FUNCTION		
MMSE **The Mini Mental Status Exam** The MMSE is copyright-protected (Folstein, Folstein & McHugh, 1975; Halverson & Chan, 2004; Powsner & Powsner, 2005)	▶ Measures orientation, registration, attention and calculation, recall, and language ▶ 30 items screen for cognitive loss and quantify cognitive function ▶ Information is obtained through a series of questions and commands ▶ Rating: One point is given for each correct answer ▶ Scoring: 24–30 [no cognitive impairment]; 18–23 [mild cognitive impairment]; 0–17 [severe cognitive impairment]	▶ Will not detect subtle memory loss in well-educated patients ▶ Does not diagnose dementia or delirium ▶ Those with low intelligence, limited education, poor socioeconomic status, or from other cultures may do poorly in the absence of cognitive impairment ▶ May underestimate cognitive impairment among those with moderate to severe psychiatric illness ▶ Not sensitive for frontal lobe impairment (executive dysfunction)
MOCA* **Montreal Cognitive Assessment** (Nasreddine, Phillips, Bédirian, Charbonneau, Whitehead, Collin, et al. 2009)	▶ Measures cognitive dysfunction by assessing attention and concentration, executive function, visuospatial function, naming, memory, attention, language, visuoconstructional skills, conceptual thinking, calculation, abstraction, delayed recall, and orientation ▶ Rating: Variable ▶ Scoring: A score of 26 or greater is normal	Clinician-administered ▶ Administration requires specific instructions; scoring can be cumbersome and somewhat subjective ▶ If the individual has less than a 12th-grade education, give one additional point
SPMSQ* **Short Portable Mental Status Questionnaire** (Fan, 1994; Roccaforte, Burke, & Wengel, 1994)	▶ Assessment of orientation, memory, general knowledge, and subtraction ▶ 10 questions [e.g., What is the date today? Where were you born?] are administered either during direct interview or over the telephone. ▶ Rating: One point for each correct answer ▶ Scoring: More than three incorrect answers indicates dementia; the more incorrect answers, the more severe the cognitive impairment	Clinician-administered ▶ Rapid, simple, and repeatable ▶ Those with low intelligence, limited education, poor socioeconomic status. or from other cultures may do poorly in the absence of cognitive impairment ▶ May underestimate cognitive impairment among those with moderate to severe psychiatric illness

* indicates public domain

CONTINUED ▶

ASSESSMENT OF ACUTE AND CHRONIC DISEASE STATES   125

TABLE 5–4. CONTINUED ▶

ASSESSMENT TOOLS	CHARACTERISTICS	COMMENTS
DEPRESSION		
BDI-2 Beck Depression Inventory (Aben, Verhey, Lousberg, Lodder, & Honig, 2002; Halverson, & Chan, 2004; STABLE National Coordinating Counsel, 2008; Valente & Saunders, 2005)	▶ Presence and impact of depressive symptoms during the previous week, including attitude and characteristic symptoms of depression ▶ 21 questions focusing on self-dissatisfaction, vegetative symptoms, inhibition, fatigability, hopelessness, and suicide wish ▶ Rating: 0 [no problem] to 3 [severe problem] ▶ Scoring: < 10 [normal]; 11–17 [mild depression]; 18–23 [moderate depression]; 24+ [severe depression]	▶ Self-reported or clinician-administered ▶ Age 13 and older; both genders; validated in diverse cultures and in a variety of comorbid conditions ▶ Sensitivity > 90% ▶ Must be purchased from a variety of online sources
CCSD* Cornell Scale for Depression in Dementia (Alexopoulos, Abrams, Young, & Shamoian, 1988)	▶ Used to assess the signs and symptoms of major depression in patients with co-occurring dementia ▶ A semistructured interview, covering 19 items, first with an informant and then the patient, regarding the presence of signs and symptoms of depression over the previous week ▶ Rating: from 0 [absent symptoms] to 2 [severe] ▶ Scoring: < 6 (absence of significant depressive symptoms); 8–17 (probable major depression); > 18 (definite depressive symptoms)	▶ Self-reported and clinician observation ▶ The clinician both evaluates content and makes direct behavioral observations ▶ Look back over the last week ▶ http://qmweb.dads. state.tx.us/Depression/ CSDD.htm
GDS* Geriatric Depression Scale (Halverson & Chan, 2004;Valente & Saunders, 2005)	▶ Assesses the presence of depression in those over 65 ▶ 30 simple yes or no questions [short form has 15 questions] addressing cognitive complaints, orientation, self-image, losses, agitation, obsessive traits, and overall motivation ▶ Rating: 0 [no] or 1 [yes] ▶ Scoring: 0–9 [normal]; 10–19 [mild depression]; 20–30 [severe depression]	▶ Self-reported or clinician-administered ▶ Age 65 and older; both genders; diverse cultural groups ▶ Does not assess for somatic complaints ▶ Cognitive impairment may negatively affect test validity ▶ Major depression: sensitivity 84%; specificity 95% ▶ Minor depression: sensitivity 70%; specificity 80%
HAM-D* Hamilton Rating Scale for Depression (Hamilton, 1960)	▶ Measures the severity of depressive symptoms in patients with primary depressive illness ▶ Several versions with 17–21 questions; 17 item version is the most commonly used ▶ Scoring: 0–7 [no depression]; 8–13 [mild depression]; 14–18 [moderate depression]; 19–22 [severe depression]; 23+ [very severe depression]	▶ Self-reported or clinician-administered ▶ Concurrent somatic illnesses can render score inaccurate ▶ Standard depression outcome measure for the FDA and National Institute of Mental Health

* indicates public domain

CONTINUED ▶

TABLE 5-4. SELECTED ASSESSMENT TOOLS CONTINUED ▶

ASSESSMENT TOOLS	CHARACTERISTICS	COMMENTS
PHQ-9* Patient Health Questionnaire (Kroenke, Spitzer, Williams, Monahan, & Lowe, 2007; STABLE National Coordinating Counsel, 2008)	▶ Multipurpose instrument for screening, diagnosing, monitoring, and measuring the severity of depression during the last two weeks ▶ Nine diagnostic criteria are included; both symptom frequency and severity are measured ▶ Rating: 0 [symptom not present at all] to 3 [nearly every day] ▶ Scoring: 5 [mild depression]; 10 [moderate]; 15 [moderately severe]; 20 [severe depression]	▶ Self-reported or clinician-administered ▶ Brief, lending itself to clinical use ▶ Scores > 10: sensitivity 88%; specificity 88% ▶ http://www.cqaimh. org/stable.html
PHQ-2* Patient Health Questionnaire (Family Practice Notebook, n.d.; Kroenke, Spitzer, Williams, Monahan, & Lowe, 2007; STABLE National Coordinating Counsel, 2008)	▶ Presence and frequency of depressed mood and anhedonia over the last two weeks ▶ In the past 2 weeks how often have you been bothered by: ▷ Little interest or pleasure in doing things? ▷ Feeling down, depressed or hopeless? ▶ Rating: 0 [not at all] to 3 [nearly every day] ▶ Scoring: A score of 3 is considered positive ▶ If positive, administer the PHQ-9	▶ Self-reported or clinician-administered ▶ Adults; both genders ▶ Reduces evaluation to two screening questions that are easily incorporated into routine symptom inquiry ▶ A score of 3 has a sensitivity of 82.9%, specificity of 90% ▶ A screening tool only ▶ http://www.cqaimh.org/ pdf/STABLE_toolkit.pdf
QIDS* Quick Inventory of Depressive Symptomatology (Rush, Trivedi, Ibrahim & Carmody, 2003)	▶ 16-item screening tool used to assess the severity of depressive symptoms	▶ Self- and clinician-administered versions are available ▶ Assesses *DSM-IV* symptom criteria for major depressive episode ▶ Can be used to screen for depression but is more commonly used to measure the severity of symptoms ▶ http://www.ids-qids.org/ tr-english.html
SDS* Zung Self-Rating Depression (Halverson & Chan, 2004; Zung, 1965)	▶ Assessment of mood, appetite, suicidal thoughts ▶ Measures the degree of depression in previously diagnosed patients ▶ Rating: 20 statements, 10 positively stated and 10 negatively stated; the patient is asked to rate from 1 [little of the time] to 4 [most of the time] ▶ Scoring: 0-50 [normal range]; 51-59 [mild depression]; 60-69 [moderate to marked depression]; 70+ [severe depression]	▶ Self-reported or clinician-administered ▶ Age 13 and older; both genders, validated in diverse cultures ▶ Sensitivity: 70-90%; specificity: 90%

* indicates public domain

CONTINUED ▶

ASSESSMENT OF ACUTE AND CHRONIC DISEASE STATES 127

TABLE 5–4. CONTINUED ▶

ASSESSMENT TOOLS	CHARACTERISTICS	COMMENTS
RADS [child] RADS-2 [adolescent] Reynolds Adolescent Depression Inventory (Sharp & Lipsky, 2002)	▶ 30 questions, written in present tense, at a 3rd-grade reading level ▶ Focus is on dysphoric mood; anhedonia and negative affect; negative self-evaluation; somatic complaints	Self-reported or clinician-administered ▶ RADS: children age 8–12; written at the 2nd-grade level ▶ RADS-2: adolescents age 13–20; written at the 3rd-grade level ▶ Scales can be purchased through a variety of online sources
DISABILITY		
SDS* Sheehan Disability Scale (STABLE National Coordinating Counsel, 2008)	▶ Assessment of the degree of functional impairment in three domains: work or school, social, and family life ▶ A 10-point visual analog scale is used ▶ There is no cut-off score and therefore it is best used over time to monitor response to treatment	▶ Self-reported or clinician-administered ▶ Has been used in the following mental disorders: alcohol dependence, drug dependence, general anxiety disorder, major depressive disorder, obsessive compulsive disorder, and panic disorder ▶ Sensitivity 83%; specificity 69% ▶ http://www.cqaimh.org/ pdf/STABLE_toolkit.pdf
MANIA / HYPOMANIA		
Kiddie-SADS Kiddie Schedule for Affective Disorders and Schizophrenia The Kiddie-SADS is copyright- protected but can be used free of charge in nonprofit agencies and for research (Kaufman, Birmaher, Brent, Rao, & Rian, 1996)	▶ Assesses current and past psychopathology in children and adolescents, including major depression, dysthymia, mania, hypomania, cyclothymia, bipolar disorders, schizoaffective disorders, schizophrenia, schizophreniform disorder, brief reactive psychosis, panic disorder, agoraphobia, separation anxiety disorder, avoidant disorder of childhood and adolescence, simple phobia, social phobia, overanxious disorder, generalized anxiety, obsessive compulsive disorder, attention deficit hyperactivity disorder, conduct disorder, oppositional defiant disorder, enuresis, encopresis, anorexia nervosa, bulimia, transient tic disorder, Tourette disorder, chronic motor or vocal tic disorder, alcohol abuse, substance abuse, posttraumatic stress disorder, and adjustment disorders ▶ Technical and complex rating and scoring	▶ Clinician interview of parent(s) and the child through summary ratings of parent(s), other family members, school, medical and psychiatric records ▶ Considered a diagnostic tool for a variety of childhood illnesses ▶ Complex assessment process, time-consuming, requiring objective assessments ▶ Copies for use in non-profit facilities or in research can be obtained from http:// www.wpic.pitt.edu/ ksads/ksads-pl.pdf

* indicates public domain

CONTINUED ▶

TABLE 5-4. SELECTED ASSESSMENT TOOLS CONTINUED ▶

ASSESSMENT TOOLS	CHARACTERISTICS	COMMENTS
MDQ* **Mood Disorder Questionnaire** (Hirschfeld, Holzer, Calabrese, Weissman, Reed, Davies, et al., 2003; STABLE National Coordinating Counsel, 2008;)	▶ Screening for the presence and past episodes of mania or hypomania ▶ Three questions: The first includes 13 symptoms associated with bipolar disorder; the second assesses symptom clustering; and the third evaluates symptom-generated functional impairment ▶ Rating: Yes or no responses ▶ Scoring: Positive if seven or more of the 13 items in question one are present *and* question two is answered yes *and* question three garners a "moderate problem" or "serious problem" response	▶ Self- or clinician-administered ▶ Efficient method to *screen* for mania and hypomania ▶ Is better when scoring bipolar I [depression and mania] than bipolar II or bipolar NOS ▶ Outpatient mood disorder clinic: sensitivity 73%; specificity 90% ▶ Outpatient clinic treating depression: sensitivity 58%; specificity 93% ▶ http://www.cqaimh.org/pdf/STABLE_toolkit.pdf
YMRS* **Young Mania Rating Scale** (Massachusetts General Hospital, 2010; Young, Biggs, Ziegler, & Meyer, 1978)	▶ Used to assess the severity of mania in those previously diagnosed ▶ Items: Elevated mood; increased motor activity and energy; sexual interest; sleep; irritability; speech; language and thought; content; disruptive and aggressive behavior; appearance; and insight ▶ Range: 0-60 ▶ Score: Adults: 12 [mania] Children: 25 [mania], 20 [hypomania]; score > 13 warrants further assessment	▶ Self-reported or clinician observation ▶ Adults: 11 items (reflect over last 48 hours) ▶ Children: P-YMRS (parent form) ▶ http://www.psych.uic.edu/csp/images/stories/physicians/rating%20scales/YMRS.pdf
OBSESSIVE COMPULSIVE		
CY-BOCS* **Children's Yale-Brown Obsessive Compulsive Scale** (Massachusetts General Hospital, 2010)	▶ The CY-BOCS is a 10-item scale with two subscales one for obsessions and the other for compulsions ▶ Subscales score the frequency, distress, interference, resistance, and control over either obsessions or compulsions ▶ Rating: 0-4, with higher numbers indicating greater severity of symptoms	▶ Self-reported or clinician-administered ▶ Age 6-14
YBOCS* **Yale-Brown Obsessive Compulsive Scale** (Massachusetts General Hospital, 2010; Scahill, Riddle, McSwiggin-Hardin, Ort, King, Goodman, et al., 1997)	▶ 10-item scale rating both the type and severity of symptoms in OCD during the previous 48 hours ▶ Rating: Varies by question ▶ Scoring: Add each item score; higher total score indicates increased severity ▶ The clinician assesses symptom severity by having the patient identify the three obsessions and compulsions that are most distressing and focusing on them during the interview	▶ Self-reported or clinician-administered ▶ Age 14 and older ▶ Most commonly used scale for OCD ▶ Considered the gold standard for assessment of obsessive-compulsive symptoms; commonly used in research and for assessing obsessive compulsive symptoms

* indicates public domain

CONTINUED ▶

ASSESSMENT OF ACUTE AND CHRONIC DISEASE STATES 129

TABLE 5–4. CONTINUED ▶

ASSESSMENT TOOLS	CHARACTERISTICS	COMMENTS
PSYCHOSIS		
BPRS* **Brief Psychiatric Rating Scale** (Overall & Gorham, 1962)	▶ Assessment of psychopathology (including positive, negative, and affective psychopathology) in patients suspected of having schizophrenia ▶ Evaluation is based on a clinical interview and behavior observation during the prior 2–3 days ▶ Domains include somatic complaints, anxiety, emotional withdrawal, conceptual disorganization, guilt feelings, tension, mannerisms and posturing, grandiosity, depressive mood, hostility, suspiciousness, hallucinatory behaviors, motor retardation, uncooperativeness, unusual thought content, and blunted affect ▶ Rating: 0 [not present] to 6 [extremely severe] ▶ Scoring: 0–9 [negative]; 10–20 [possible SAD]; 21+ [SAD likely]	▶ Clinician-administered ▶ Age 18 and older; both genders ▶ The most widely used rating scale in psychiatry ▶ Not for screening or diagnosis ▶ Sole purpose is rating the current clinical picture through evaluation of symptom severity over time
PANSS* **Positive and Negative Syndrome Scale** (Kay, Fiszbein, & Opler, 1987)	▶ Used to measure changes in symptom intensity in patients with psychosis and schizophrenia ▶ 30 symptoms are identified including 7 positive, 7 negative, and 16 general psychopathology items; the rating period includes the prior week ▶ Rating: 1 [absence of symptom] to 7 [extreme symptomatology] ▶ Scoring: Positive and negative scales range 7–49; 16–112 for general psychopathology; composite scale is obtained by subtracting the negative from the positive score, rendering a bipolar index with a range of –42 to +42	▶ Self-reported or clinician-administered ▶ Age 18 and older; both genders ▶ Considered the gold standard in studies of treatment efficacy ▶ http://www.femonline.org/content/downloads/39/PANSS%20Scoring%20Criteria.pdf
SUICIDE / RISK ASSESSMENT		
SPS **Suicide Probability Scale** (Valente & Saunders, 2005)	▶ Rapid measure of suicide risk in adolescents and adults, used to differentiate those likely to attempt suicide from those unlikely to attempt it ▶ Over time, can be used to monitor changes in suicidality ▶ 36 feeling and behavior statements, divided into four subscales: hostility, hopelessness, suicidal ideation, and negative self-evaluation ▶ Rating: Symptom presence is rated 1 [none or little of the time] to 4 [present almost all the time] ▶ Scoring: The higher the score, the greater the suicide risk	▶ Self-reported or clinician-administered ▶ Age 13 and older ▶ Does not consider lethality or intent

* indicates public domain

CONTINUED ▶

TABLE 5-4. SELECTED ASSESSMENT TOOLS CONTINUED ▶

ASSESSMENT TOOLS	CHARACTERISTICS	COMMENTS
TREATMENT ASSESSMENT		
CIWA-Ar* **Clinical Institute Withdrawal Assessment of Alcohol Scale, Revised** (Bayard, McIntyre, Hill, & Woodside, 2004; Sullivan, Sykora, Schneiderman, Naranjo, & Sellers,1989)	▶ Quantify the severity of alcohol withdrawal syndrome, establish medication dosing, and monitor response to treatment over time ▶ Nine items rating symptoms on a scale from 0 [none] to 7 [severe]; one additional question assessing orientation and sensorium ▶ Scoring: Maximum score is 67; typically, scores less than 10 do not warrant intervention	▶ Clinician-administered ▶ Other medical or psychiatric conditions can mimic withdrawal ▶ Medical conditions and medications can mask withdrawal
COWS* **Clinical Opiate Withdrawal Scale** (Wesson, 2003)	▶ Quantify the severity of withdrawal syndrome, establish medication dosing, monitor response to treatment over time ▶ Used for induction of Suboxone ▶ Scoring: 5–12 [mild]; 13–24 [moderate]; 25–36 [moderate to severe]; 36+ [severe withdrawal]	

* indicates public domain

CASE STUDY

A 22-year-old college student presents to the clinic for assistance with complaints of frequent headaches, generalized body aches, difficulty concentrating, and insomnia. She has been losing weight over the past few weeks and is unable to study or concentrate in class. She states that she feels "sick" but denies any other recent illnesses. She has an unremarkable history, has no chronic illnesses, and takes no routine medications. She is a moderate social drinker and does not smoke. Recent stressors include a heavy course load and a recent disappointment at failing to be accepted for membership in a sorority on campus. She denies family history for mental illness and talks at great length about why she believes she is "sick, not crazy." There are many issues to consider in assessing this patient.

▶ What additional assessments would you make at this time?

▶ What specific diagnostic and laboratory tests would you order, and why?

▶ What, if any, specific physical findings would you look for?

▶ What communication strategies would you use to facilitate assessment of this patient?

▶ What milieu considerations would precede your interactions with her?

REFERENCES

Anandarajah, G., & Hight, E. (2001). Spirituality and medical practice: Using the hope questions as a practical tool for spiritual assessment. *American Family Physician, 63*(1), 81–88.

American Nurses Association. (2007). *Scope and standards of psychiatric–mental health clinical nursing practice.* Washington, DC: American Nurses Association.

American Psychiatric Association. (2000a). *Diagnostic and statistical manual of mental disorders* (4th ed., text rev.). Washington, DC: American Psychiatric Association.

American Psychiatric Association. (2000b). *Practice guidelines for the treatment of patients with major depressive disorder.* Washington, DC: American Psychiatric Association.

American Psychiatric Association. (2006). *Practice guideline for psychiatric evaluation of adults.* Washington, DC: American Psychiatric Association.

American Psychiatric Association, Work Group on Eating Disorders. (2000). Practice guideline for the treatment of patients with eating disorders. *American Journal of Psychiatry, 157*(Suppl. 1), 1–39.

Bakerman, S. (2002). *ABCs of interpretive laboratory data* (4th ed.). Greenville, NC: Interpretive Laboratory Data.

Bickley, L. S. (2007). *Bates' guide to physical examination and history taking* (9th ed.). Philadelphia: Lippincott.

Bryson, S. E., & Smith, I. M. (1998). Epidemiology of autism: Prevalence, associated characteristics, and service delivery. *Mental Retardation and Developmental Disabilities Research Reviews, 4,* 97–103.

Clinical Evidence Organization. (2000). *Clinical evidence international sourcebook.* London: BMJ Publishing Group.

Davidson, J. R. (2000). Trauma: The impact of post-traumatic stress disorder. *Journal of Psychopharmacology, 14*(Suppl. 1), S5–S12.

Faulkner, G. (2000). *Behavioral outcomes and guidelines sourcebook.* New York: Faulkner & Gray.

Fombonne, E. (1998). Epidemiology of autism and related conditions. In F. R. Volkmar (Ed.), *Autism and pervasive developmental disorders* (pp. 32–63). Cambridge, England: Cambridge University Press.

Haddow, J. E., Palomaki, G. E., Allan, W. C., Williams, J. R., Knight, G. J., & Gagnon, J. (1999). Maternal thyroid deficiency during pregnancy and subsequent neuropsychological development of the child. *New England Journal of Medicine, 341,* 549–555.

Hoyert, D. L., Kochanek, K. D., & Murphy, S. L. (1999). *Deaths: Final data for 1997–99* (National Vital Statistics Report 47[19], DHHS Publication No. 99-1120). Hyattsville, MD: National Center for Health Statistics.

Margolin, G., & Gordis, E. B. (2000). The effects of family and community violence on children. *Annual Review of Psychology, 51,* 445–479.

National Institute of Health. (2013). *Clear communication: A NIH Health Literacy Initiative.* Retrieved from www.nih.gov/clearcommunication/culturalcompetency.htm

National Institute of Mental Health. (2006). *The numbers count: Mental disorders in America.* Retrived from www.nimh.nih.gov

O'Reilly, D. J. (2000). Thyroid function tests: Time for reassessment. *British Medical Journal, 320,* 1332–1334.

Pop, V. J., Kuijpens, J. L., van Baar, A. L., Verkerk, G., van Son, M. M., & de Vijlder, J. J. (1999). Low maternal free thyroxine concentrations during early pregnancy are associated with impaired psychomotor development in infancy. *Clinical Endocrinology, 50,* 149–155.

Sadock, B., & Sadock, V. (2007). *Kaplan and Sadock's synopsis of psychiatry* (10th ed.). New York: Lippincott Williams & Wilkins.

Schatsburg, A., Cole, J., & DeBattista, C. (2007). *Manual of clinical psychopharmacology* (6th ed.).Washington, DC: American Psychiatric Association.

Shea, C. A., Pelletier, L., Poster, E. C., Stuart, G. W., & Verhey, M. P. (1999). *Advanced practice nursing in psychiatric mental health care.* St. Louis, MO: Mosby.

Strub, R. (2000). *The mental status examination in neurology.* Philadelphia: Oxford University Press.

Stuart, G. W., & Laraia, M. T. (2004). *Principles and practice of psychiatric nursing* (8th ed.). St. Louis, MO: Mosby.

Weissman, M. M., Bland, R. C., & Canino, G. J. (1999). Prevalence of suicide ideation and suicide attempts in nine countries. *Psychological Medicine, 29*(1), 9–17.

Wolraich, M. L., Hannah, J. N., Baumgaertel, A., & Feurer, I. D. (1998). Examination of *DSM-IV* criteria for attention deficit/hyperactivity disorder in a countywide sample. *Journal of Developmental and Behavioral Pediatrics, 19,* 162–168.

CHAPTER 6

PHARMACOLOGICAL PRINCIPLES

Psychopharmacology, one of the most active and developing areas of psychiatric research, is the use of psychotropic medication to treat psychiatric disorders (Sadock & Sadock, 2007). Psychiatric–mental health nurse practitioners (PMHNPs) must have a thorough understanding of the science and art of prescribing—of the pharmacokinetic and pharmacodynamic actions of a given drug, as well as the patient's motivation to take the drug. The basic pharmacological principles are discussed in this chapter.

CONCEPTS IN PHARMACOLOGICAL MANAGEMENT

▶ *Pharmacology:* Study of what drugs do and how they do it

▶ *Pharmacokinetics*: Study of what the body does to drugs; includes absorption, distribution, metabolism, and excretion

▶ *Pharmacodynamics*: Study of what drugs do to the body; target sites for drug actions include receptors, ion channels, enzymes, and carrier proteins.

Pharmacokinetics

▶ *Absorption*: Method and rate at which drugs leave the site of administration

  ▸ With oral medications, absorption normally occurs in the small intestine and then in the liver.

▶ *Distribution*: Occurs after the drug leaves the systemic circulation and enters the interstitium and cells

  ▸ Drugs are redistributed in organs according to their fat and protein content.

» Most psychotropic medications are lipophilic and highly protein-bound. Only the unbound (free) portion of the drug is active. Therefore, people with low protein (albumin) levels, such as in malnutrition, wasting, or aging, can potentially have toxicity (see below) from an increased amount of free drug. People with high fat-to-lean body mass ratio (as in older adults) will have erratic amounts of active drug in their system.

▶ *Metabolism*: Process by which the drug becomes chemically altered in the body.

▶ *First-pass metabolism*: Process by which the drug is metabolized by P-450 enzymes in the intestines and liver prior to going to the systemic circulation.

▶ *Elimination*: Process by which the drug is removed from the body.

▶ *Half-life (T ½)*: Time needed to clear 50% of the drug from the plasma.

» The half-life also determines the dosing interval and the length of time to reach a steady state.

▶ *Steady state*: Point at which the amount of drug eliminated between doses is approximately equal to the dose administered.

» Drugs usually are administered once every half-life to achieve a steady state.

» It takes approximately 5 half-lives to achieve a steady state and 5 half-lives to completely eliminate a drug.

▶ Alterations in pharmacokinetics

» Hepatic cytochrome P450 enzyme interactions can induce or inhibit the metabolism of certain drugs, thus changing their desired concentration levels (Table 6–1)

» First-pass metabolism activity in young children varies by drug substrate, but may exceed rates of adolescents and adults

TABLE 6–1. CYTOCHROME P450 INHIBITORS AND INDUCERS

INHIBITORS	INDUCERS
▶ buproprion	▶ carbamazepine
▶ clomipramine	▶ hypericum (St John's Wort)
▶ cimetidine	▶ phenytoin
▶ clarithromycin	▶ phenobarbital
▶ diltiazem	▶ tobacco
▶ duloxetine	
▶ erythromycin	
▶ floroquinolones	
▶ grapefruit juice	
▶ ketoconazole	
▶ nefazodone	
▶ SSRIs	

▶ Enzyme inducers can decrease the serum level of other drugs that are substrates of that enzyme, thus possibly causing subtherapeutic drug levels.

▶ Enzyme inhibitors can increase the serum level of other drugs that are substrates of that enzyme, thus possibly causing toxic levels.

▶ Liver disease will affect liver enzyme activity and first-pass metabolism, resulting in possible toxic plasma drug levels.

► Kidney disease or drugs that reduce renal clearance, such as nonsteroidal anti-inflammatory drugs (NSAIDs), may increase serum concentration of drugs that are excreted by the kidneys (such as lithium).

► Older adults are more sensitive to psychotropics because of their decreased intracellular water, protein binding, low muscle mass, decreased metabolism, and increased body fat concentration.

► Most psychotropics are lipophilic and highly protein-bound. Thus, because older adults have more body fat and less protein, they are more likely to develop toxicity due to accumulation and erratic blood levels of drug.

Pharmacodynamics

► Target sites for drug actions include *receptors*. Several types of pharmacodynamics involving receptors are

- *Agonist effect*: Drug binds to receptors and activates a biological response

- *Inverse agonist effect*: Drug causes the opposite effect of agonist

- *Partial agonist effect*: Drug does not fully activate the receptors

- *Antagonist effect*: Drug binds to the receptor but does not activate a biological response

► Another site for drug actions is *ion channels,* which exist for many ions such as sodium, potassium, chloride, and calcium and can be open at some times and closed at other times. Neurotransmitters or drugs may be excitatory or inhibitory depending on the type of ion channel they gate.

- *Excitatory response*: Depolarization; involves the opening of sodium and calcium channels with these ions going into the cell

- *Inhibitory response*: Repolarization; involves the opening of chloride channels with chloride going into the cell, potassium leaving, or both

► Another site for drug actions is *enzymes,* which are important for drug metabolism and play an important role in the chemical alteration of the drug. Some drugs (e.g., monoamine oxidase inhibitors [MAOIs]) inhibit the action of a particular enzyme, thus increasing the availability of the neurotransmitter.

► Another site for drug actions is *carrier proteins* or *reuptake pumps,* which transport neurotransmitters out of the synapse and back into the presynaptic neuron to be recycled or reused. Some drugs will inhibit reuptake pumps such as selective serotonin reuptake inhibitors (SSRIs), thus increasing the synaptic availability of the neurotransmitter.

Other Terminology

► *Potency*: Relative dose required to achieve certain effects

► *Therapeutic index*: Relative measure of the toxicity or safety of a drug; ratio of the median toxic dose to the median effective dose

- Drugs with a high therapeutic index (divalproex, 50–125) have a high margin of safety; that is, the therapeutic dose and the toxic dose are far apart.

- Drugs with a low therapeutic index (lithium, 0.5–1.2) have a low margin of safety; that is, the therapeutic dose and the toxic dose are close together.

► *Tolerance*: The process of becoming less responsive to a particular drug as it is administered over time.

► *Tachyphylaxis:* An acute decrease in the therapeutic response

PMHNP ROLE OF PHARMACOLOGICAL MANAGEMENT

▶ Pharmacological management process:

- ▸ Make a diagnosis and identify the target symptoms.

- ▸ Consider the phase of illness (such as acute, relapse, recurrence).

- ▸ Assess prior personal and family history of response to certain medications.

- ▸ Assess the patient's motivation for and any misgivings about treatment

- ▸ Identify potential interactions between the current prescribed medications.

- ▸ Identify cultural implications of certain drugs.

- ▸ Discuss the risks and benefits of the treatment.

- ▸ Document informed consent and the patient's understanding of target symptoms, benefits, risks, and alternatives to treatment.

- ▸ Monitor response and side effects.

▶ Follow-up and role of the PMHNP

- ▸ Use of standards of care:

  - ▷ Assist in determining length of treatment.

  - ▷ Do relapse planning.

  - ▷ It is helpful and advised to use standardized clinical rating scales to establish the patient's baseline and to monitor progress or decompensation over time. Screening tests also will aid in making a diagnosis and ruling out other disorders.

- ▸ Common screening tests for mood disorders include

  - ▷ Beck Depression Inventory (BDI; Beck, Ward, Mendelson, Mock, & Erbaugh, 1961)

  - ▷ Mood Disorder Questionnaire (MDQ; Hirschfeld & Holzer, 2003)

  - ▷ Positive and Negative Symptom Scale (PANSS; Kay & Fiszbein, 1987)

  - ▷ Brief Psychosis Rating Scale (BPRS; Overall & Gorham, 1962)

- ▸ It is important to recognize the large body of evidence-based data supporting the combined use of pharmacological and nonpharmacological treatments as offering psychiatric patients the best possibility for significant clinical improvement.

- ▸ Nonadherence is a common problem with all chronic illness, including psychiatric disorders, and should be a continuous focus of concern for the PMHNP.

- ▸ Common medications used in the clinical management of psychiatric disorders and usually prescribed by the PMHNP are identified in Table 6–2.

- ▸ A Drug Enforcement Administration (DEA) number is required for prescription of controlled substances.

  - ▷ Schedule of controlled substances

- Schedule I
  - Nonmedicinal substances
  - High abuse potential
  - Used for research purposes only
  - Not legally available by prescription
  - Examples include heroin or marijuana
- Schedule II
  - Medicinal drugs in current use
  - High potential for abuse and dependency
  - Written prescription allowed
  - No telephone orders allowed
  - No refills allowed on prescription
  - Examples include morphine sulfate, codeine, fentanyl, methadone, hydromorphone (Dilaudid), oxycodone (Oxycontin)
- Schedule III
  - Medicinal drugs with less abuse potential than Schedule II drugs
  - Still greater potential for abuse than Schedule IV drugs
  - Telephone orders if followed by written prescription
  - Prescription must be renewed every 6 months
  - Refills limited to 5
  - Examples include appetite suppressants, butalbital, testosterone
- Schedule IV
  - Medicinal drugs with less abuse potential than Schedule III drugs
  - Examples include dextropropxyphene (Darvon), pentazocine (Talwin), benzodiazepines (such as alprazolam [Xanax], chlordiazepoxide [Librium], clonazepam [Klonopin], diazepam [Valium], clorazepate [Tranxene], lorazepam [Ativan]), modifinil [Provigil], phenobarbital, zolpidem [Ambien], eszopiclone [Lunesta], temazepam [Restoril]}.
- Schedule V
  - Medicinal drugs with the lowest abuse potential
  - Handled in manner similar to noncontrolled drugs
  - Examples include loperamide (Imodium), buprenorphine (Buprenex), cheratussin (Robitussin) with codeine, promethazine (Phenergan) with codeine.

138 PSYCHIATRIC–MENTAL HEALTH NURSE PRACTITIONER REVIEW MANUAL, 3RD EDITION

TABLE 6-2. MEDICATIONS COMMONLY USED IN THE CLINICAL MANAGEMENT OF PSYCHIATRIC DISORDERS

Medications Used to Treat Schizophrenia and Other Psychotic Disorders	
Typical antipsychotics	▶ Haloperidol (Haldol), haloperidol decanoate (Haldol Decanoate) ▶ Loxapine (Loxitane) ▶ Thioridazine (Mellaril) ▶ Molindone (Moban) ▶ Thiothixene (Navane) ▶ Fluphenazine (Prolixin), fluphenazine decanoate (Prolixin Decanoate) ▶ Mesoridazine (Serentil) ▶ Trifluoperazine (Stelazine) ▶ Chlorpromazine (Thorazine) ▶ Perphenazine (Trilafon)
Atypical antipsychotics	▶ Clozapine (Clozaril) ▶ Ziprasidone (Geodon) ▶ Risperidone (Risperdal) ▶ Quetiapine (Seroquel) ▶ Olanzapine (Zyprexa) ▶ Aripiprizole (Abilify) ▶ Paliperidone (Invega) ▶ Iloperidone (Fanapt) ▶ Asenipine (Saphris) ▶ Lurasidone (Latuda)
Medications Used to Treat Mood Disorders and Bipolar Affective Disorders	
Mood stabilizers	▶ Valproic acid (Depakene) ▶ Divalproex sodium (Depakote) ▶ Lithium carbonate (Eskalith, Lithobid, Lithonate, Lithotabs) ▶ Lamotrigine (Lamictal) ▶ Carbamazepine (Tegretol) ▶ Carbamazepine ER (Equetro) ▶ Oxcarbazepine (Trileptal: off label)
Medications Used to Treat Mood Disorders and Bipolar Affective Disorders	
Mood stabilizers	▶ Valproic acid (Depakene) ▶ Divalproex sodium (Depakote) () ▶ Lithium carbonate (Eskalith, Lithobid, Lithonate, Lithotabs) ▶ Lamotrigine (Lamictal) ▶ Carbamazepine (Tegretol) ▶ Carbamazepine ER (Equetro) ▶ Oxcarbazepine (Trileptal) (off label)

CONTINUED ▶

PHARMACOLOGICAL PRINCIPLES **139**

TABLE 6–2. CONTINUED ▶

Medications Used to Treat Mood Disorders, Unipolar Affective Disorders, and Depressive Disorders	
Tricyclics (TCAs)	▶ Clomipramine (Anafranil) ▶ Amoxapine (Asendin) ▶ Amitriptyline (Elavil) ▶ Desipramine (Norpramin) ▶ Nortriptyline (Pamelor) ▶ Doxepin (Sinequan) ▶ Trimipramine (Surmontil) ▶ Imipramine (Tofranil) ▶ Protriptyline (Vivactil)
Serotonin selective reuptake inhibitors (SSRIs)	▶ Citalopram (Celexa) ▶ Fluvoxamine (Luvox) ▶ Paroxetine (Paxil) ▶ Paroxetine mesylate (Pexeva) ▶ Fluoxetine (Prozac) ▶ Sertraline (Zoloft) ▶ Escitalopram (Lexapro)
Monoamine oxidase inhibitors (MAOIs)	▶ Phenelzine (Nardil) ▶ Tranylcypromine sulfate (Parnate) ▶ Selegiline transdermal (EMSAM)
Other agents	▶ Trazodone (Desyrel) ▶ Venlafaxine (Effexor) ▶ Desvenlafaxine (Pristiq) ▶ Mirtazapine (Remeron) ▶ Nefazodone (Serzone) ▶ Bupropion (Wellbutrin) ▶ Duloxetine (Cymbalta)

Medications Used to Treat Anxiety Disorders	
Benzodiazepines (BNZs)	▶ Lorazepam (Ativan) ▶ Clonazepam (Klonopin) ▶ Chlordiazepoxide (Librium) ▶ Oxazepam (Serax) ▶ Clorazepate (Tranxene) ▶ Alprazolam (Xanax)
Anxiolytics	▶ Buspirone (BuSpar)
Other agents	▶ Propranolol (Inderal) ▶ Atenolol (Tenormin)

Medications Used to Treat Attention Deficit Disorder and Attention Deficit Hyperactivity Disorder	
Stimulants	▶ Amphetamine/dextroamphetamine (Adderall) ▶ Dexmethylphenidate (Focalin) ▶ Dextroamphetamine (Dexedrine) ▶ Methylphenidate (Ritalin) ▶ Methylphenidate (Concerta) ▶ Lisdexamfetamine dimesylate (Vyvanse)
Other agents	▶ Guanfacine (Intuniv) ▶ Clonidine (Kapvay) ▶ Atomoxetine (Strattera) ▶ Antidepressants such as desipramine (Norpramin), venlafaxine (Effexor), and bupropion (Wellbutrin) are also used in the clinical management of ADHD.

Other Pharmacological Considerations

▶ It is vital to be aware of the teratogenic nature of many psychotropic agents. It is important to discuss the risks versus the benefits of medications during pregnancy.

- Possible risks of psychotropic medications during pregnancy include

    ▷ Feeding difficulties

    ▷ Transient agitation or sedation

    ▷ Premature labor

    ▷ Drug discontinuation symptoms

    ▷ Teratogenic effects of certain psychotropics

- Possible risks of not taking psychotropic medications during pregnancy include

    ▷ Recurrence of symptoms

    ▷ Adverse effects on mother–infant bonding

    ▷ Poor maternal self-care

▶ Federal Drug Administration (FDA) pregnancy ratings for medications

- **A:** Controlled studies show no risk

- **B:** No evidence of risk in humans

- **C:** Risk cannot be ruled out

- **D:** Positive evidence of risk

- **X:** Absolutely contraindicated in pregnancy

▶ Teratogenic risks of common psychiatric medications

- Benzodiazepines: Floppy baby syndrome, cleft palate

- Carbamazepine (Tegretol): Neural tube defects

- Lithium (Eskalith): Epstein anomaly

- Divalproex sodium (Depakote): Neural tube defects, specifically spina bifida,

▶ Some common medications can induce depression or mania (see Table 6–3)

TABLE 6-3. MEDICATIONS THAT INDUCE DEPRESSION OR MANIA

MEDICATIONS THAT INDUCE DEPRESSION	MEDICATIONS THAT INDUCE MANIA
▶ Beta blockers ▶ Steroids ▶ Interferon ▶ Isotretinoin (Accutane) ▶ Some retroviral drugs ▶ Neoplastic drugs ▶ Benzodiazepines ▶ Progesterone	▶ Steroids ▶ Disulfiram (Antabuse) ▶ Isoniazid (INH) ▶ Antidepressants in persons with bipolar disorder

▶ Remember that some medications can *possibly* cause a false urinary drug screen result.

PHARMACOLOGICAL PRINCIPLES **141**

TABLE 6–4. MEDICATIONS THAT CAN CAUSE FALSE POSITIVE DRUG SCREEN

FALSE POSITIVE FOR	DRUG RESPONSIBLE
Amphetamines	► Stimulants (i.e., amphetiamine/dextroamphetamine [Adderall], methylphenidate [Ritalin]) ► Bupropion (Wellbutrin) 　► Fluoxetine (Prozac) 　► Trazodone 　► Ranitidine 　► Nefazodone (Serzone) 　► Nasal decongestants 　► Pseudoephedrine
Alcohol	► Valium
Benzodiazepines	► Sertraline (Zoloft)
Cocaine	► Amoxicillin ► Most antibiotics ► NSAIDs
Heroin or morphine	► Quinolones ► Rifampin ► Codeine ► Poppy seeds
Methadone or PCP	► Over-the-counter cough medicine (such as Nyquil) ► Dextromethorphan

CASE STUDY

Jane, a 74-year-old patient whom the PHMNP has been seeing for depression, presented at her appointment with complaints of tremors, diaphoresis, headache, and nausea over the past week. She is currently being prescribed amitriptyline (50 mg q h.s.), which was increased at her last visit, and sertraline (100 mg q.d.). She denies depression but admits to increased confusion and memory problems.

► What is your biggest pharmacological concern with the combination of medication the patient is being prescribed?

► What would be your plan of action?

► What pharmacokinetics should you keep in mind when treating older adults?

REFERENCES

American Psychiatric Association. (2000). *Practice guidelines for the treatment of patients with major depressive disorder.* Washington, DC: American Psychiatric Association.

Antai-Otong D. (Ed). (2003). *Psychiatric nursing: Biological and behavioral concepts.* New York: Delmar.

Beck, A. T., Ward, C. H., Mendelson, M., Mock, J., & Erbauh, J. (1961). An inventory for measuring depression. *Archives of General Psychiatry, 4,* 561–571.

Boyd, M. A. (2002). *Psychiatric nursing: Contemporary practice* (2nd ed.). Philadelphia: Lippincott.

Dipiro, J. T., Talbert, R. L., & Yee, G. C. (Eds.). (2002). *Pharmacotherapy: A pathophysiological approach* (5th ed.). New York: McGraw-Hill.

Fuller, M., & Sajatovic, M. (2005). *Lexi-Comp's psychotropic drug information handbook (mental health).* Cleveland, OH: Lexi-Comp.

Hirschfeld, R., & Holzer, C. (2003). Validity of the mood disorder questionnaire: A general population study. *American Journal of Psychiatry, 160,* 178–180.

Kay, S. R., & Fiszbein, A. (1987). The positive and negative syndrome scale for schizophrenia. *Schizophrenia Bulletin, 13,* 261–275.

Merck. (2012). *Principles of drug treatment in children.* Retrieved from http://www.merckmanuals.com/professional/pediatrics/principles_of_drug_treatment_in_children/overview_of_drug_treatment_in_children.html

Overall, J. E., & Gorham, C. R. (1962). The brief psychiatric rating scale. *Psychological Reports, 10,* 790–812.

Rapuri, S., Ramaswamy, S., Madaan, V., Rasimas, J., & Krahn, L. (2006). "WEED" out false positive urine drug screens. *Current Psychiatry, 5*(8), 107–110.

Sadock, B., & Sadock, V. (2007). *Kaplan and Sadock's synopsis of psychiatry* (10th ed.). New York: Lippincott Williams & Wilkins.

Schatsburg, A., Cole, J., & DeBattista, C. (2007). *Manual of clinical psychopharmacology* (6th ed.). Washington, DC: American Psychiatric Association Press.

Stahl, S. (2006). *Essential psychopharmacology: The prescriber's guide.* New York: Cambridge University Press.

CHAPTER 7

NONPHARMACOLOGICAL TREATMENT

This chapter discusses nonpharmacological interventions such as individual psychotherapies, group therapy, family therapies, and complementary and alternative therapies. Because medications alone do not treat a person's environmental or interpersonal stressors and his or her responses to these stressors, an integrated approach is the most beneficial in treating mental illnesses. Although some people seek counseling for self-discovery, the most common issues for individual therapy are:

► Losses

► Interpersonal conflicts

► Symptomatic presentations such as panic, phobias, and negativity

► Unfulfilled expectations at life transitions

► Characterological issues such as narcissism or aggressiveness

Confidentiality may be broken when there is increased potential for self-harm or harm to others, in cases of abuse of children, older adults, or people with disabilities, when the therapist determines that the patient needs hospitalization, and when patients request that their information be released to a third party.

INDIVIDUAL THERAPY

► Psychoanalytic Therapy

    » Originated by Sigmund Freud (1856–1939), who believed that behavior is determined by unconscious motivations and instinctual drives (see also Chapter 3)

    » Promotes change by the development of greater insight and awareness of maladaptive defenses

- Attends to past developmental and psychodynamic factors, which shape present behaviors

▶ Cognitive Therapy

  - Originated by Aaron Beck (born 1921)

  - Purports that external events do not cause anxiety or maladaptive responses

  - States that a person's expectations, perceptions, and interpretations of events cause anxiety

  - Allows patients to view reality more clearly through an examination of their central distorted cognitions

  - Goal is to change patients' irrational beliefs, faulty conceptions, and negative cognitive distortions

▶ Behavioral Therapy

  - Originated by Arnold Lazarus (born 1932)

  - Focuses on changing maladaptive behaviors by participating in active behavioral techniques such as exposure, relaxation, problem-solving, and role-playing

▶ Dialectical Behavioral Therapy

  - Originated by Marsha Linehan (born 1943)

  - Commonly used with patients with borderline personality disorder

  - Focuses on emotional regulation, tolerance for distress, self-management skills, interpersonal effectiveness, and mindfulness, with an emphasis on treating therapy-interfering behaviors

  - *Goals*

    ▷ Decrease suicidal behaviors

    ▷ Decrease therapy-interfering behaviors

    ▷ Decrease emotional reactivity

    ▷ Decrease self-invalidation

    ▷ Decrease crisis-generating behaviors

    ▷ Decrease active passivity

    ▷ Increase realistic decision-making

    ▷ Increase accurate communication of emotions and competencies

▶ Existential Therapy

  - Originated by Viktor Frankl (1905–1997)

  - A philosophical approach in which reflection on life and self-confrontation is encouraged

- Emphasizes accepting freedom and making responsible choices

- States that a basic dimension of humans includes finding meaning and purpose in life—"Why am I here? What is my purpose?"

- Goals are to live authentically and to focus on the present and on personal responsibility

► Humanistic Therapy

- Originated by Carl Rogers (1902–1987)

- Also known as *person-centered therapy*

- Concepts include self-directed growth and self-actualization; people are born with the capacity to direct themselves toward self-actualization

- Each individual has the potential to actualize and find meaning

INTERPERSONAL THERAPY

- Originated by Gerald L. Klerman (1928–1992) and Myrna M. Weissman (born 1940)

- Evidence-based therapy with focus on interpersonal issues that are creating distress

- Time-limited, active, focused on the present and on interpersonal distress

- Developed to treat aspects of depression and is effective for adults and adolescents

- Has been applied to treat interpersonal distress related to other disorders; bipolar, substance use, and eating disorders

► Eye Movement Desensitization and Reprocessing (EMDR)

- Originated by Francine Shapiro (born 1948)

- A form of behavioral therapy

- Involves the use of bilateral stimulation—moving the eyes back and forth, alternating tapping on hand or knee, or sounds in ears

- Most commonly used in posttraumatic stress disorder

- Goal is to achieve adaptive resolution

- *Desensitization phase:* The patient visualizes the trauma, verbalizes the negative thoughts or maladaptive beliefs, and remains attentive to physical sensations. This process occurs for a limited time while the patient maintains rhythmic eye movements. He or she is then instructed to block out negative thoughts; to breathe deeply; and then to verbalize what he or she is thinking, feeling, or imagining.

» *Installation phase:* The patient installs and increases the strength of the positive thought that he or she has declared as a replacement of the original negative thought.

» *Body Scan:* The patient visualizes the trauma along with the positive thought and then scans his or her body mentally to identify any tension within.

GROUP THERAPY

▶ Benefits

» Increases insight about oneself

» Increases social skills

» Is cost-effective

» Develops sense of community

▶ Irvin Yalom (born 1931) was the first person to put a theoretical perspective on group work and identified 10 curative factors that differentiate group therapy from individual therapy.

1. *Instillation of hope:* Participants develop hope for creating a different life. Members are at different levels of growth; thus, they gain hope from others that change is possible.

2. *Universality:* Participants discover that others have similar problems, thoughts, or feelings and that they are not alone.

3. *Altruism:* This results from sharing oneself with another and helping another.

4. *Increased development of socialization skills:* New social skills are learned, and maladaptive social behaviors are corrected. The group can provide a "natural laboratory."

5. *Imitative behaviors:* Participants are able to increase their skills by imitating the behaviors of others.

6. *Interpersonal learning:* Interacting with others increases adaptive interpersonal relationships.

7. *Group cohesiveness:* Participants develop an attraction to the group and other members as well as a sense of belonging.

8. *Catharsis:* Participants experience catharsis as they openly express their feelings, which were previously suppressed.

9. *Existential factors:* Groups enable participants to deal with the meaning of their own existence.

10. *Corrective refocusing:* Participants reexperience family conflicts in the group, which allows them to recognize and change behaviors that may be problematic.

► Group Phases

- *Pregroup phase*: The leader considers the direction and framework of the group.

  ▷ Purpose

  ▷ Goals

  ▷ Membership criteria

  ▷ Membership size

  ▷ Pregroup interview

  ▷ Informed consent

- *Forming phase*: Members are concerned about self-disclosure and being rejected. Goals and expectations are identified, and boundaries are established. The development of trust and rapport is very important.

- *Storming phase*: Members are resistant and may begin to use testing behaviors. Issues related to inclusion, control, and affection begin to surface. Leaders' tasks are to allow expression of both positive and negative feelings, assist the group in understanding the underlying conflict, and examine nonproductive behaviors.

- *Norming phase*: Resistance to the group is overcome by members. A strong attraction to the group and others emerges. Open and spontaneous communication occurs, and the group norms are established.

- *Performing phase*: The group's work becomes more focused. There is creative problem-solving, and solutions begin to emerge. Experiential learning takes place. Group energy is directed toward completion of goals.

- *Adjourning phase*: Preparation is made to end the group. (Remember that the work of termination begins during the first stage of the group.) Both members and leaders express their feelings about each other and termination. A discussion and overview of what has been learned, as well as what issues still need to be worked on, takes place.

► Reminiscence Therapy

- Characterized by a progressive return of memories of past experiences

- Used with older adults

- Enables participants to search for meaning in their lives and strive for some resolution of past interpersonal and intrapsychic conflicts.

FAMILY THERAPIES

▶ Family system concepts

- A *system* is any unit structured on feedback—such as the family.

- The process by which all family members operate together is referred to as the *family system.*

- Family systems theory is based on the idea that one could not understand any family member (part) without understanding how all family members operate together (system).

- The family system operates based on a set of rules that may be overt or covert.

- *Boundaries:* Barriers that protect and enhance the functional integrity of families, individuals, and subsystems. System boundaries can be physical or psychological.

  ▷ Types of boundaries

  - *Clearly defined boundaries:* Maintain individual's separateness while emphasizing belongingness

  - *Rigid or inflexible boundaries:* May lead to distant relationships and to disengagement

  - *Diffuse boundaries:* Blurred and indistinct boundaries; lead to enmeshment

- *Circular causality:* An ongoing feedback loop; a series of actions and reactions that maintain a problem. Individuals and emotional problems are best understood within the context of relationships and through assessing interactions within an entire family.

- *Family homeostasis:* Tendency of families to resist change and to maintain a steady state

- *Morphogenesis:* A family's tendency to adapt to change when changes are necessary

- *Morphostasis:* A family's tendency to remain stable in the midst of change

▶ Family Systems Therapy

- Originated by Murray Bowen (1913–1990), who believed that an individual's problematic behavior may serve a function or purpose for the family or be a symptom of dysfunctional patterns.

- Focus is on chronic anxiety within families.

- Treatment goals are to increase the family member's awareness of their function within the family and to increase levels of *self-differentiation* (the level at which one's sense of self-worth is not dependent on external relationships, circumstances, or occurrences).

  ▷ *Triangles:* Dyads that form triads to decrease stress; the lower the level of family adaptation, the more likely a triangle will develop

▷ *Nuclear family emotional system:* Level of differentiation of the parents usually equal to the level of differentiation for the entire family

▷ *Multitransmission process:* Dysfunction present over several generations

▷ *Family projection process:* Parents transmitting their own level of differentiation on the most susceptible child

▷ *Emotional cutoffs:* Attempting to break contact with the family of origin

▷ *Sibling position:* Influences interactions and personality characteristics

▶ Structural Family Therapy

  ▹ Originated by Salvador Minuchin (1913–1990), who placed emphasis on how, when, and to whom family members relate in order to understand and then change the family's structure.

  ▹ An individual's symptoms are rooted in the context of family transaction patterns. The symptom is a function of the health of the whole family and is maintained by structural problems in the system.

  ▹ The main treatment goal is to produce a structural change in the family organization to more effectively manage problems—changing transactional patterns and family structure.

    ▷ *Family structure:* An invisible set of functional demands that organize the way members interact with each other, made up of subsystems (e.g., marital, parental, sibling), coalitions (e.g., two members joining forces against a third member), and boundaries

    ▷ *Structural mapping* (genogram): Mapping relationships using symbols to represent overinvolvement, conflict, coalitions, and so forth

    ▷ *Hierarchies:* Distribution of power

▶ Experiential Therapy

  ▹ Originated by Virginia Satir (1916–1988)

  ▹ Behavior is determined by personal experience and not by external reality.

  ▹ Focus is on being authentic, on freedom of choice, on human validation, and on experiencing the moment.

  ▹ Treatment goals are to develop authentic, nurturing communication and increased self-worth of each family member; overall goal is growth rather than symptom reduction alone.

  ▹ It does not focus on particular techniques.

▶ Strategic Therapy

  ▹ Originated by Jay Haley (1923–2007)

  ▹ Focus is that symptoms are viewed as metaphors and reflect problems in the hierarchal structure. Symptoms are a way to communicate metaphorically within a family.

- Treatment goal is to help family members behave in ways that will not perpetuate the problem behavior.
- Interventions are problem-focused. Strategic therapy is more symptom-focused than structural therapy.
- Strategic family therapists are concerned mainly with those techniques that change the sequence of interactions that is maintaining the problem.
- Techniques are straightforward directives, paradoxical directives, and reframing belief systems.
    - *Straightforward directives:* Tasks that are designed in expectation of the family member's compliance
    - *Paradoxical directives:* A negative task that is assigned when family members are resistant to change and the member is expected to be noncompliant (use this technique with caution)
    - *Reframing belief systems:* Problematic behaviors are relabeled to have more positive meaning (e.g., *jealousy* reframed to *caring*)

▶ Solution-Focused Therapy

- Originated by Steve deShazer (1940–2005), Bill O'Hanlon (born 1952) and Insoo Berg (1934–2007)
- Focus is to rework for the present situation solutions that have worked previously.
- Treatment goal is effective resolution of problems through cognitive problem-solving and use of personal resources and strengths.
- Techniques include the use of miracle questions, exception-finding questions, and scaling questions.
    - *Miracle questions:* "If a miracle were to happen tonight while you were asleep, and tomorrow morning you awoke to find that the problem no longer existed, what would be different?" "How would you know the miracle took place?" "How would others know?"
    - *Exception-finding questions:* Directing individuals to a time in their life when the problem did not exist, which helps them move toward solutions by assisting them in searching for any exceptions to the pattern. "Was there a time when the problem did not occur?"
    - *Scaling questions:* "On a scale of 1–10, with 10 being very anxious and depressed, how would you rate how you are feeling now?" This is useful for highlighting small increments of change.

COMPLEMENTARY AND ALTERNATIVE THERAPIES (CAMS)

- CAMs deal with the connection between the mind and the body and are viewed as holistic health care (dealing with the biopsychosocial and spiritual components of the patient).
- In 1998, the National Institute of Health established The National Center for Complementary and Alternative Medicine (NCCAM) with a mission to study CAM therapies with a goal to improve health (http://nccam.nih.gov/).
  - *Complementary therapies:* Used in addition to traditional medical practices
  - *Alternative therapies:* Used in place of traditional medical practices
  - *Integrative therapies:* Recent term used to describe the use of traditional complementary therapies
- Why people use CAMs
  - Desire for more control over decision-making
  - Decreased insurance coverage, therefore making the use of CAMs cheaper
  - Preference for natural rather than synthetic medications
  - Increased cost of prescriptions and services
  - Failure of conventional medications
- Mind–body interventions
  - Guided imagery
  - Meditation
  - Yoga
  - Biofeedback
- Biologically based therapies
  - Herbal products
  - Vitamins
  - Supplements
  - Aromatherapy
- Manipulative and body-based therapies
  - Acupressure and acupuncture
  - Massage
  - Reflexology

- ► Acupressure and acupuncture
  - ▹ Based on the basic tenet of Chinese medicine that vital energy *(chi)* flows along specific pathways that have many points and that manipulating these points, by either hands or needles, corrects imbalances. This occurs by stimulating or removing blockages to energy flow.
  - ▹ Thought to produce effects by regulating the nervous system and aiding the activity of endorphins and immune system cells at different sites in the body
  - ▹ Also thought to alter brain chemistry by changing the release of neurohormones and neurotransmitters.
- ► Biofeedback
  - ▹ A process providing a person with visual or auditory information about the autonomic physiologic functions of his or her body, such as blood pressure, muscle tension, and brain wave activity
  - ▹ The person learns to consciously control these processes, which were previously regarded as involuntary.
  - ▹ Uses
    - ▹ Stress-related symptoms (e.g., anxiety)
    - ▹ Pain
    - ▹ Insomnia
    - ▹ Neuromuscular problems (e.g., migraines, muscular tension, tension headaches, Raynaud's disease, urinary incontinence)
    - ▹ Neurobehavioral disorders
    - ▹ Enhancement of healing
    - ▹ Athletic and work performance
  - ▹ Desired outcome
    - ▹ Positive change in baseline measures
    - ▹ Demonstrated skill at self-regulation
    - ▹ Improvement in symptoms
    - ▹ Improved use of skills in daily life
    - ▹ Reduction of muscle bracing
    - ▹ Increased sense of self-efficacy
- ► Aromatherapy
  - ▹ Therapeutic use of plants or oils to obtain many therapeutic effects, such as analgesic, psychological, and antimicrobial benefits
  - ▹ In psychiatry, olfactory stimulation used to elicit feelings or memories during psychotherapy

► Herbal products and supplements

  ▸ Relies on plants to cure illnesses and maintain health

  ▸ Similar to prescription medications, many plants contain active compounds that produce physiological effects

  ▸ Food and Drug Administration (FDA) approval not required; thus, no uniform standards for quality control or potency

  ▸ Common supplements and interactions include:

    ▹ Omega-3 fatty acids

      ▸ Used for attention-deficit hyperactivity disorder, dyslexia, cognitive impairment, dementia, cardiovascular disease, asthma, lupus, and rheumatoid arthritis

      ▸ Interacts with warfarin (Coumadin), increasing anticoagulant effect (patients cautioned to stop using before surgery)

    ▹ Sam-e

      ▸ Used for depression, osteoarthritis, and liver disease

      ▸ May cause hypomania, hyperactive muscle movements, and possible serotonin syndrome

    ▹ Tryptophan

      ▸ Used for depression, obesity, insomnia, headaches, and fibromyalgia

      ▸ Found in high concentrations in turkey

      ▸ Increased risk of serotonin syndrome with use of serotonin reuptake inhibitors (SSRIs), monoamine oxidase inhibitors (MAOIs), and St. John's wort

    ▹ Vitamin E

      ▸ Used for enhancing the immune system and protecting cells against effects of free radicals

      ▸ Used for neurological disorders, diabetes, and premenstrual syndrome

      ▸ Interacts with warfarin, increasing anticoagulant effect; antiplatelet drugs; and statins, increasing additive effect and risk of rhabdomyolysis.

    ▹ Melatonin

      ▸ Used for insomnia, jet lag, shift work, and cancer

      ▸ Sets timing of circadian rhythms and regulates seasonal responses

      ▸ Interacts with aspirin, nonsteroidal antiinflammatory drugs (NSAIDs), beta blockers, corticosteroids, valerian, kava kava, and alcohol

      ▸ Can inhibit ovulation in large doses.

▷ Fish oil

» Used for bipolar disorder, hypertension, lowering triglycerides, and decreasing blood clotting

» Interacts with warfarin, aspirin, NSAIDs, garlic, and ginkgo

» May alter glucose regulation.

» Most herbals are secreted in breast milk and are contraindicated during lactation and should also be avoided during pregnancy.

» Common herbals with psychoactive effects include:

▷ *Black cohosh:* Menopausal symptoms, premenstrual syndrome, dysmenorrhea

▷ *Belladonna:* Anxiety

▷ *Catnip:* Sedation

▷ *Chamomile:* Sedation, anxiety

▷ *Ginkgo:* Delirium, dementia, sexual dysfunction caused by SSRIs

▷ *Ginseng:* Depression, fatigue

▷ *Valerian:* Sedation

▶ Massage

» Believed to increase blood circulation, improve lymph flow, improve musculoskeletal tone, and have tranquilizing effect on the mind

▶ Meditation

» Consciously directing one's attention to alter one's state of consciousness

» Produces physiological effects such as decreased heart rate, blood pressure, and respiratory rate; decreased anxiety; and increased alpha brain waves

▶ Reflexology

» Stimulates the body's natural healing power through massaging the feet, hands, and ears

» Based on the concept of alleviating tension by cleaning crystalline deposits under the skin that may interfere with the natural flow of the body's energy

» Based on the mapping of body parts on the soles and sides of the feet, hands, and ears

» Treats disorders related to the represented body parts by application of pressure

» Used for back pain, migraines, infertility, sleep disorders, digestive disorders, and stress-related conditions

▶ Macrobiotics

» Use of a specific diet in attempt to live in harmony with nature

» Foods classified as yin (cold and wet) and yang (hot and dry)

» Goal is to keep the yin and yang in balance

► Yoga

   » Originated in Indian philosophy

   » Combines mind and body connection

   » Uses breathing, physical movements, and meditation

CASE STUDY

You are a psychiatric mental health nurse practitioner psychotherapist working with Judy, who has depression. In session, Judy states, "Nothing good ever happens to me, I'm just a failure and should accept that people at work think I'm inadequate to do my job."

► What cognitive and behavioral techniques would be helpful for Judy?

► What type of distortions does Judy have?

REFERENCES

Brown, J., & Christensen, D. (1999). *Family therapy: Theory and practice* (2nd ed.). Pacific Grove, CA: Brooks/Cole.

Corey, G. (2005). *Theory and practice of counseling and psychotherapy* (7th ed.). Belmont, CA: Thompson, Brooks/Cole.

Corey, M., Corey, G., & Corey, C. (2010). *Groups: Process and practice* (8th ed.). Pacific Grove, CA: Brooks/Cole.

Goldenberg, I., & Goldenberg, H. (2004). *Family therapy: An overview* (6th ed.). Stamford, CT: Wadsworth.

Hawks, J., & Moyad, M. (2003). CAM: Definition and classification overview. *Urologic Nursing, 23*(3), 221–223.

Kazdin, A. E., & Weisz, J. R. (2003). *Evidence-based psychotherapies for children and adolescents.* New York: Guilford Press.

Long, L., Huntley, A., & Ernst, E. (2001). Which complementary and alternative therapies benefit which conditions? A survey of the opinions of 223 professional organizations. *Complementary Therapy in Medicine, 9*(3), 178–185.

Nichols, N. P., & Schwartz, R. C. (2003). *Family therapy: Concepts and methods* (6th ed.). Boston: Allyn & Bacon.

Sadock, B., & Sadock, V. (2007). *Kaplan and Sadock's synopsis of psychiatry* (10th ed.). New York: Lippincott Williams & Wilkins.

Sholevar, G. P., & Schwoeri, L. D. (Eds). (2003). *Textbook of family and couples therapy: Clinical applications.* Arlington, VA: American Psychiatric Press.

Snyder, M., & Lindquist, R. (Eds). (2010). *Complementary & alternative therapies in nursing* (6th ed.). New York: Springer.

Wheeler, K. (2008). *Psychotherapy for the advanced practice psychiatric nurse.* St. Louis, MO: Mosby Elsevier.

Yalom, I. (2005). *Theory and practice of group psychotherapy* (5th ed.). New York: Basic Books.

CHAPTER 8

DEPRESSIVE DISORDERS, GRIEF AND BEREAVEMENT STATES, AND BIPOLAR DISORDERS

This chapter reviews the mood disorders and evidence-based practice guidelines that psychiatric–mental health nurse practitioners (PMHNPs) utilizes in treating patients who have these disorders. Mood disorders are the most common of all psychiatric illnesses

It has become increasingly common for mood disorders to be treated in primary care settings, and often patients first present in such settings because of the high degree of somatic symptomatology that accompanies these disorders.

Sadness is a common, normal human emotion. PMHNPs caring for patients who present for evaluation of depression must distinguish between normal levels of sadness and pathological levels that are symptomatic of an underlying brain-based illness called major depression. Major depression requires treatment and generally will not fully abate without therapeutic intervention. Untreated, major depression predisposes people to other serious health problems, so pathological levels of depression should not go untreated.

SADNESS AS A COMMON EMOTIONAL STATE

► Sadness, one of the most common human emotions, exists on a continuum ranging from the absence of depression at one end to pathological levels that produce significant symptoms of a psychiatric disorder called major depression at the other.

► Cultural differences affect behavioral manifestations of depression.

- Mild depression can be a healthy reaction to life stressors that motivates a person to deal with events and emotions
  - Sadness can be pathological if it
    - Is disproportionate to events and sustained over a significant time period.
    - Significantly impairs normal social functioning (e.g., occupational, social, school, relational).
    - Significantly impairs normal somatic functioning (e.g., loss of appetite, altered sleep, altered self-care activities, altered sexual functioning).
    - Is apparently unrelated to any identifiable event or situation in a person's life.

MAJOR DEPRESSIVE DISORDER (MDD)

Description
- Is one of the most common psychiatric disorders and represents the primary unipolar affective disorder
- Is a complex brain-based illness with a primary characteristic of a persistent disturbance in mood
- Represents an excessive or distorted degree of sadness and manifests with behavioral, affective, cognitive, and somatic symptoms
- May have a known precipitating event, situation, or concern but often occurs without any precipitating stressor identified
- Significantly interferes with daily functioning and goal attainment
- Has complex genetic, biochemical, and environmental etiological factors

Etiology
- Multiple theories of the etiology of depression range from psychological to neurobiological.
- Theories are categorized as psychodynamic, cognitive–behavioral, and biological.
- Psychodynamic theories
  - Object Loss Theory (Ronald Fairbairn, D. W. Winnicott, Harry Guntrip)
    - This theory assumes that early psychological developmental issues lay the foundation for depressive responses in later life; that the accomplishment of the first stage of development in which the child is able to form relationships is normal; and that, during the second stage of development, the child experiences traumatic separation from significant objects of attachment (usually a maternal object).
    - Loss may be related to maternal death, illness, or emotional lack of availability and is unexpected and overwhelming.

▷ Depth of loss produces constellation of responses dominated by separation anxiety, grief, mourning, and despair.

▷ This critical object loss event predisposes the child to respond in similar ways to any future losses or significant separation.

» Aggression-Turned-Inward Theory (Sigmund Freud)

▷ This theory assumes that early psychological developmental issues lay the foundation for depressive responses in later life; that the accomplishment of the first stage of development in which the child is able to form relationships is normal; and that, during the second stage of development, the child experiences the loss of the significant mothering individual.

▷ The loss can be a real or imagined and is unexpected and overwhelming.

▷ The loss may be related to maternal death, illness, or emotional lack of availability or to the birth of a new sibling and the child's perception of losing undivided, individualized attention from the mother. The child's initial reaction is anger; however, the child feels unsafe to express this anger openly and directly. This may relate to the child's fearing further loss if he or she responds with anger or his or her subjective perception that anger is unacceptable.

▷ The child uses defense mechanisms to deal with conflict created by desire for the love object but co-occurring with anger for the love object.

▷ Instead of anger being expressed outward at the maternal figure, it turns inward because it is more acceptable and safer to be angry at oneself than at the mother.

▷ Anger at oneself is rationalized as the child assumes that loss of the mother was related to something bad that he or she did rather than to the caregiver's actions.

▷ Excessive guilt becomes a manifestation of the process of dealing with aggression experienced with the loss of the mother's attention.

▷ A similar emotional reaction (such as low self-esteem, excessive guilt, inability to cope with anger, self-destructive impulses) occurs as an adult whenever a loss is experienced.

» Cognitive Theory (Aaron Beck)

▷ This theory represents a cognitive diathesis–stress model in which developmental experiences sensitize a person to respond to stressful life events in a depressed manner.

▷ This theory assumes that people with a tendency to be depressed think about the world differently than nondepressed people and that depressed people are more negative and believe that bad things are going to happen to them because of their own personal shortcomings and inadequacies.

▷ This thinking promotes low self-esteem and beliefs that the person deserves to have bad things happen to him or her and promotes pessimistic perceptions about the world at large and about his or her future, as well as globalizing the negativity to all events, situations, and people in his or her life.

▷ When confronted by stressful events, these people tend to appraise them and the potential consequences in a negative, hopeless manner and therefore are more depressed than people with different cognitive styles.

▸ Learned Helplessness-Hopelessness Theory (M. Seligman)

▷ This theory is a modified aspect of cognitive theory, which assumes that a person becomes depressed due to perceptions of lack of control over life events and experiences. These perceptions are learned over time, especially as the person perceives others seeing him or her as inadequate.

▷ Perceptions of lack of control lead to the person not adapting or coping.

▷ The person's behavior becomes passive and nonreactive because of self-perceptions of personal characteristics of being helpless, hopeless, and powerless.

► Biological theories

▸ Genetic predisposition

▷ There is a clear genetic predisposition to depressive disorders; one assumption is a polygenic single nucleotide polymorphism (SNP) disorder.

▷ Having a depressed parent is the single strongest predictor of depression. Children of depressed parents are 3 times more likely to experience MDD in their lifetimes than the general population and have a 40% chance of having a depressive episode before age 18 years.

▷ The earlier the age of onset for MDD and the more severe the symptoms, the more likely it is that a person has a strong genetic load for depression.

▸ Endocrine dysfunction

▷ MDD has symptoms that suggest endocrine abnormalities as part of the etiologic picture.

▷ Neurovegetative symptoms commonly seen in MDD (e.g., sleep disturbances, appetite disturbances, libido disturbances, lethargy, anhedonia) are related to functions of the hypothalamus and pituitary and the hormones they secrete.

▷ A high incidence of postpartum mood disturbances is suggestive of endocrine dysfunction.

▷ Deregulation of *hypothalamic–pituitary–adrenal axis* (HPA, which controls the physiological response to stress and consists of interconnected feedback pathways among the hypothalamus, pituitary gland, and the adrenal glands) is another theory of an endocrine basis for MDD. In this theory, MDD is presumed to be, at least in part, a result of an abnormal stress response related to HPA dysregulation.

▸ The HPA functions in response to stress.

▸ The hypothalamus releases corticotropin-releasing hormone (CRH), which then stimulates the pituitary to release adrenocorticotropic hormone (ACTH). This then stimulates the adrenals to release cortisol.

- Hyperactivity of the HPA has been shown to be present in people with MDD, as have possible elevated cortisol levels.
- Over time, elevated cortisol levels damage the central nervous system (CNS) by altering neurotransmission and electrical signal conduction.
- Evidence supports that cortisol over time can cause changes in size and function of brain tissue.
  - HPA dysregulation is the rationale and scientific basis for the dexamethasone suppression test (DST), a screening test for depression, which has proved to be too nonspecific and is not commonly used in clinical practice.
- Abnormalities of neurotransmitter function
  - All of the following are possible neurotransmitter function abnormalities causing depression:
    - Dysregulation of one or more biogenic amine neurotransmitters: dopamine, serotonin, norepinephrine
    - Low levels of endogenous catecholamines in specific areas of the brain
      - Serotonin levels were shown to be low in postmortem studies on people who commit suicide and in people with MDD.
    - Low level of precursor tryptophan
    - Low levels of serotonin metabolite 5HTIAA
    - Receptor sensitivity for neurotransmitters set unusually high in specific areas of the brain
      - A stronger neurotransmitter receptor cascade is required to induce neuronal activity.
    - Low density of receptor sites in specific areas of the brain
    - Hypometabolism in specific areas of the brain regulating mood, appetite, and cognition
    - Complexity of brain functions imply that the etiology of complex disorders such as MDD involves the relative balance of available neurotransmitters and not just a low level of one neurotransmitter.
- Structural brain changes
  - Neuroimaging has shown consistent abnormalities in certain structures of the brain in people with chronic and severe depression.
    - Hypovolemic hippocampus
    - Hypovolemic prefrontal cortex–limbic striatal regions
  - MDD is a common comorbidity in people who have experienced brain damage, including damage from stroke and trauma.

- Chronobiological theory
    - Desynchronization of circadian rhythms produces the symptom constellation collectively called MDD.
    - Circadian rhythms control biological processes that are frequent problems in depressed persons.
        - Interrupted sleep–rest cycle
        - REM abnormalities
        - Frequent waking
        - Intensified dreaming
        - Diurnal variations to circadian-related behaviors
        - Decreased arousal and energy levels
        - Decreased activity patterns
        - Increased cortisol secretion
        - Increased emotional reactivity

Incidence and Demographics

- ▶ MDD is a common illness, with approximately 5% of the U.S. population ages 18 and older in a given year, or 9.9 million U.S. adults, having the disorder..

- ▶ MDD is the leading cause of disability in the United States and is the most common psychiatric illness seen in primary care practices; however, only 50% of people with MDD ever receive treatment.

- ▶ MDD can occur at any age; however, the average age of onset is mid-20s.

- ▶ During reproductive years, the lifetime risk for MDD varies with gender—25% for women, 12% for men; the risk is equal for the genders before puberty and after menopause.

- ▶ MDD is a greater source of morbidity for women than any other illness.

- ▶ MDD is associated with high mortality; 15% of people with MDD will die by suicide. People with MDD have a 4-times-greater risk of premature death than the normal control population.

- ▶ The disease course is variable and can involve isolated episodes separated by many years, clusters of episodes, or a severe episode with some remission of symptoms but with chronic symptoms persisting over time.

- ▶ If left untreated, an episode of symptoms of MDD usually lasts 4 months or longer.

- ▶ MDD tends to be a chronic, recurrent illness.

- ▶ One year after initial diagnosis of MDD, symptoms often persist.
    - 40% of patients have significant enough symptoms to meet full *DSM-IV* (American Psychiatric Association, 2000a) criteria for MDD.
        - 20% of patients do not meet full *DSM-IV* criteria but still have a significant symptom level that impairs functioning.
        - 40% have no symptoms.

▶ The number of prior episodes predict the likelihood of future episodes (Judd, Paulus, & Schettler, 2000).

▶ There is approximately a 60% risk of a second episode in people with first-episode MDD.

    ▹ There is approximately a 70% risk of a third episode after the second.

    ▹ There is approximately a 90% risk of a fourth episode after the third.

Risk Factors

▶ Genetic loading

    ▹ Family history, especially a first-degree relative

▶ Prior episode of MDD

▶ Female gender

▶ Postpartum period

▶ Medical comorbidity

▶ Single marital status

▶ Significant environmental stressors, especially multiple losses

Prevention and Screening

▶ Provide at-risk family education.

▶ Provide community education to help reduce stigma, to convey signs and symptoms of illness, and to emphasize the treatment potential for control of symptoms.

▶ Provide significant screening efforts to help recognize, intervene, and initiate treatment early.

▶ Provide healthcare provider education to facilitate early recognition and effective treatment.

▶ Significant and protracted prodromal symptom period usually noted before full onset of illness.

Assessment

History

▶ Detailed history of present illness, including time frame, progression, and any associated symptoms

▶ Social history, including present living situation, marital status, occupation, spirituality; education, alcohol, tobacco, and illicit drug use

▶ Medication use, including prescription, over-the-counter, alternative, supplements, and home remedies

▶ Recent medical illness or surgery

▶ Initial and periodic functional history and assessment

- ▶ Validation of history with family member
- ▶ Initial presentation: often manifests as vague somatic complaints
  - ▸ Bodily aches, pains
  - ▸ Headaches
  - ▸ Muscle pains
  - ▸ Lack of energy
  - ▸ Gastrointestinal problems
- ▶ When mood is the presenting complaint, often patient word choice is vague or indirect.
  - ▸ The person may describe mood as *depressed, discouraged, sad, "blue," "blah,"* or *"down in the dumps."*
  - ▸ Irritable mood is a frequent subjective state validated by a significant person in the patient's life.
- ▶ Characteristic low energy is seen, so assess for individual activity intolerance without other apparent cause.
  - ▸ Anhedonia is almost always present to some degree.
  - ▸ Sleep disturbance is almost always present.
    - ▷ Typically problems occur with middle or terminal insomnia.
    - ▷ Hypersomnia can be present.
    - ▷ Diurnal variations can be present.
  - ▸ A prodromal episode consisting of a high level of subjective anxiety and mild depressive symptoms often develops over days to weeks before onset of a full episode.
  - ▸ Women often report symptoms occurring in fixed pattern several days before onset of menses, so assess menstrual history. Assess for symptom changes in the per- and post-menopausal periods.
  - ▸ Psychotic features can be present, so always assess for their presence.
- ▶ Assess for patient's symptoms according to diagnostic criteria for MDD:
  - ▸ Anhedonia or a depressed mood, or both
    - ▷ Depressed mood most of the day, nearly every day, as indicated by subjective reports or observations of others
    - ▷ In children, irritable mood
  - ▸ Marked anhedonia in all or almost all activities of daily living
    - ▷ At least 3 or more significant symptoms present during the same 2-week period that represent a change in previous functioning
    - ▷ Significant, unintentional weight loss or gain of more than 5% of body weight; with increased appetite and usually a concurrent craving for specific foods, such as carbohydrates or sweets
  - ▸ Hypersomnia or insomnia nearly every day

- Psychomotor agitation or retardation
- Fatigue or loss of energy
- Self-deprecating comments or thoughts
- Feelings of worthlessness or excessive or inappropriate guilt nearly every day
- Decreased concentration and memory
- Recurrent morbid thoughts or suicidal ideation
- Symptoms that begin within 2 months of significant loss such as death of a loved one and do not persist beyond 2 months are generally considered bereavement and not MDD.

Physical Exam

▶ There are no specific physical findings.

▶ People with certain other disorders (such as diabetes, myocardial infarction, carcinomas, stroke) have a statistically significant increased risk for MDD.

- Prognosis for treatment of other disorders is poor if MDD is not recognized and effectively treated.

▶ Patients with MDD may have trouble participating in assessments related to the cognitive problems of the disorder.

- Impaired ability to report chronological timeline of illness
- Poor decision-making
- Slowed thought processes
- Requires focus assessment

▶ Patients with MDD often have psychomotor findings.

- Agitation
- Retardation

Mental Status Exam

▶ Appearance

▶ Unkempt

▶ Tired-looking

▶ Clothing showing little attention or care about how the person looks

▶ Dark-colored, loose-fitting clothing

▶ Significant weight change from baseline

▶ Speech

- Underproductive
- Blocking
- Slowed response times
- Monotonal intonation

▶ Affect
- Constricted or blunted
- Sad, tearful
- Anxious
- Irritable

▶ Mood
- Sad
- "Depressed"
- Anxious
- Irritable

▶ Thought process
- Usually organized but may be disorganized if psychosis present
- Slowing
- Distractible
- Ruminative

▶ Thought content
- Morbid preoccupation
- Suicidal ideation exists on continuum of severity:
  - Guilt for not being able to overcome the depression or for what they are "putting loved ones through"
  - Thoughts that others would be better off if the person was "gone"
  - Transient recurrent thoughts of suicide
  - Nonspecific thoughts of active action to commit suicide
  - Specific plan for committing suicide
  - Specific plan with timeline for completion
  - Specific plan with acquisition of the means to carry out plan (suicidal motivation differs for different patients)

▶ Despair

DEPRESSIVE DISORDERS, GRIEF AND BEREAVEMENT STATES, AND BIPOLAR DISORDERS   167

- Desire to give up struggle
- Attempt to end significant emotional pain
- Lack of any visible options for dealing with stressors, hopeless, helpless
- Anger and frustration with poor impulse control
  - Research evidence supports that it is not possible to predict accurately whether or when a person will attempt suicide (see Table 8–1 for review of suicide assessment).

TABLE 8-1. ASSESSING FOR SUICIDAL BEHAVIOR

Past history of suicide in family or suicide attempts in patient or family
Negativity and morbidity
Suicidal ideation currently
Plan and intent for suicide action
Means and access to commit suicide
Perceived social supports
Lethality of intended suicide action ▸ *High lethality:* Jumping from significant height, gun, hanging ▸ *Moderate lethality:* Overdose of toxic agents (such as aspirin, sleeping pills) ▸ *Low lethality:* Superficial wrist cutting, breath-holding
Impulsivity
Substance abuse or dependence
History of psychiatric disorder

- ▶ Suicide risk especially high for persons with certain symptoms or history:
  - Presence of psychotic symptoms
  - History of past attempts
  - History of first-degree relative who committed suicide
  - Concurrent substance abuse or dependency
  - Current serious health problem (see below for clinical management of suicidality)
- ▶ Orientation
  - Patient is usually oriented to person, place, and time unless psychosis present.
- ▶ Memory
  - Usually impaired recent and short-term memory
- ▶ Concentration
  - Usually significantly impaired

- ▶ Abstraction
  - ▸ Abstract ability on proverb testing usually intact
  - ▸ If concrete, assess for other psychotic findings
- ▶ Judgment
  - ▸ Impaired for self-welfare

Diagnostic Studies

- ▶ No specific lab findings specific to MDD exist
- ▶ CBC, chemistry profile, thyroid function tests, or B_{12} level to rule out metabolic causes or unidentified conditions; consider referral for sleep study if snoring, apnea, or suspicion of other sleep disorder
- ▶ Drug toxicity screening, if indicated by history
- ▶ Depression related to a differential diagnosis
  - ▸ Endocrine disorders
    - ▷ Hypothyroidism
    - ▷ Diabetes
    - ▷ Hyperaldosteronism
  - ▸ Cushing's or Addison's disease
  - ▸ Neurological disorders
    - ▷ Stroke
    - ▷ Epilepsy
    - ▷ Dementia
    - ▷ Huntington's disease
    - ▷ Sleep apnea
  - ▸ Wilson's disease
  - ▸ Neoplasms
  - ▸ Head trauma
  - ▸ Multiple sclerosis
  - ▸ Parkinson's disease
- ▶ Cardiac disorders
  - ▸ Myocardial infarction
  - ▸ Congestive heart failure
  - ▸ Hypertension

- ▶ Infectious and inflammatory states
  - ▹ Mononucleosis
  - ▹ AIDS
  - ▹ Pneumonia: viral and bacterial
  - ▹ Systemic lupus erythematous
  - ▹ Temporal arteritis
  - ▹ Tuberculosis
- ▶ Nutritional disorders
  - ▹ Pernicious anemia
  - ▹ Pellagra
- ▶ Other disorders
  - ▹ Fibromyalgia
  - ▹ Chronic fatigue syndrome
  - ▹ Bereavement or grief reaction
  - ▹ Electrolyte imbalance
  - ▹ Uremia and other renal conditions
- ▶ Psychiatric disorders
  - ▹ Anxiety disorders
  - ▹ Eating disorders
  - ▹ Bipolar affective disorder
  - ▹ Substance dependence–related disorders
- ▶ Medications that can cause altered mood states as side effects
  - ▹ Steroids
  - ▹ Estrogen compounds
  - ▹ Antihypertensive agents
  - ▹ Anti-Parkinson's agents
  - ▹ Antineoplastic agents
  - ▹ Antibacterial and antifungal agents
  - ▹ Analgesics

Clinical Management

▶ The top goal in the acute phase of MDD is ensuring patient safety.

▶ A general consideration is to rule out or treat any conditions that may contribute to depression and cognitive impairment.

▶ Assess for the acuity level of patient presentation.

▶ Reasons for brief hospitalization during acute episodes of MDD:

  ▪ Ensure patient safety

  ▪ Initiate medication change, when doing so as an outpatient poses undue risk

  ▪ Restabilize on medication

  ▪ Monitor suicidality

  ▪ Ensure patient compliance with treatment to reach stabilization

▶ Clinical management during nonacute episodes occurs most often in community settings.

  ▪ Obtain baseline labs before initiation of treatment.

    ▷ Pharmacological clinical management

    ▷ Nonpharmacological management (psychotherapy)

Pharmacologic Treatment

▶ Consider non-pharmacological measures (pyschotherapy, exercise, relaxation, bright light exposure) as first-line treatment for mild symptoms of depression

▶ Inform client that therapeutic effect may take at least 4 to 6 weeks.

▶ Once started, continue antidepressants for a minimum of 6 to 12 months.

  ▪ If patient has more than two prior episodes of MDD, consider continuing antidepressants indefinitely.

▶ Not all symptoms of MDD will respond to pharmacological interventions.

  ▪ Identify clear, measurable target symptoms and educate the patient about these symptoms (see Table 8–2).

  ▪ Research has found that the most effective intervention is a combination of medication and psychotherapy

  ▪ Antidepressant rebound is common when stopping antidepressants abruptly, particularly when drugs with short half-lives are involved

  ▪ Antidepressants may induce mania or mixed mania in susceptible persons

  ▪ All antidepressants have "black box" warning regarding suicidality for children, adolescents, and young adults

DEPRESSIVE DISORDERS, GRIEF AND BEREAVEMENT STATES, AND BIPOLAR DISORDERS **171**

TABLE 8-2. TARGET SYMPTOMS OF ANTIDEPRESSANT TREATMENT

Depressed mood
Sleep–rest disturbances
Anxiety
Irritability
Impaired concentration
Impaired memory
Appetite disturbance
Agitation
Anhedonia

▶ Classes of antidepressants

    ▷ Selective serotonin reuptake inhibitors (SSRIs)

        ▷ Action primarily to increase serotonin levels in CNS by inhibiting their presynaptic reuptake

        ▷ See Table 8–3 for examples

    ▷ Tricyclic antidepressants (TCAs)

        ▷ Elevate serotonin and norepinephrine levels primarily by inhibiting their presynaptic reuptake

        ▷ See Table 8–4 for examples and Table 8–6 for dietary precautions

    ▷ Monoamine oxidase inhibitors (MAOIs)

        ▷ Elevate serotonin and norepinephrine levels primarily by inhibiting MAO, the enzyme that breaks down monoamine neurotransmitters

        ▷ See Table 8–5 for examples

    ▷ Serotonin norepinephrine reuptake inhibitors (SNRIs)

        ▷ Inhibit dual reuptake of norepinephrine and serotonin

        ▷ Action very selective on neurotransmitters

        ▷ Elevate serotonin and norepinephrine levels by inhibiting their presynaptic reuptake

        ▷ See Table 8–7 for examples

    ▷ Norepinephrine dopamine reuptake inhibitors (NDRIs)

        ▷ Inhibits dual reuptake of norepinephrine and dopamine

        ▷ Action very selective on neurotransmitters

        ▷ Elevates dopamine and norepinephrine levels by inhibiting their presynaptic reuptake

        ▷ See Table 8–7 for examples

- Serotonin agonist and reuptake inhibitors (SARIs)

  ▷ Dual action

  ▷ Agonist of serotonin 5HT-2 receptors

  ▷ Action very selective on neurotransmitters

  ▷ Elevates serotonin levels by inhibiting serotonin reuptake

  ▷ See Table 8–7 for examples

- The various antidepressants differ markedly in characteristics such as

  ▷ Cost

  ▷ Side-effect profile

  ▷ Safety in overdose

  ▷ Safety in patients with other disorders

  ▷ Drug–drug interactions

  ▷ Cytochrome P-450 liver effects

► To achieve best control of symptoms, match patient's symptom profile to the pharmacodynamic and pharmacokinetic properties of specific antidepressant agents.

SSRIs

► First-line treatment for moderate symptoms. Consider non-pharmacological treatment for mild, first episode symptoms.

- Serious side effects are rare

- Much safer in overdose than TCAs

- Also effective for panic disorder, obsessive–compulsive disorder, bulimia, generalized anxiety disorder, social phobia, posttraumatic stress disorder, and premenstrual dysphoric disorder

DEPRESSIVE DISORDERS, GRIEF AND BEREAVEMENT STATES, AND BIPOLAR DISORDERS **173**

TABLE 8-3. ANTIDEPRESSANTS: SELECTIVE SEROTONIN REUPTAKE INHIBITORS (SSRIs)

AGENT	BRAND NAME	DOSAGE FORMS & DAILY DOSAGE	SIDE EFFECTS	COMMENTS
Citalopram (SSRI)	Celexa	Tablet, 20–40 mg/day	► Sedation ► Sexual dysfunction ► Agitation ► Yawning ► GI disturbances ► Weight gain	► Pregnancy Category C ► Lactation Category L2 ► 2011 warning about prolonged QTc interval in doses above 40 mg and in those susceptible to prolonged QTc
Escitalopram (SSRI)	Lexapro	Tablet, 10–20 mg/day	► Somnolence ► Headache ► Sexual dysfunction ► GI disturbances	► Pregnancy Category C ► Lactation Category L3
Fluoxetine (SSRI)	Prozac	Capsule, tablet, liquid, 20–80 mg/day	► Insomnia ► Headache ► GI disturbances ► Sexual dysfunction	► Long half-life ► Pregnancy Category C ► Lactation L2 ► Discontinuation syndrome unlikely
Fluvoxamine (SSRI)	Luvox	Tablet, 100–300 mg/day	► Sedation ► Sexual dysfunction ► Agitation ► GI disturbances	► Doses above 150 mg should generally be given b.i.d. ► Pregnancy Category C ► Lactation Category L2
Paroxetine (SSRI)	Paxil CR/ Pexeva	Tablet, liquid, 20–60 mg/day	► Headache ► GI disturbances ► Somnolence ► Sexual dysfunction	► Pregnancy Cateogry D ► Lactation Category L2 ► Discontinuation syndrome very common
Sertraline (SSRI)	Zoloft	Tablet, 50–200 mg/day	► Sexual dysfunction ► GI disturbances ► Somnolence ► Headache	► Pregnancy Category C ► Lactation Category L2

TCAs

▶ Considered second-line drugs for treating MDD (see Table 8–4)

▶ Affect many neurotransmitters, leading to more side effects and possibly poor adherence

  ▸ *Anticholinergic:* Dry mouth, blurred vision, constipation, memory problems (from muscarinic receptor blockade)

  ▸ *Antiadrenergic:* Orthostatic hypotension (from alpha 1 receptor blockade)

  ▸ *Antihistaminergic:* Sedation and weight gain (from histamine receptor blockade)

  ▸ EKG changes and cardiac dysrhythmias possible; avoid in patients known to have susceptibility (personal or family history). Monitor EKG before treatment and annually in older adults.

▶ Unsafe in many co-occurring disorders (such as cardiac disease)

▶ Known to induce hypomania in susceptible patients

▶ Have well-identified serum blood levels that guide dosing (particularly nortriptyline) and predict toxicity

  ▸ Are inexpensive and available in generic forms

▶ Anticholinergic properties may be highly problematic but may also be useful in those who have significant bowel irritability

▶ Avoid abrupt withdrawal because of significant discontinuation syndrome

▶ Avoid prescribing to people who are at high risk for suicide; *lethal dose is 1,000 mg or more (a week's supply of an average dose)*

▶ Combination of TCAs with MAOIs can cause lethal serotonin syndrome, hypertensive crisis, or both; adhere to 2-week washout period (5 weeks for fluoxetine) before switching between the two classes of medications.

▶ Use caution if the person is taking both a TCA and an SSRI, because the SSRI can elevate TCA concentrations because of pharmacodynamic or pharmacokinetic interactions. Monitor TCA levels.

DEPRESSIVE DISORDERS, GRIEF AND BEREAVEMENT STATES, AND BIPOLAR DISORDERS **175**

TABLE 8-4. TRICYCLIC ANTIDEPRESSANTS (TCAs)

AGENT	BRAND NAME	DOSAGE FORMS & DAILY DOSAGE	COMMENTS
Amitriptyline	Elavil	Tablet, IM 50–300 mg/day	Also used for chronic pain (particularly neuropathic), insomnia
Clomipramine	Anafranil	Capsule, 100–250 mg/day	Approved for obsessive–compulsive disorder; 250 mg/day maximum because of increased seizure risk
Desipramine	Norpramin	Tablet, capsule, 100–300 mg/day	Also used for attention-deficit hyperactivity disorder (off label for peds and for ADHD)
Doxepin	Sinequan	Capsule, liquid, 100–300 mg/day	Also used for insomnia
Imipramine	Tofranil	Tablet, capsule, IM, 100–300 mg/day	Also used for enuresis and separation anxiety
Nortriptyline	Pamelor	Capsule, liquid, 50–150 mg/day	Also used for enuresis and attention deficit hyperactivity disorder
Protriptyline	Vivactil	Tablet, 15–60 mg/day	
Trimipramine	Surmontil	Capsule, 100–300 mg/day	

MAOIs

▶ Normally are never first- or second-line agents for MDD because of dangerous food and drug interactions (see Tables 8–5 and 8–6).

  ▹ *Hypertensive crisis* occurs when MAOIs are taken in conjunction with foods containing *tyramine*, a dietary precursor to norepinephrine.

  ▹ When MAO is inhibited, tyramine exerts a strong vasopressor effect— stimulating the release of catecholamines, epinephrine, and norepinephrine, which can increase blood pressure and heart rate.

  ▹ Hypertensive crisis is life-threatening and cannot be reversed unless more MAO is produced by the body.

    ▹ *Hypertensive crisis* and death also can occur when MAOIs are taken in conjunction with certain medications:

      ▹ Meperidine

      ▹ Decongestants

      ▹ TCAs

      ▹ Atypical antipsychotics

      ▹ St. John's wort

- L-tryptophan

- Stimulants and other sympathomimetics

- Asthma medications

- Symptoms of hypertensive crisis:

  ▷ Sudden, explosive-like headache, usually in occipital region

  ▷ Elevated blood pressure

  ▷ Facial flushing

  ▷ Palpitations

  ▷ Pupillary dilation

  ▷ Diaphoresis

  ▷ Fever

- Treatment of hypertensive crisis:

  ▷ Discontinue the MAOI.

  ▷ Give phentolamine (binds with norepinephrine receptor sites, blocks norepinephrine).

  ▷ Stabilize fever.

  ▷ Reevaluate the person's diet and adherence, and reiterate medication guidelines as necessary.

  ▷ People on MAOIs must follow a *tyramine-free diet* and must avoid many medications, including most over-the-counter cold and allergy preparations.

- Combining an MAOI with a serotonergic agent is contraindicated, because this may cause serotonin syndrome.

► Symptoms of serotonin syndrome

- Agitation, restlessness

- Rapid heart rate and elevation in blood pressure

- Headache

- Sweating, shivering, and goose bumps

- Myoclonic jerking and loss of coordination

- Confusion, fever, seizures, unconsciousness

► There is little safety in overdose.

► Side-effect profile and stringent dietary restrictions often lead to poor patient adherence

► Clinically significant side effects of MAOIs include

- Insomnia

- Hypertensive crisis

DEPRESSIVE DISORDERS, GRIEF AND BEREAVEMENT STATES, AND BIPOLAR DISORDERS **177**

- ▹ Weight gain

- ▹ Anticholinergic side effects

- ▹ Lightheadedness and dizziness

- ▹ Sexual dysfunction

► MAOIs are unsafe in many co-occurring disorders

► MAOIs are inexpensive, and most come in generic form

TABLE 8-5. MONOAMINE OXIDASE INHIBITORS (MAOIs)

DRUG	BRAND NAME	DOSAGE FORMS & DAILY DOSAGE	COMMENTS
Isocarboxazid	Marplan	Tablet, 100–60 mg/day	► Also used for panic disorder, phobic disorders, selective mutism
Phenelzine	Nardil	Tablet, 45–90 mg/day	► *Caution:* Requires low tyramine diet; sympathyomimetic agents
Tranylcypromine	Parnate	Tablet, 20–50 mg/day	► Divided dosing: b.i.d. and q.i.d.
Selegiline	EMSAM	Transdermal patch, 6–12 mg	► No dietary restrictions with 6-mg dosage; may need higher dose to see antidepressant effect

TABLE 8-6. TYRAMINE-FREE DIETARY CONSIDERATION

CATEGORY OF FOOD	SPECIFIC FOODS TO AVOID
Cheeses	Aged cheeses such as blue, brie, camembert, and Roquefort
Meat	Smoked, aged, and cured meats such as sausages, pastrami, and salami
Fish	Smoked, aged, and cured fish such as pickled herring and salted fish
Beverages	Any aged and fermented beverages such as wine, chianti, aged liquors, whiskey, beer (tap and unpasteurized), and alcohol-free beers; caffeine
Other	Bean curd, soy bean paste, sauerkraut, soy sauce, miso soup, yeast extract, chocolate, MSG, nuts, and bananas

OTHER ANTIDEPRESSANTS

► Other antidepressants used in the treatment of MDD are SNRIs, NDRIs, SARIs and others. See Table 8–7.

TABLE 8-7. OTHER ANTIDEPRESSANT AGENTS

DRUG	BRAND NAME	DOSAGE FORMS & DAILY DOSAGE	SIDE EFFECTS	COMMENTS
Bupropion (NDRI)	Wellbutrin	Tablet, 150–450 mg/day	▸ Headache ▸ Nervousness ▸ Tremors ▸ Tachycardia ▸ Insomnia ▸ Decreased appetite	▸ Contraindicated if patient has seizures, eating disorder ▸ SR offers b.i.d. dosing ▸ XL offers once-daily dosing ▸ Can increase energy level ▸ Also used for attention-deficit hyperactivity disorder and smoking cessation
Bupropion SR/XL	Wellbutrin SR	Sustained release, 150–400 mg/day Extended release, 150–450 mg/day		▸ Caution with caffeine and in people with panic disorder
Vilazodone	Viibryd	Tablet, 10–40 mg/day	▸ Gastrointestinal ▸ dizziness ▸ drowsiness ▸ restlessness/ jitteriness	▸ Start at 10 mg q.d. and increase by no more than 10 mg every week until target dose of 40 mg is reached ▸ 3A4 (primarily) substrate
Mirtazapine (NaSSA)	Remeron	Tablet, 15–45 mg/day	▸ Sedation ▸ Weight gain ▸ Increased cholesterol	▸ Inverse relationship between dosage and sedation
Nefazodone (SARI)	Serzone	Tablet, 300–600 mg/day	▸ Headache ▸ Drowsiness ▸ GI disturbances	▸ *Must* monitor LFTs ▸ Can cause liver failure ▸ Safer in overdose than TCAs ▸ q.h.s. or b.i.d. dosing ▸ Potent P450 3A4 inhibitor
Trazodone (SARI)	Desyrel	Tablet, 200–600 mg/day	▸ Sedation ▸ Nausea ▸ Headache ▸ hypotension	▸ Safer in overdose than TCAs ▸ Priapism possible ▸ Not well tolerated at antidepressant dosage because of sedation ▸ Most commonly used as hypnotic at 50–200 mg/h.s. ▸ May prolong QTc interval
Venlafaxine (SNRI)	Effexor, Effexor XR	Capsule (XR), tablet, 75–375 mg/day XR, 75–225 mg/day	▸ Diaphoresis ▸ Headache ▸ Dizziness ▸ GI disturbances	▸ Can raise BP ▸ q.d. for XR capsules ▸ b.i.d.–t.i.d. dosing for tablets ▸ Full SNRI effect at doses at or above 150 mg ▸ Safer in overdose than TCAs ▹ Has *significant* discontinuation syndrome if stopped abruptly
Duloxetine (SNRI)	Cymbalta	Capsule, 30–120 mg	▸ Dizziness ▸ Headache ▸ GI disturbances	▸ Once-daily dosing ▸ Can elevate BP ▸ Can elevate liver function tests ▹ Has *significant* discontinuation syndrome if stopped abruptly

DEPRESSIVE DISORDERS, GRIEF AND BEREAVEMENT STATES, AND BIPOLAR DISORDERS **179**

► Psychotic features can be present with MDD.

 ▸ Routinely assess for the presence of psychotic symptoms during periods of symptom exacerbation

 ▸ Features are usually mood congruent

 ▸ Can be managed with short-term use of antipsychotic medications (see Chapter 10)

► Comorbidities are common and include various medical conditions (as noted earlier in the chapter) as well as psychiatric comorbidities such as panic disorder, obsessive–compulsive disorder, and substance abuse or dependence.

 ▸ Altered appetite and sleep–rest patterns predispose clients with MDD to decreased overall health status.

 ▸ Increased mortality exists in people with MDD.

Nonpharmacologic Treatment

► Electroconvulsive therapy (ECT)

 ▸ Grand mal seizure induced in anesthetized person

 ▸ Usual course is 6 to 12 treatments

 ▸ Mechanism of action:

  ▹ Neurotransmitter theory: Increases dopamine, serotonin, and norepinephrine

  ▹ Neuroendocrine theory: Releases hormones such as prolactin, thyroid-stimulating hormone, pituitary hormones, endorphins, and adrenocorticotropic hormone

  ▹ Anticonvulsant theory: Exerts an anticonvulsant effect, which then produces an antidepressant effect.

 ▸ Situations in which ECT is used:

  ▹ Patient preference

  ▹ Need for rapid response because of severity of illness

  ▹ Risk of other treatment outweighs risk of ECT

  ▹ Treatment resistance

 ▸ Possible contraindications:

  ▹ Cardiac disease

  ▹ Compromised pulmonary status

  ▹ History of brain injury or brain tumor

  ▹ Anesthesia medical complications

- Adverse effects:
  - Possible cardiovascular effects
  - Systemic effects (e.g., headaches, muscle aches, drowsiness)
  - Cognitive effects (e.g., memory disturbance and confusion)
- ▶ Transcranial magnetic stimulation (TMS)
  - Option for those patients who have not had adequate response to medications and psychotherapy (treatment-resistant depression)
  - Involves placement of small wire coil on scalp to conduct electrical current, creating a magnetic field through the tissues of the head
  - Preformed in office setting, without anesthesia
  - Sessions typically last 40 minutes and typical course is 5 sessions per week for 6 weeks
  - Side effects are minimal but may include headache, scalp discomfort, tingling or twitches to facial muscles, lightheadedness, and hearing discomfort from procedure noise
  - Seizures, although rare, have been reported
- ▶ Vagal nerve stimulation (VNS)
  - Option for those patients who have not had adequate response to medications and psychotherapy (treatment-resistant depression)
  - Pacemaker-like device implanted in left side of chest to stimulate left branch of nerve; transcutaneous devices being tested.
  - Generally done as outpatient procedure, but anesthesia is required
  - Side effects generally occur as the pulse generator is stimulating and include: voice changes, hoarseness, cough, throat or neck pain, chest spasms, dyspnea on exertion, tingling of skin, dysphagia
  - Intended for use along with traditional treatments
- ▶ Phototherapy
- ▶ Individual therapy
  - Cognitive–behavioral therapy (CBT)
    - Modify perceptions
    - Decrease negativity
    - Increase sense of internal control
    - Enhance coping skills
    - Modify environmental factors contributing to illness

- Brief therapy (solution-focused therapy)
  - Focus on precipitant stressor
  - Cope with immediate impact of MDD on personal life
  - Modify contributory environmental factors
- Group therapy
  - Improve decision-making
  - Improve socialization skills
  - Improve assessment of individual strengths
  - Gain new coping skills
- Family therapy
  - Enhance family coping
  - Improve knowledge base
  - Plan for relapse
  - Gain insight into effects of MDD on family
  - Undertake psychoeducation for family members about the illness state of MDD

When to Consult, Refer, Hospitalize

Clinical Management of Suicidality

- ▶ Pay significant attention to positive assessments for suicidality.
- ▶ Always assume patient is serious when he or she vocalizes suicidal thoughts.
- ▶ Identify current stressors that may be contributing to crisis.
  - Generally do not manage in community setting during acute suicidal ideation periods unless patient is able to make a "no harm" agreement.
- ▶ Consider hospitalization.
- ▶ Consider mobilizing available social resources.
  - Risk factors for suicide:
    - Ages 45 or older if male
    - Ages 55 or older if female
    - Divorced, single, or separated
    - White
    - Living alone
    - Psychiatric disorder
    - Physical illness

▷ Substance abuse

▷ Previous suicide attempt

▷ Family history of suicide

▷ Recent loss

▷ Male gender

Special Considerations

Children

▶ Core symptoms of MDD are the same for children. However, some symptoms are more pronounced in children.

- ▸ Irritability

- ▸ Somatic complaints

- ▸ Social withdrawal

    ▷ Some core symptoms are *less common* in children before onset of puberty:

    - ▸ Psychosis

    - ▸ Motor retardation

    - ▸ Hypersomnia

    - ▸ Increased appetite

- ▸ MDD often has a strong separation anxiety component in children.

- ▸ Children usually do not respond well to tricyclics; however, they do respond well to SSRIs.

    ▷ All antidepressants indicated for children, adolescents, and young adults carry a black box warning about an increase in suicidal thoughts; monitor closely for suicidal thoughts, behavior, agitation, and aggression in children taking antidepressants.

Special Considerations

Older Adults

▶ Persons with MDD admitted to a long-term-care facility have significantly shorter life spans than the control population.

- ▸ 65% are more likely to die within the first year in a long-term-care facility.

▶ Cognition and memory symptoms of MDD in the older adult population often are confused with dementia-related symptoms (pseudodementia).

▶ In dementia, there is usually a premorbid history of slowly declining cognition.

► In MDD, cognitive changes have a relatively acute onset and are significant when compared to premorbid functioning.

► It is important to complete a functional assessment for older adults.

  » Determines the degree to which the person's abilities and performance match the demands of his or her life

  » Determines the impact of illness on overall functioning

  » *Skill deficit*: Inability to perform a functional skill despite the physical ability, as in dementia

  » *Performance deficit*: Ability to perform a functional skill but lacks the motivation to do so, as in depression

► Reasons for performing functional assessment:

  » To correctly diagnose (for example, to differentiate depression from dementia)

  » To track patient improvement or decompensation

  » To help families set realistic expectations.

► Components of functional assessment:

  » Activities of daily living (ADLs): Basic self-care skills, such as bathing, dressing, eating, and toileting

  » Instrumental activities of daily living (IADLs): Complex activities needed for independent functioning, such as shopping, cooking, driving, and housekeeping

  » Executive functioning: Judgment and planning; ability to maintain calendar, manage money and appointments, and prioritize activities

► The degree of change over time and the speed of change are better observed with objective recording and when the assessment is measured at intervals such as every 6 months.

Follow-up

► Follow-up care practices for the PMHNP to consider

  » Include in patient teaching the goals, risks, benefits, and potential side effects of medication treatment.

  » Continuously monitor patient's response to medication; the treatment goal is complete remission of symptoms.

  » Teach patients the symptoms of depression and that it is a chronic illness; establish a relapse plan for all patients.

  » Assess for suicidality during every patient contact.

  » Assess for the presence of psychotic symptoms during every patient contact.

- Assess and manage patient for side effects of treatment, including sexual side effects, in an attempt to increase medication compliance.

- Observe all patients treated with antidepressants for development of *serotonin syndrome* (overstimulation of serotonin receptors usually caused by drug–drug interactions).

► Drug combinations that can cause serotonin syndrome:

- SSRIs and MAOIs

- Drug and herbal interactions

- SSRIs and St. John's wort

► Symptoms of serotonin syndrome:

- Autonomic instability

- Altered sensorium

- Restlessness

- Agitation

- Myoclonis

- Hyperreflexia

- Hyperthermia

- Diaphoresis

- Tremor

- Chills

- Diarrhea and cramps

- Ataxia

- Headache

- Insomnia

► Remember to monitor for adverse effects over time.

► Some SSRIs are known to increase blood glucose and contribute to hyperlipidemia, and others may elevate liver function tests.

► Discontinue SSRIs slowly to prevent *discontinuation syndrome.*

► Symptoms of discontinuation syndrome:

- Flulike symptoms

- Fatigue and lethargy

- Myalgia

- Decreased concentration

- Nausea and vomiting

- Impaired memory

- Paresthesias, including "shock-like" sensations

- Irritability

- Anxiety

- Insomnia

- Crying without provocation

- Dizziness and vertigo

► Risk factors for discontinuation syndrome:

- Medications with short half-life

- Abrupt discontinuation

- Noncompliant, irregular use pattern

- High dose range

- Long-term treatment

- Prior history of discontinuation syndrome

  ▷ Whenever possible, discontinue all antidepressants slowly.

    - Rapid discontinuation of TCAs can cause *cholinergic rebound syndrome*:

      ▷ Nausea

      ▷ GI upset

      ▷ Diaphoresis

      ▷ Myalgias, especially of neck muscles

► Expected course of MDD

- Evidence indicates the best treatment outcomes if medications are used in conjunction with appropriate therapy.

- Evidence indicates that patients should take an antidepressant agent for at least 12 months after remission of symptoms.

- Patients who have had 2 or more episodes of MDD usually require lifelong medication.

DYSTHYMIC DISORDER

Description

▶ A disorder similar to MDD but with less acute symptoms; with a more protracted, chronic disease course; and without any manifestations of psychotic symptoms

▶ Less discrete episodes of illness than MDD

▶ Symptoms often go undetected and therefore untreated for years

▶ Vegetative symptoms (e.g., sleep, appetite, weight changes) much less common in dysthymic disorder than in MDD

Etiology

▶ Similar to MDD

Incidence and Demographics

▶ Affects 5.4% of the U.S. population ages 18 or older, or 10.9 million Americans.

▶ People with dysthymia have an increased risk for developing MDD; 15% to 25% of people diagnosed with dysthymic disorder will have a lifetime episode of MDD.

▶ In people with onset of symptoms before age 21, there is a 75% likelihood that they will have a lifetime episode of MDD.

▶ Women are 2 to 3 times more likely to develop dysthymic disorder than men.

Risk Factors

▶ Genetic predisposition

▶ A first-degree relative with MDD

▶ A first-degree relative with dysthymic disorder

▶ Female gender

Prevention and Screening

▶ At-risk family education

▶ Community education

▶ Stigma reduction

▶ Signs and symptoms of illness

▶ Treatment potential for control of symptoms

▶ Early recognition, intervention, and initiation of treatment

▶ Because of chronic nature of disorder, symptoms become a part of patients' day-to-day existence and often go unreported unless solicited by direct questioning

▶ Aggressive screening procedure required.

DEPRESSIVE DISORDERS, GRIEF AND BEREAVEMENT STATES, AND BIPOLAR DISORDERS   187

Assessment

History
- ▶ Assess for the following:
  - ▹ Chronically depressed mood that occurs for most of the day, more days than not, for at least 2 years
  - ▹ Prominent presence of low self-esteem, self-criticism, and a perception of general incompetence compared to others
  - ▹ Other common symptoms:
    - ▷ Low energy and fatigue
    - ▷ Poor concentration
    - ▷ Difficulty with decision-making
    - ▷ Feelings of hopelessness
    - ▷ Feelings of inadequacy
    - ▷ Mild anhedonia
    - ▷ Social withdrawal
    - ▷ Brooding about past issues
    - ▷ Subjective irritability or anger
    - ▷ Decreased productivity and activity
  - ▹ Less common symptoms:
    - ▷ Alteration in appetite
    - ▷ Alteration in sleep–rest patterns

Physical Exam
- ▶ Similar to MDD

Mental Status Exam
- ▶ Similar to MDD
- ▶ Usually no vegetative findings
- ▶ Mood described as *sad, "down for all of my life"*

Diagnostic Studies
- ▶ Nonspecific
- ▶ Polysomnographic findings
  - ▹ Similar to those found in MDD

Differential Diagnosis
- ▶ Similar to MDD

Clinical Management

Pharmacologic Treatment

▶ Because of increased risk for development of MDD, dysthymia is usually treated with antidepressant medications in a manner similar to MDD.

Nonpharmacologic Treatment

▶ Similar to MDD

▶ Often good clinical outcomes with just nonpharmacological treatment if patient is willing.

Common Comorbidities

▹ MDD is often superimposed on dysthymia ("double depression").

▹ The subjective worsening of symptoms or onset of new symptoms such as vegetative ones often brings the person into treatment.

▹ When dysthymia precedes MDD, clinical management is more complex and outcomes can be less positive.

▹ Dysthymic disorder is associated with personality disorders.

  ▷ Borderline

  ▷ Histrionic

  ▷ Narcissistic

  ▷ Avoidant

  ▷ Dependent

Special Considerations

▶ Similar to MDD

▶ In children, prevalence rates of dysthymia are equal for boys and girls.

▶ Associated with several childhood disorders

  ▹ Attention-deficit hyperactivity disorder

  ▹ Conduct disorder

  ▹ Anxiety disorders

  ▹ Learning disorders

  ▹ Mental retardation

▶ Period of symptoms required for diagnosis is only 1 year in children, compared with 2 years for adults

▶ In children, the mood usually described as *irritable* rather than *sad* but may report both irritability and sadness

▶ Low self-esteem, poor social skills, and pessimism

Follow-up

▶ Similar to MDD

GRIEF AND BEREAVEMENT

Description

▶ Involve a wide range of normal responses that can become abnormal and excessive

▶ Involve normative emotional, cognitive, and behavioral reactions to death or loss of a significant individual or object

▶ Unlike in major depression, self-esteem is usually preserved in the grieving individual

▶ Involve nonnormative psychological responses to an identifiable stressor that can result in the development of clinically significant emotional or behavioral symptoms

    ▸ Stressor encompassing elements of perceived loss

    ▸ Develops *within 3 months* of stressor

        ▷ Single event

        ▷ End of relationship

        ▷ Death of relative or partner

        ▷ Recurring event

            ▸ Living with person with terminal illness

        ▷ Developmental event

            ▸ Leaving home to go away to school

            ▸ Getting married

            ▸ Becoming a parent

            ▸ Retiring from work

▶ PMHNP assessment is needed to separate normal, healthy grieving from pathological grieving, which may represent an adjustment disorder or major depression. The PMHNP must consider:

    ▸ Severity of response

    ▸ Duration of response

    ▸ Effects of response on normal daily functioning

    ▸ Person's perceptions of impact of stressor

▶ When severity or duration is excessive, the grieving may be abnormal.

    ▸ In the absence of other significant clinical symptoms, grief usually is classified as ajustment disorder.

    ▸ Adjustment disorder with depressed mood

    ▸ Adjustment disorder with anxiety

- Adjustment disorder with mixed anxiety and depression
- Adjustment disorder with disturbed conduct

Etiology

▶ Significant loss

▶ Limited coping skills

▶ Limited social supports

Incidence and Demographics

▶ Normal grief is universally experienced.

▶ Grief is common in older adults as their social sphere begins to decrease.

▶ 20% of older adults who lose a spouse experience depression within the first year of that loss.

▶ There is a 2%–8% lifetime prevalence for adjustment disorder in the U.S. population.

▶ Grief occurs in 12% of general hospital patients.

▶ Grief occurs in 50% of cardiac patients after cardiac surgery.

Risk Factors

▶ Limited social network

▶ Poor physical health

▶ Limited coping skills

Prevention and Screening

▶ Ask about losses.

▶ Identify at-risk persons.

▶ Do preventative counseling.

▶ Begin early recognition, intervention, and initiation of treatment.

- Routine screening at all health care settings.

Assessment

▶ Often patients will not disclose grieving or bereavement issues unless directly asked.

History

▶ Assess for the following:

- Recent losses
- Anniversary dates of past losses
- Reaction to loss

- Functional impairment
- Social and family support systems
- Insomnia
- Anorexia
- Presence of dysfunctional coping
  - Suicidal thoughts
  - Substance abuse
  - Denial

Physical Exam
- Nonspecific

Mental Status Exam
- Depressed mood
- Anxious affect
- Crying uncontrollably

Diagnostic Studies
- CBC, chemistry profile, thyroid function tests, and B_{12} level to rule out metabolic causes or unidentified conditions
- Drug toxicity screening, if indicated by history

Differential Diagnosis
- Normal grieving
- Major depressive disorder (MDD)
- Anxiety disorders (see Chapter 9)
- Substance-related disorders (see Chapter 12)

Management

Pharmacologic Treatment
- If needed
  - Short-term use of anti-anxiety agents
- Benzodiazepines
  - Short-term use of sleep-induction agents
- Tricyclic or other sedating antidepressants
- Antihistamines

Nonpharmacologic Treatment

- ▶ Encourage expression of grief and loss
- ▶ Use support groups
- ▶ Offer community resources
- ▶ Offer psychoeducation on grief reactions and responses
- ▶ With significant functional impairment, consider psychotherapy (e.g., crisis therapy, brief solution-focused therapy, CBT)

Special Considerations

- ▶ Can occur at any age
- ▶ Older adults at greater risk because of higher numbers of losses that may become cumulative in their impact.

Follow-up

- ▶ Follow up weekly during acute period
- ▶ Monitor for development of MDD
- ▶ Monitor for impact on general health
- ▶ Maintain supportive follow-up over time
- ▶ Be sensitive to nontraditional losses that may be significant to the person:
  - ▹ Loss of a pet
  - ▹ Loss of status in work or school setting

BIPOLAR (BP) DISORDER

Description

- ▶ Complex brain-based illness with a primary characteristic of disturbance in mood
- ▶ Mood disturbance often of both polarities:
  - ▹ Depressive
  - ▹ Expansive or manic
- ▶ Several patterns:
  - ▹ Single-polarity symptoms only (mania)
  - ▹ Cyclic symptom patterns of alternating polarity—manic symptoms alternating with depressive symptoms
  - ▹ Mixed, co-occurring symptoms
- ▶ Represents an excessive or distorted degree of sadness or elation, or both
- ▶ Manifests with behavioral, affective, cognitive, and somatic symptoms

► May have precipitating event, situation, or concern but often occurs without any precipitating stressor identified

► Has complex genetic, biochemical, and environmental etiological factors

Etiology

► Multiple theories ranging from psychological to neurobiological

► Probable multifactorial etiological profile

  ▸ Biological theories

    ▷ GABA deregulation

    ▷ Increased noradrenergic activity

    ▷ Voltage-gated ion channel abnormalities

    ▷ Abnormalities lead to abnormal balances of intracellular and extracellular levels of neurotransmitters, which then cause subsequent disruption of electric signal transmission in brain regions

    ▷ Kindling: Process of neuronal membrane threshold sensitivity dysfunction

      ▸ Long-lasting, epileptogenic changes induced by daily subthreshold brain stimulation

      ▸ Brain becomes overly sensitive to electrical stimuli

      ▸ Neuronal misfiring occurs

      ▸ Process becomes automatic; neuronal firing occurs even without stimuli.

Incidence and Demographics

► Less common than MDD

► 0.7% of general population at risk

► Affects 2.3 million American adults; 1.2% of the U.S. adult population older than age 18

► Mean age of onset is early 20s

► May present in childhood (rare) or adolescent years.

► Prevalence for males and females is the same

Risk Factors

► Genetic loading

  ▸ Family history of first-order relative having MDD or BP disorder

  ▸ 24% increased risk if relative has BP disorder Type I (see below)

  ▸ 5% increased risk if relative has BP disorder Type II (see below)

  ▸ 25% increased risk if relative has MDD

  ▸ For BP disorder Type II, similar to MDD

Prevention and Screening

▶ At-risk family education

▶ Community education

    ▸ Stigma reduction

    ▸ Signs and symptoms of illness

    ▸ Treatment potential for control of symptoms

▶ Early recognition, intervention, and initiation of treatment

    ▸ Significant and protracted prodromal symptom period usually noted before full onset of illness

    ▸ Usually mild manifestations of criteria symptoms before full clinical syndrome is apparent

    ▸ The longer time between onset of symptoms and diagnosis, the more difficult to interrupt cyclicity of illness

    ▸ Depressive episodes predominate, making misdiagnosis common

Assessment

History

▶ Assess for the following:

    ▸ Detailed history of present illness, including time frame, progression, and any associated symptoms

        ▷ Social history, including present living situation; marital status; occupation; education; and alcohol, tobacco, and illicit drug use

        ▷ Medication use, including prescription, over-the-counter, alternative, supplements, and home remedies

    ▸ Initial and periodic functional history and assessment

    ▸ Corroborative information from family member when possible

    ▸ Diagnostic criteria

        ▷ Period of abnormally or persistently elevated, expansive, or irritable mood, lasting for at least 1 week

        ▷ Mood episode has rapid development and escalation of symptoms over a few days

        ▷ Often precipitated by significant environmental stressor

        ▷ Mood disturbance may result in brief psychotic symptoms

        ▷ Manic episodes last days to several months

        ▷ Briefer duration and ending more abruptly than major depressive episodes

        ▷ In 60% of people, a major depressive episode immediately precedes or follows the manic episode

        ▷ Persistence of other suggestive symptoms:

- Decreased need for sleep
- Feels rested after 3 hours sleep on average
- Usually a marked difference from normal baseline sleep pattern
- Inflated self-esteem
- Grandiosity
- Increased goal-directed activities
- Excessive involvement in pleasurable activities with a high potential for painful consequences
- Unrestrained buying sprees
- Sexual indiscretions
- Unsound business ventures
- Excessive substance use or abuse
- Highly recurrent depressive episodes
  - Recurrent shifts in polarity
    - Major depressive episode shifting to a manic episode
    - Manic episode shifting to a major depressive episode
    - Major depressive episode shifting to a mixed episode
  - Expansive or elated mood symptoms
    - Manic
  - Symptoms as described above
  - Hypomanic
    - Similar to mania
    - More brief in duration
    - Episode not as severe as mania
    - Does not require hospitalization
    - Does not cause significant functional impairment
- Two common types
  - Type I
    - Clinical history characterized by occurrence of one or more manic or mixed episodes
  - Type II
    - Clinical history characterized by occurrence of one or more major depressive episodes accompanied by at least one ~~manic or~~ hypomanic episode

- In a small subset of people with BP disorder, the recurrent shifts in polarity can occur more frequently—*rapid cycling*
  - Occurrence of 4 or more mood episodes during the previous 12 months
  - Mood episodes are either major depressive or manic
  - Other than occurring more frequently, mood episodes are same as nonrapid-cycling episodes
  - 20% of people with BP disorder have rapid cycling
  - Most rapid cyclers are women (90%)
- Identifying rapid cycling is important.
- Antidepressants may accelerate the cycling.
- Persons with rapid cycling have a poorer prognosis.

Physical Exam
- Nonspecific
- Clinical findings consistent with thyroid dysfunction

Mental Status Exam
- Appearance
  - Psychomotor restlessness or agitation
  - Frequent change of dress
  - Prone to bright-colored, often sexualized dress
  - Dramatic or flamboyant dress usually out of character for person when compared to nonsymptomatic periods
- Speech
  - Rapid
  - Loud
  - Pressured
  - Difficult to interrupt
  - Joking, irrelevantly amusing
  - Word clanging in severely ill patients
- Affect
  - Labile
  - Irritable
  - Overly theatrical and dramatic
- Mood
  - Euphoric
  - Cheerful

- High
- Expansive
- Irritable
► Thought process
  - Thoughts racing
  - Flight of ideas
  - Thoughts disorganized and incoherent in severely ill patients
► Thought content
  - Inflated self-esteem
  - Indiscriminate enthusiasm
  - Inflated sense of abilities bordering on delusional
  - Increased sexual content
► Orientation
  - Fully oriented
► Memory
  - Impaired short-term
  - Impaired recall
► Concentration
  - Highly distractible
► Abstraction
  - Generally abstractive
  - Can be concrete on proverb testing during psychotic episodes
► Judgment
  - Poor
  - Prone to imprudent behavioral choices with potential for negative consequences
► Insight
  - The person usually does not recognize that he or she is ill
  - Resists treatment options

Diagnostic Studies
► CBC, chemistry profile, thyroid function tests, and B_{12} level to rule out metabolic causes or unidentified conditions
► Drug toxicity screening if indicated by history

Differential Diagnosis

▶ If first onset of manic symptoms occurs after age 40, most likely symptoms are caused by another medical condition

▶ Many medical conditions mimic manic symptoms:

- Endocrine disorders

- Hyperthyroidism

- Intoxication or withdrawal from illicit drug use:

  ▷ Amphetamines

  ▷ Cocaine

  ▷ Hallucinogens

  ▷ Opiates

- Medications:

  ▷ Captopril

  ▷ Cimetidine

  ▷ Corticosteroids

  ▷ Cyclosporine

  ▷ Disulfiram

  ▷ Hydralazine

  ▷ Isoniazid

▶ Mania can be precipitated by treatment of MDD or other unipolar mood disorders.

- Antidepressants

- ECT

- Light therapy

Management

▶ Rule out or treat any conditions that may contribute to current symptom manifestation

▶ Assess and identify patient's level of acuity

▶ Determine severity of illness

▶ Determine duration of illness

▶ Ascertain history of response to treatment

▶ During acute manic episodes or significant depressive episodes, patient may require brief hospitalization

- To ensure patient safety

- To ensure patient adherence with treatment to reach stabilization

- To rapidly stabilize on medication

▶ Clinical management during nonacute episodes occurs most often in community settings

Pharmacologic Treatment

► Pharmacologic management should never entail the use of an antidepressant agent if a mood-stabilizing agent is not in place.

  ▹ Especially important in patients who are rapid-cycling

  ▹ Well known to precipitate manic polarity shift

  ▹ Can worsen the kindling process

► Mood-stabilizing agents

  ▹ Commonly used pharmacologic agents

    ▹ Lithium carbonate

      ▹ Gold standard for treating manic episodes

      ▹ Evidence of antisuicidal effects

      ▹ Action largely unknown

      ▹ Long history of use; drug profile well established

      ▹ Evidence exists showing some effectiveness on depressive symptoms as well as on manic symptoms

      ▹ Has many clinically significant side effects; patients on this drug require careful monitoring (see Table 8–8)

      ▹ Narrow therapeutic window

      ▹ Therapeutic effect and potential for adverse side effects monitored by use of serum lithium level

    ▹ Drawn as trough level

    ▹ 12 hours post-dose

    ▹ Therapeutic serum range 0.5 to 1.2 mEq/L

    ▹ Level greater than 1.2 mEq/L increases risk for toxic side effects

  ▹ Need baseline labs before initiation of lithium to ensure safety and efficacy

    ▹ Thyroid panel

    ▹ Serum creatinine

    ▹ Blood urea nitrogen (BUN)

    ▹ Urinalysis

    ▹ CBC

    ▹ ECG for patients older than age 50

      ▹ Rapid-cycling patients seldom respond to lithium monotherapy

      ▹ Must educate patient (and significant others) about side effects and signs and symptoms of lithium toxicity

    ▹ Anticonvulsant mood-stabilizing agents

▷ Anticonvulsant medication (see Table 8–9)

▷ Divalproex sodium considered gold standard for rapid-cycling pattern

▷ Action reduces kindling

▷ Response to treatment with lithium or anticonvulsant medications is 1 to 2 weeks

TABLE 8-8. CLINICALLY SIGNIFICANT SIDE EFFECTS OF LITHIUM

ORGAN SYSTEM AFFECTED	CLINICAL FINDING
Endocrine	▶ Weight gain ▶ Impaired thyroid functioning ▶ Impaired parathyroid functioning
Central nervous system	▶ Fine hand tremors ▶ Fatigue ▶ Fasciculations ▶ Mental cloudiness ▶ Headaches ▶ Coarse hand tremors with toxicity ▶ Nystagmus
Dermatological	▶ Maculopapular rash ▶ Pruritus ▶ Acne
Gastrointestinal	▶ GI upset ▶ Diarrhea ▶ Vomiting ▶ Cramps ▶ Anorexia
Renal	▶ Polyuria with related polydipsia ▶ Diabetes insipidus ▶ Edema ▶ Microscopic tubular changes
Cardiac	▶ T-wave inversions ▶ Dysrhythmias
Hematological	▶ Leukocytosis

TABLE 8-9. DRUGS FOR BIPOLAR DISORDER

AGENT	BRAND NAME	DAILY DOSAGE	THERAPEUTIC PLASMA LEVEL	SIDE EFFECTS	COMMENTS
Lithium carbonate	Eskalith Lithobid	1,200–2,400 mg/day (acute) 900–1,200 mg/day (maintenance)	0.8–1.2 mEq/L 0.6–1.2 mEq/L	► *Common:* Nausea, fine hand tremors, increased urination and thirst ► *Toxicity:* Slurred speech, confusion, severe GI effect	► Established standard treatment for bipolar disorder ► Risk of hypothyroidism ► Avoid in pregnancy, especially 1st trimester ► Monitoring kidney functioning is essential ► Concurrent use of NSAIDs and ACEIs may double lithium level
Carba-mazepine	Tegretol	10–20 mg/kg/day	6–12 mcg/mL	► *Rare:* Agranulocytosis, aplastic anemia ► *Common:* Nausea, dizziness, sedation, headache, dry mouth, constipation, skin rash	► Hepatic enzyme inducer ► Monitor LFTs ► Alternative to lithium or valproic acid ► Avoid in pregnancy, especially in 1st trimester
Valproic acid, divalproex sodium	Depakene, Depakote	15–40 mg/kg/day	50–125 mcg/mL	► *Common:* Nausea, diarrhea, abdominal cramps, sedation, tremor ► *Rare:* Increased liver enzymes	► Depakote minimizes GI effects ► More effective than lithium for rapid cycling and mixed bipolar ► Loading dose: 20 mg/kg ► Avoid in pregnancy, especially 1st trimester
Lamotrigine	Lamictal	25–200 mg/day	Blood monitoring not necessary	► *Common:* Dizziness, ataxia, somnolence, diplopia, nausea, headache, hepatotoxicity ► *Rare:* Life-threatening rashes, leukopenia	► Helps in depressive phase of bipolar affective disorder ► Monitor for blood dyscrasia; titrate dosages slowly

Nonpharmacologic Treatment

- ► Somatic treatments
  - ▸ Treatment as previously discussed for MDD episodes
- ► Therapies
  - ▸ Treatment as previously discussed for MDD episodes
- ► During acute phase of manic episode:
  - ▸ Monitor and help patient meet nutritional needs.
  - ▸ Help patient meet sleep and rest needs
  - ▸ Monitor safety
- ► During less acute periods:
  - ▸ CBT
  - ▸ Behavioral therapies
  - ▸ Interpersonal therapies
  - ▸ Supportive groups
  - ▸ Milieu therapy
    - ▷ Provides for structure and safety needs
    - ▷ Provides socialization and interpersonal support
    - ▷ Encourages independence
- ► Patient and family education
  - ▸ Explain underlying pathology of illness
  - ▸ Discuss signs and symptoms
  - ▸ Help identify strategies for living with illness
  - ▸ Help understand and make decisions regarding care options
    - ▷ Relapse prevention plan
    - ▷ Overall health promotion

Common comorbidities

- ► Hypothyroidism
- ► Substance abuse

General health considerations

- ► High-risk activities from manic behavior
  - ▸ Sexual
    - ▷ Patient education for sexually transmitted infections (STIs)
    - ▷ Assessment and monitoring for STIs

- Financial and legal
    - ▷ Patient access community resources
- ▶ Nutritional counseling
- ▶ Patient health education

Special Considerations

- ▶ Adolescent manic episodes present differently from adult episodes.
    - More psychotic features
    - Often associated with antisocial behavior
    - Often associated with substance abuse
    - Prodromal period of significant behavioral problems
        - ▷ School truancy
        - ▷ Failing grades

Follow-up

- ▶ Patients initially should be seen weekly to titrate medications and monitor serum blood levels of pharmacological agents.
- ▶ Treatment duration and success rates vary with individual characteristics and motivation.
- ▶ Patients and significant others should be taught symptoms of mania and depression and that the disorders are chronic illnesses.
- ▶ Relapse is common and occurs frequently.
- ▶ Relapse plans need to be developed.
- ▶ Patient teaching should include risk, benefits, potential side effects, and signs and symptoms of medication toxicity.
- ▶ Educate about potential dietary and fluid intake effects on lithium level
    - Lithium and divalrpoex sodium are teratogenic.
    - Women of child-bearing years need effective contraceptive care while on BP disorder treatment medication.
- ▶ Routine use of lab tests to monitor for therapeutic serum levels of anticonvulsants and lithium is needed.
    - Routine evaluation of CBC, renal function, and thyroid function is needed for patients taking lithium long term.
- ▶ Assessment for suicidality should occur during every patient contact.
- ▶ All patients should be observed for development of adverse effects of pharmacological treatment.
    - Standardized rating scales help to monitor clinical status, establish baseline functioning, and monitor disorder course over time: Young Mania Rating Scale (YMRS; Young, Biggs, Ziegler, & Meyer, 1978)

CYCLOTHYMIC DISORDER

Description
▶ Chronic, fluctuating mood disorder whose symptoms are similar to but less severe than BP disorder

▶ Numerous periods of hypomanic and dysthymic symptoms.

Etiology
▶ Similar to BP disorder.

Incidence and Demographics
▶ Lifetime prevalence 0.4% to 1%

▶ Insidious onset

▶ Chronic course

▶ Begins early in life

▶ 15% to 50% of persons with cyclothymic disorder subsequently develop BP disorder.

Risk Factors
▶ Genetic loading

▶ Family history

▶ BP disorder Type I

▶ Substance abuse

Prevention and Screening
▶ At-risk family education

▶ Community education

　» Stigma reduction

　» Signs and symptoms of illness

　» Treatment potential for control of symptoms

▶ Early recognition, intervention, and initiation of treatment

　» Significant and protracted prodromal symptom period usually noted before full onset of illness

　» The longer the time period between onset of symptoms and diagnosis, the more difficult to interrupt cyclicity of illness.

Assessment

History

► Assess for the following:

  ▸ Fluctuating mood episodes

  ▸ Affected people can function well during hypomanic episodes

  ▸ May experience clinically significant distress or impaired function related to cyclicity

  ▸ Unpredictable mood changes

    ▷ Often regarded by others as *temperamental, moody, unpredictable, inconsistent,* and *unreliable*

  ▸ No psychotic episodes

Physical Exam

► Similar to MDD and BP disorder

Mental Status Exam

► Similar to MDD and BP disorder but with less severity of symptoms

Diagnostic Studies

  ▸ Similar to MDD and BP disorder

Differential Diagnosis

► Nonpsychiatric

  ▸ Similar to MDD and BP disorder

► Psychiatric

  ▸ BP disorder

  ▸ Dysthymia

  ▸ Substance abuse

Management

Pharmacologic Treatment

► Similar to MDD and BP disorder

► Because of increased risk for development of BP disorder, commonly treated with medication

Nonpharmacologic Treatment

▶ Similar to MDD and BP disorder

Special Considerations

▶ Usually begins in adolescence

▶ Onset in later life usually suggests general medical condition such as multiple sclerosis

Follow-up

▶ Similar to MDD and BP disorder

CASE STUDY

Mary, a 35-year-old homemaker and mother of two children, presents to her primary care provider accompanied by her husband with complaints of lack of energy and inability to sleep that are getting progressively worse. The symptoms are affecting her ability to take care of her children and the household. Her husband reports that she often has crying spells, is not eating well, and cannot seem to concentrate. When questioned further, her husband said that she has mentioned not wanting to live, but he thought that she was just having a bad day.

Past Medical History

▶ Seasonal allergies and stress-induced asthma

▶ No significant surgical history, except for a tonsillectomy when she was a child

▶ Normal pregnancies and deliveries

▶ No chronic health problems identified

Family History

▶ Significant for grandmother and father, who had "breakdowns"

▶ Father had alcoholism

Social History

Mary is a homemaker and has two children, ages 8 and 10. She and her husband moved to the area 6 months ago. She does not smoke or use drugs but drinks socially. She has an MA degree in English and had planned to go back to school to get her teaching certificate when her children began high school.

Mental Status Exam

Patient appears clean but somewhat disheveled. Hair is not combed or washed. She appears very tired. She avoids eye contact, talks very softly, and is slow to respond to questions. She hardly moves during the interview. Affect is constricted and sad. She says has no energy, and her mood is "very sad." She does not hear voices or have hallucinations. Her thoughts are appropriate and organized. She does admit to having episodic thoughts of suicide and has a vague plan to ingest an overdose of aspirin, acetaminophen, and alcohol when the children are with their father but has no clear timeline or planned intent. She is unable to do serial number testing and shows impaired short-term memory. She exhibits a few problems with immediate recall. She has difficulty concentrating but no difficulty with abstractions. She is oriented times 3, and shows good judgment and insight. She has above-average intelligence.

Current Medications

Mary takes cetirizine for allergies and is now on ethinyl estradiol/norgestimate contraceptive pills.

Labs

- ► Platelets 230/mm^3
- ► WBC 6,000/mm^3
- ► Hematocrit 40%, hemoglobin 13.0
- ► NA 140, K 4.0, Cl 101, CO_2 26, BUN 15, creatinine 0.9, glucose 102
- ► TSH 1.1, T3 179, T4 1.3.

There are several issues to consider in planning care for Mary:

- ► What is the most probable diagnosis?
- ► What further assessment is needed?
- ► What target symptoms does the patient display that are consistent with the probable diagnosis?
- ► What medications would be considered?
- ► If patient had psychotic features with her depression, how would this change the treatment plan?
- ► How would the plan differ if patient had a heart condition and was taking no other medications?

REFERENCES

Agency for Health Care Policy and Research. (1993). *Depression in primary care treatment of major depression* (Clinical Practice Guideline 5, AHCPR Publication No. 93-0551). Rockville: U.S. Department of Health and Human Services.

American Psychiatric Association. (1998). *Practice parameters for the assessment and treatment of children and adolescents with bipolar disorder.* Washington, DC: American Psychiatric Association.

American Psychiatric Association. (2000a). *Diagnostic and statistical manual of mental disorders* (4th ed., text rev.). Washington, DC: Author.

American Psychiatric Association. (2000b). *Practice guidelines for the treatment of patients with major depressive disorder.* Washington, DC: Author.

Beck, A. (1979). *Cognitive therapy of depression.* New York: Guilford Press.

Beck, A. T., Ward, C. H. Mendelson, M., Mock, J., & Erbaugh, J. (1961). An inventory for measuring depression. *Archives of General Psychiatry, 4,* 561–571.

Beydoun, A. (2001). Innovative treatment strategies with anticonvulsants: A focus on bipolar disorder. *Primary Psychiatry, 8*(6), 49–52.

Birmaher, B., Brent, D. A., & Benson, R. S. (1998). Summary of the practice parameters for the assessment and treatment of children and adolescents with depressive disorders. *Journal of the American Academy of Child and Adolescent Psychiatry, 37,* 1234–1238.

Freidrich, M. (1999). Lithium: Proving its mettle for 50 years. *Journal of the American Medical Association, 281,* 2271–2275.

George, M. S., Wassermann, E. M., Williams, W. A., Callahan, A., Ketter, T. A., Basser, P., & Post, R. M. (1995). Daily repetitive transcranial magnetic stimulation (rTMS) improves mood in depression. *Neuroreport, 6,* 1853–1856.

Ghaemi, S. N. (2001). Bipolar disorder and antidepressants: An ongoing controversy. *Primary Psychiatry, 6*(2), 28–34.

Giles, D. E., Kupfer, D. J., Rush, A. J., & Roffwarg, H. P. (1998). Controlled comparison of electrophysiological sleep in families of probands with unipolar depression. *American Journal of Psychiatry, 155,* 192–196.

Gloaguen, V., Cottraux, J., Cucherat, M., & Blackburn, I. M. (1998). A meta-analysis of the effects of cognitive therapy in depressed patients. *Journal of Affective Disorders, 49*(1), 59–62.

Green, J. (2001). Helping patients understand depression and its treatment. *Primary Psychiatry, 8*(11), 49–53.

Hirschfeld, R., Holzer, C., Calabrese, J., Weissman, M., Reed, M., Davies, M., Hazard, E. (2003). Validity of the mood disorder questionnaire: A general population study. *American Journal of Psychiatry, 160,* 178–180.

Hoyert, D. L., Kochanek, K. D., & Murphy, S. L. (1998). *Deaths: Final data for 1997* (National Vital Statistics Report, DHHS Publication No. PHS-99-1120). Hyattsville, MD: National Center for Health Statistics.

Kimrell, T., Little, R., & Dunn, T. (1999). Frequency dependence of antidepressant response to left prefrontal repetitive transcranial magnetic stimulation (rTMS) as a function of baseline cerebral glucose metabolism. *Biological Psychiatry, 46,* 1603–1613.

Klein, D. N., Schwartz, J. E., & Rose S. (2000). Five-year course and outcome of dysthymic disorder: A prospective, naturalistic follow-up study. *American Journal of Psychiatry, 157,* 931–939.

Lowe-Ponsford, F. L., & Nutt, D. J. (2001). Pathophysiology of depression. *Primary Psychiatry, 8*(11), 43–48.

McBride, A., & Austin, J. (1996). *Psychiatric mental health nursing: Integrating the behavioral and biological sciences.* Philadelphia: W. B. Saunders.

McQuade, R., & Young, A. (2000). Future therapeutic targets in mood disorders: The glucocorticoid receptor. *British Journal of Psychiatry, 177,* 390–395.

Monroe, S. M., Rohde, P., & Seeley, J. R. (1999). Life events and depression in adolescence: Relationship loss as a prospective risk factor for first onset of major depressive disorder. *Journal of Abnormal Psychology, 108,* 606–614.

Ornstein, S., Stuart, G., & Jenkins, R. (2000). Depression diagnosis and antidepressant use in primary care practices. *Journal of Family Practice, 49*(1), 68–71.

Saeed, M. (2001). Assessment and management of the suicidal patient in the managed care era. *Primary Psychiatry, 8*(6), 38–45.

Shaffer, D., & Craft, L. (1999). Methods of adolescent suicide prevention. *Journal of Clinical Psychiatry, 60*(Suppl. 2), 70–74.

Spencer, T., Biederman, J., & Wilens, T. (1999). Attention-deficit/hyperactivity disorder and comorbidity. *Pediatric Clinics of North America, 46,* 915–927.

Stuart, G. W., & Laraia, M. (2004). *Principles and practice of psychiatric nursing* (8th ed.). St. Louis, MO: Mosby.

Young, R. C., Biggs, J. T., Ziegler, V. E., & Meyer, D. A. (1978). A rating scale for mania: Reliability, alidity, and sensitivity. *British Journal of Psychiatry, 133,* 429-435.

CHAPTER 9

ANXIETY DISORDERS

This chapter reviews the psychiatric–mental health nurse practitioner's (PMHNP's) evaluation of and treatment of people who have anxiety disorders. Anxiety disorders are among the most common of all psychiatric illnesses, and can initially manifest as a number of physical illness states. Often only after extensive, unnecessary assessment and diagnostic evaluation is a patient's problem correctly identified as an anxiety disorder. Because of the high degree of somatic symptomatology, it is common for patients to present to a primary care setting and thus receive initial care from a primary care provider.

Anxiety is a very common and normal human emotion. PMHNPs caring for patients who present for evaluation of anxiety must be able to distinguish between normal levels of anxiety and pathological levels that are symptomatic of an underlying brain-based illness. Pathological levels of anxiety require treatment and generally will not fully abate without therapeutic intervention. Untreated high levels of anxiety predispose people to other serious health problems; therefore, pathological levels of anxiety should not go untreated (Narrow, Rae, & Regier, 1998).

NORMAL EMOTION OF ANXIETY

- ► Anxiety is one of the most common human emotions.
- ► Anxiety exists on a continuum ranging from the absence of anxiety at one end to pathological levels that produce significant symptoms of psychiatric disorder at the other (see Table 9–1).
- ► Anxiety can be a normal, healthy reaction to life stressors that motivates a person to deal with events and emotions.
- ► Anxiety can be pathological if it is disproportionate to events, if it is sustained over a significant time frame, if it significantly impairs functioning, or if it is apparently unrelated to any identifiable event or situation in a person's life.

► High pathological levels of anxiety interfere with perceptions, memory, judgment, and motor responses.

► Cultural differences can affect behavioral manifestations of anxiety.

 ▸ "Ataques de nervios" is a Latino cultural syndrome usually provoked by disruptions in family bonds and may be manifested by trembling, crying, and screaming. The attacks are usually experienced in the presence of others and the person often feels relief afterward.

 ▸ "Khyal" (wind) attacks are a common manifestation among Cambodian and other Asian cultures, and commonly manifest in neck soreness and tinnitus.

► Older adults often express anxiety as somatic concerns and anxiety disorders may overlap with medical conditions

► Psychotherapy is the first-line treatment for children and adolescents who are diagnosed with an anxiety disorder

► The role of the PMHNP in assessing anxiety is to separate normal vs. pathological levels of anxiety, to intervene to lower the level of anxiety, and to improve overall functioning.

TABLE 9-1. ASSESSING LEVELS OF ANXIETY

LEVEL OF ANXIETY	DEFINITION	PHYSIOLOGICAL SIGNS & SYMPTOMS	PSYCHOLOGICAL SIGNS & SYMPTOMS
Level I. Mild	Normative level experienced by all, which functions to motivate	Vital signs normal, pupils constricted, minimal increase in muscle tone	Perceptual field broadened, heightened awareness of environment
Level II. Moderate	Normative level experienced by most in response to significant stressors	Vital signs normal, mild increased heart rate, moderate increase in muscle tone	Subjective feeling of tension or worry, narrowed perceptions
Level III. Severe	Pathological level	Autonomic nervous system triggered, flight-or-fight response, pupils dilated, vital signs increased, diaphoresis, muscles rigid, hearing decreased, pain threshold increased, urinary frequency, diarrhea	Perceptual field greatly narrowed, difficulty with problem-solving, distorted perception of time, selective inattention, dissociative sensations, automatic behavior
Level IV. Panic	Pathological level	Severe symptoms markedly increased: patient is pale, hypotensive, has poor eye-hand coordination, muscle pains, marked decrease in hearing, dizziness, shortness of breath	Scattered perceptions, unable to attend to environmental stimuli, illogical thinking, may exhibit hallucinations or delusions

ANXIETY DISORDERS

Description

▶ Anxiety disorders are the most common group of psychiatric disorders and are characterized by the degree of anxiety experienced by the patient, by the duration and severity of the anxiety, and by the typical behavioral manifestation of anxiety observed in the patient. Anxiety ranges from acute states to chronic disorders and is accompanied by multiple somatic symptoms.

▶ Patients most often present first in primary care settings with nonspecific physical concerns.

  » Often confused with cardiac and respiratory disorders, so careful differential diagnostic assessment is essential.

▶ Frequent comorbidity exists with substance abuse, depression, and eating disorders

  » Symptoms significantly impair functioning and occur more days than not for a period of at least 6 months, with the patient reporting little or no volitional control over the symptoms.

  » Nine specific anxiety disorders are identified in the *DSM-IV-TR* (American Psychiatric Association, 2000) and are described in more detail in this chapter.

Etiology

▶ Multiple theories range from psychological to neurobiological; however, more likely there is a multifactorial etiological profile.

  » Psychodynamic Theory

    ▷ This theory is based on work of Sigmund Freud (1856–1939), who believed that anxiety initially occurs in response to the stimulation of birth and need of the infant to adapt to the changed environment.

    ▷ Subsequent anxiety results from intrapsychic conflict.

    ▷ The process of unconscious repression of sexual drive is at the core of much of the conflict.

    ▷ Conflict exists between instinctual needs of the *id* and the *superego (conscience)*; anxiety signals the individual of the need to deal with the id–superego conflict.

    ▷ Conflict is unconscious, but anxiety is consciously perceived.

    ▷ Conflict entails fear of punishment and of doing wrong.

    ▷ Defense mechanisms are unconsciously used by the patient to deal with the conflict.

    ▷ The behavioral manifestations of anxiety disorders stem from the pathological overuse of defense mechanisms.

- Interpersonal Theory

  - This theory is based on work of Harry Stack Sullivan (1892–1949), who believed that humans are goal-directed toward attainment of satisfaction and security needs.

  - Satisfaction and security needs are normally met in interpersonal interactions.

  - Anxiety arises when a person's needs are unmet.

    - Anxiety is first experienced in an infant's interactions with his or her mother.

    - Subsequent anxiety arises because of interpersonal conflict.

    - Conflict occurs when a person perceives his or her needs will not be met because of rejection, feelings of inferiority, or inability to engage with significant others.

  - Sense of self becomes based on the person's perception of how others view him or her.

- Neurobiological Theory

  - Pathological levels of anxiety result from neurobiological deficits in normal brain functioning.

  - Deficits are genetically mediated by and involve predominantly the limbic system, midline brainstem area, and sections of the cortex.

  - Deficits predispose the person to abnormal stress responses, with hyperactivity of autonomic nervous system causing symptoms such as increased heart rate and blood pressure, diaphoresis, papillary dilation, tremors, and increased respiratory rate.

  - Problems with the hypothalamic pituitary adrenal (HPA) axis:

    - Threat is perceived, and amygdala signals the hypothalamus to secrete corticotrophin-releasing hormone (CRH).

    - The amygdala also activates the sympathetic nervous system to start the fight-or-flight response.

    - The pituitary is stimulated to release adrenocorticotropic hormone (ACTH).

    - The adrenal glands are then stimulated to release cortisol, which shuts off the alarm system and restores the body to homeostasis.

  - In anxiety disorders, the amygdala may not be able to shut off the response (overactive amygdala), or there may not be enough cortisol to stop the fight-or-flight response.

  - Neurobiological deficits result in low levels of the neurotransmitter GABA (gamma-aminobutyric acid), the chemical responsible for inhibitory responses of neurons, and in high levels of norepinephrine, the chemical associated with the fight-or-flight response

  - Neurotransmitters involved in suppressing the HPA axis are serotonin and GABA.

Incidence and Demographics

▶ Anxiety disorders are common, with a lifetime prevalence of 28.8% among the general U.S. population.

▶ Except for obsessive–compulsive disorder (OCD) and social phobia, anxiety disorders are more common in girls and women than in boys and men.

▶ Most anxiety disorders manifest in adolescence and early adulthood (Narrow, Rae, & Regier, 1998).

▶ Median age at onset is 11 years of age.

Risk Factors

▶ Genetic loading (National Institute of Mental Health, Genetics Workgroup, 1998)

▹ A first-degree relative of a person with panic disorder is up to 8 times more likely than general population to develop panic disorder.

▹ If a first-degree relative of a person developed panic disorder before age 20, that person is up to 20 times more likely than general population to develop panic disorder.

▶ Limited range of coping skills

▶ History of trauma

▶ High levels of parental distress affect a child's ability to cope with traumatic devents

Prevention and Screening

▶ At-risk family education

▶ Community education

▹ Stigma reduction

▹ Signs and symptoms of illness

▹ Treatment potential for control of symptoms

▶ Early recognition, intervention, and initiation of treatment

▹ Teach at-risk persons to recognize and manage anxiety levels.

▹ Help at-risk persons reduce anxiety through improved coping activities.

Assessment

History

▶ Assess for the following:

▹ Detailed history of present illness, including time frame and progression, any associated symptoms

▹ Social history, including present living situation; marital status; occupation; education level

- Medication use, including prescription, over-the-counter, alternative, supplements, and home remedies

- People initially may be more troubled by, and complain more often of, physical symptoms and may not identify anxiety as a concern.

- Explore the patient's subjective sensations of being nervous, tense, worried, anxious, or stressed out.

- Identify current environmental stressors as experienced by the patient.

- Determine if anxiety is normative or pathological.

▶ *Pathological* levels of anxiety indicative of underlying anxiety disorder:

- Anxiety is perceived of as distressing and out of the control of the person.

- Anxiety is unlinked and not seen as caused by life events.

- Anxiety is accompanied by somatic complaints, which is more uncommon in normal anxiety levels.

- Anxiety interferes with social, occupational, and recreation activities and with activities of daily living.

  ▷ Determine the level of the patient's anxiety using the 4-point scale of mild to panic levels (1 = mild to 4 = panic; see Table 9–1).

  ▷ Use standardized rating scales such as the Hamilton Rating Scale for Anxiety (HAM-A; Hamilton, 1959) for establishing and monitoring the patient's anxiety level over time.

  ▷ Assess general level of health and presence of concomitant illnesses.

  ▷ Assess for *dysfunctional coping*

  - Alcohol use and abuse

  - Illicit substance use and abuse

  - Caffeine use

  - Increased nicotine use.

  - Misuse of anti-anxiety medications

  ▷ Assess for specific *psychological symptoms of anxiety:*

  - Fear of dying, losing one's mind, or a sense of unreality

  - Belief that he or she is very ill, with no findings to support this belief

  - Narrowed perceptions

  - Limited eye contact

Physical Exam

▶ Possible physical manifestations:

- Pupillary dilation

- Tachycardia

- Increased muscle tone

- Headaches
- Hypertension
- Motor restlessness
- Diaphoresis
- Palpitations, often with tightness of chest
- GI problems
- Dizziness or light-headedness

Mental Status Exam

▶ Appearance
- Psychomotor restlessness
- Tremors
- Handwringing

▶ Speech
- Over-productive
- Rapid
- Distractible speech patterns
- Thought-blocking

▶ Affect
- Anxious
- Worried
- Tearful

▶ Mood
- Nervous
- Worried

▶ Thought process
- Overall organized
- Goal-directed
- Redirectable

▶ Thought content
- Thematic for worry
- Mild perseveration on topics of concern

▶ Orientation
- Usually fully oriented

- Memory
  - Impaired short-term and immediate memory
  - Forgetful
- Concentration
  - Inattentive
  - Decreased concentration
- Abstraction
  - Abstract on proverbs and similarities.
- Judgment
  - Intact
- Insight
  - Intact or limited insight

Diagnostic Studies

- Obtain baseline labs such as CBC, chemistry profile, thyroid function tests, and B_{12} level to rule out metabolic causes or unidentified conditions
- Obtain drug toxicity screening if indicated by history
- In some cases, patients may have labs reflecting compensated respiratory alkalosis:
  - Decreased carbon dioxide levels
  - Decreased bicarbonate levels
  - Normal pH

Differential Diagnosis

- Many medical conditions can cause worry, fear, and normal levels of anxiety (see Table 9–2).
- Ensure that patient symptoms meet criteria for anxiety disorders.

TABLE 9-2. MEDICAL CONDITIONS THAT MAY MIMIC ANXIETY DISORDERS

GENERAL CATEGORY OF DISORDER	SPECIFIC ILLNESS
Cardiovascular	► Congestive heart failure ► Mitral valve prolapse ► Myocardial infarct ► Arrhythmias, especially tachycardic arrhythmias ► Pulmonary embolism ► Coronary artery disease
Respiratory	► Asthma ► Chronic obstructive pulmonary disorder ► Pneumonia
Endocrine	► Hyperthyroidism ► Hyperparathyroidism ► Cushing's disease
Neurological	► Seizure disorders ► Transient ischemic attacks ► Cerebral vascular accident ► Encephalitis ► Central nervous system (CNS) neoplasms
Metabolic	► Hypoglycemia ► Vitamin B deficiency ► Porphyria
Substance abuse or dependency	► Intoxication with CNS stimulants (e.g., cocaine, amphetamines, caffeine) ► Withdrawal from CNS depressants (e.g., alcohol, marijuana)

Management

► Rule out or treat any conditions that may contribute to pathological levels of anxiety.

Pharmacologic Treatment

► Most of the medications known to improve symptoms of anxiety act on the GABA system.

► Selective serotonin reuptake inhibitors (SSRIs)

  ▸ Considered *first-line agents* for chronic anxiety disorders

  ▸ Action on serotonin system and indirectly on GABA system

  ▸ Carry no risk of dependency

  ▸ Cannot be used PRN

  ▸ Clean side-effect profile

  ▸ Takes time to reach symptom control (usually 3–4 weeks)

  ▸ Best when combined with psychotherapy

    ▹ Black box warning for increased suicidality in children, adolescents, and young adults

► Benzodiazepines (BNZs)

  ▸ Potentiates the effect of GABA

  ▸ Rapid onset of action

  ▸ Can be used p.r.n.

    ▷ Limit to lowest possible dose and short-term use if possible; long-term use may lead to tolerance, dependence, memory impairment, and depression

    ▷ Use should be limited to period of excessive symptoms, period of high stress, or in unremitting symptoms

  ▸ Contraindicated in patients with history of substance dependence

  ▸ Effective but carry high risk for addiction

  ▸ BNZs with *longer half-lives* require less frequent dosing, have less severe withdrawal, and have less rebound anxiety

  ▸ BNZs with longer half-lives are more useful for continuous, moderate to severe anxiety or as bridge medication while waiting for efficacy of SSRI:

    ▷ Clonazepam (Klonopin)

    ▷ Diazepam (Valium)

  ▸ BNZs with *shorter half-lives* require more frequent dosing, have more severe withdrawal, and have more rebound anxiety:

    ▷ Alprazolam (Xanax)

    ▷ Lorazepam (Ativan)

  ▸ Advantages of BNZs with short half-lives

    ▷ BNZs with short half-lives are often useful for intermittent or infrequent moderate to severe anxiety

      ▸ Less daytime sedation

      ▸ Less drug accumulation

      ▸ Quick onset of action

      ▸ Useful for treatment of insomnia

    ▷ Disadvantages of BNZs with short half-lives:

      ▸ Increased risk of addiction

► Tricyclics (TCAs)

  ▸ Effective but affect multiple neurotransmitters causing numerous unwanted effects

  ▸ Side effects often affect compliance

► Non-BNZ anxiolytics (see Table 9–3)

  ▸ Buspirone (BuSpar)

    ▷ Must be taken regularly, not as p.r.n.

> ‣ Tiagabine (Gabitril): Off-label use

> ‣ Gabapentin (Neurontin): Off-label use

>> ▷ Usually adjunctive use with other pharmacological agent

Special Considerations

> ‣ In children, alpha-agonists are often used for anxiety.

>> ▷ Clonidine (Catapres) 0.003–0.01 mg/kg/d, off-label use

>> ▷ Guanfacine (Tenex) 0.015–0.05 mg/kg/d), off-label use

TABLE 9-3. NONBENZODIAZEPINE ANXIOLYTICS FOR ADULTS

GENERIC	BRAND	DOSAGE RANGE	SIDE EFFECTS	COMMENTS
Buspirone	Buspar	20–60 mg/daily	Dizziness, insomnia, tremors, akathisia, stomach upset, dry mouth	▶ Helpful adjunct for anxiety
Tiagabine	Gabitril	4–56 mg/daily	Dizziness, somnolence, stomach upset, tremors, dry mouth	▶ Helpful adjunct for anxiety ▶ Off-label use
Gabapentin	Neurontin	300–3,600 mg/daily	Ataxia, decreased coordination, sedation, disequilibrium	▶ Used for anxiety, neuropathic pain, fibromyalgia, and as an anti-craving ▶ Medication ▶ Off-label use

Nonpharmacologic Treatment

▶ Behavioral therapy

> ‣ Systematic desensitization

> ‣ Exposure therapy

> ‣ Relaxation therapies

> ‣ Biofeedback

▶ Cognitive–behavorial thearapy (CBT)

▶ Interpersonal therapies

▶ Community self-help groups

▶ Alternative therapies as adjunctive treatments

Special Considerations

Comorbidities

▶ Anemia

▶ Cardiac disorders, especially in patients with dysrhythmias

▶ Endocrine disorders

▹ Cushing's disease

▹ Hyperthyroidism

▹ Hypoglycemia

▶ Pulmonary conditions

▹ Chronic obstructive pulmonary disorder

▹ Asthma

▹ Pulmonary embolism

▹ Pneumothorax

▶ Adverse medication reactions

▹ Caffeine

▹ Nicotine

▹ Anticholinergics

▹ Antihistamines

▹ Antipsychotics

▹ Steroids

▹ Bronchodilators

▹ Anesthetics

▶ Mood disorders

▶ Substance abuse–related disorders

General Health Considerations

▶ Chronic anxiety is wearing on the body; therefore, assess for effects on the cardiovascular system.

▶ Perform a general assessment for a healthy lifestyle.

Follow-Up

▶ General considerations

▹ Patients should initially be seen weekly or biweekly to titrate medications.

▹ Patient teaching should include risk, benefits, and potential side effects of medication treatment.

▷ If the patient is taking BNZs, monitor for appropriate use and potential dependence.

▷ If the patient is taking SSRIs, monitor for common side effects and adverse effects.

ANXIETY DISORDERS 223

- Patients should be taught symptoms of anxiety and the fact that disorders are chronic illnesses; a relapse plan should be established for all patients.

- Assessment for suicidality should occur during symptom exacerbation periods.

- Because of frequent comorbidity with major depressive disorder, assess frequently for depression levels using standardized rating scales (see below).

- Medication should be combined with therapy to reach maximum control of symptoms.

- Patients may need encouragement to continue treatment, especially after initial symptom relief occurs.

► Standardized rating scales for anxiety disorders

- Zung's Self-Rating Anxiety Scale (Zung, 1971)

- Hamilton Rating Scale for Anxiety (HAM–A; Hamilton, 959)

- Yale–Brown Obsessive Compulsive Scale (Y–BOCS; Goodman et al., 1989).

PANIC DISORDER

Description

► Panic disorder is experienced as discrete episodes or attacks with sudden onset of intense apprehension, fearfulness, or terror, often associated with sense of impending doom.

► May be diagnosed with or without agoraphobia.

► Attacks occur without warning and in the absence of any real danger.

► Attacks build to a peak of intensity within a short, self-limiting time, usually within 10 minutes of onset.

► Panic disorder is more common in women than in men.

Assessment

History

► Assess for the following:

- Assess for *diagnostic criteria* of panic disorder:

  ▷ Discrete episode in which patient experiences 4 or more of the following symptoms having a sudden onset and peaking within 10 minute of onset:

  - Paresthesias

  - Chills or hot flushing

  - Fear of losing control or of going crazy

  - Fear of dying

  - Shortness of breath or smothering sensation

- Palpitations, pounding, or accelerated heart rate

- Chest pain, tightness, or discomfort

- Sweating

- Trembling or shaking

- Nausea or abdominal distress

▸ After first attack, persistent concern over having another attack, worry over the consequences of initial attack, or a significant behavioral change related to attack

▸ With high somatic sensations, patients are often sensitive to new somatic experiences or perceptions

▸ Often intolerant of or concerned with common side effects of medication treatments

▷ Discouraged or ashamed about "failure" to control emotions and over concern about dying when no other pathology identified

- In two-thirds of cases, major depression occurs first, followed by panic disorder symptoms

- In one-third of cases, panic disorder symptoms precede major depression symptoms.

▶ Three characteristic types

▸ Patient presentation is defined by relationship between onset of attack and presence or absence of triggers for attacks

▸ Type 1: Uncued

▷ No associated internal or external trigger

▷ Experienced as spontaneous or "out of the blue" attack

▷ May over time become cued or situationally cued (see below) or may, less commonly, remain uncued

▷ NOTE: Recurrent, unexpected, uncued attacks are required for initial fulfillment of *DSM-IV-TR* diagnostic criteria for panic disorder. If initial onset is *not* this type, consider an alternative diagnosis (e.g., phobia, posttraumatic stress disorder [PTSD], generalized anxiety disorder [GAD]; see below)

▸ Type 2: Cued

▷ Occurs immediately and invariably on exposure to or in anticipation of a situational cue or trigger.

▸ Type 3: Situationally Cued

▷ Similar to cued but is not immediate and not invariably cued to trigger.

▶ Type determined by assessment of

▸ Patient's focus of anxiety

▸ Type and number of attacks

▸ Number of situations avoided by patient

▸ Level of anxiety experienced between panic attacks

Physical Exam

▶ Nonspecific, especially when client not experiencing panic attack

▶ Nonspecific cardiac-related complaints during panic episodes often bring patient into treatment:

⊳ Chest pain

⊳ Numbness

⊳ Shortness of breath

Mental Status Exam

▶ General findings of anxiety as described earlier

▶ Findings very pronounced during panic episodes and less pronounced during nonpanic periods

▶ High level of anticipatory anxiety between panic episodes

Diagnostic Studies

▶ None specific

Differential Diagnosis

▶ Rule out general medical conditions known to produce similar symptoms, including

▹ Hyperthyroidism

▹ Hyperparathyroidism

▹ Pheochromocytosis

▹ Vestibular dysfunction

▹ Seizure disorders

▹ Cardiac arrhythmias such as SVT

▹ Use of CNS stimulants, including

⊳ Cocaine

⊳ Amphetamines

⊳ Caffeine

⊳ Another anxiety disorder such as PTSD or phobia

⊳ Separation anxiety disorder

▹ Consider general medical disorder if

⊳ First episode of panic attack symptoms occur after age 45

⊳ Panic symptoms are atypical, such as

▹ Vertigo

- Loss of consciousness
- Incontinence
- Headache
- Slurred speech
- Amnesic pattern after attacks
▶ Differentiated from other anxiety conditions by
- Sudden onset of attack
- Discrete, self-limiting nature of symptoms
- Paroxysmal symptom profile
- Level 3–4 anxiety symptoms with somatic symptoms that are experienced as distressing and severe by the patient

Management

▶ Follow guidelines of general clinical management of anxiety disorders.

Pharmacologic Treatment

▶ SSRIs

▶ BNZs, usually used for short-term symptom control

▶ Buspar effective as an adjunct to an antidepressant

▶ Other nonbenzodiazepine anxiolytic meds used as adjuncts

Nonpharmacologic Treatment

▶ CBT

▶ Individual or group therapy

▶ Exposure therapy

▶ Relaxation therapies

Special Considerations

Common Comorbidities

▶ Frequent with major depressive disorder

▶ Estimated between 10% and 65%, depending on source:

- Social phobia
- OCD
- Substance abuse

AGORAPHOBIA

Description

▶ Agoraphobia is characterized by avoidance of places or situations from which escape may be difficult or embarrassing or in which help may not be available in the event of perceived need, such as a panic attack.

> ▸ The anxiety usually leads to avoidant behavior that impairs a person's ability to travel, to work, or to carry out responsibilities of daily living.

> ▸ Differential diagnosis is assisted by the awareness that people with agoraphobia feel better and report less significant concerns with anxiety when accompanied by a trusted companion.

▶ Agoraphobia is not an independently coded *DSM-IV-TR* diagnosis and is always diagnosed in relationship to presence or absence of panic disorder.

▶ Agoraphobia most commonly occurs in conjunction with panic disorder and is labeled as *panic disorder with agoraphobia.*

▶ For patients to be diagnosed panic disorder *with agoraphobia*, they must meet the criteria for panic disorder and must experience agoraphobic anxiety about being in places or situations from which escape might be difficult or in which help may not be available in the event of a panic attack.

▶ If agoraphobia is experienced *without panic disorder*, the anxiety disorder is labeled *agoraphobia without history of panic disorder.*

Assessment

History

▶ Assess for the following:

> ▸ Clinical presentation meets *diagnostic criteria* for agoraphobia:

> > ▷ Presence of agoraphobic anxiety related to fear of developing panic-like symptoms

> > ▷ Never met criteria for panic disorder

> > ▷ Avoidant behavior as a result of the agoraphobic anxiety

Physical Exam

▶ Nonspecific for agoraphobia

Mental Status Exam

▶ Consistent with finding for anxiety

▶ Thought content consistent with criteria for agoraphobia

Diagnostic Studies

▶ Nonspecific for agoraphobia

Management

▶ Follow guidelines of general clinical management of anxiety disorders

Pharmacologic Treatment

▶ SSRIs

▶ BNZs for short-term use

▶ Beta-blockers (off-label use) for discreet episodes of social anxiety

Nonpharmacologic Treatment

▶ CBT

▶ Supportive group therapy

▶ Desensitization therapy

Common comorbidities

▶ Panic disorder

SPECIFIC PHOBIAS (SIMPLE PHOBIAS)

Description

▶ In specific phobias, patients experience a clinically significant level of marked and persistent fear that is clearly observable and is, by patient perception, clearly related to specific objects or situations.

▶ Adults, but not children, consciously recognize that the fear is excessive or unreasonable.

▶ In children, the degree of insight to the unreasonable nature of the fear increases as age increases.

Risk Factors

▶ Traumatic past exposure

  » Having been bitten by dog, having choked on food, and so forth

▶ Observation of another's trauma

  » Seeing others bitten by dog, seeing others choking on food, and so forth

▶ Excessive informational transmission

  » Repeated graphic parental warnings of dangers of certain events or situations

▶ Genetic loading

  » Having family member with specific phobia

  » Blood-injection-injury type is the most familial

▸ Subtype aggregation patterns noted within families; for example, if a patient's first-degree relative has animal subtype, the risk is highest for the patient to develop animal subtype.

Assessment

History

► Assess for the following:

▸ The content of phobias, which can vary with culture, ethnicity, and age

▷ Children manifest fear and anxiety as crying, freezing, tantrums, or excessive clinging behavior.

▷ Children normatively express a transient fear of animals and other natural objects.

▷ Phobic diagnosis should occur only when accompanied by significant functional impairment, such as full avoidance of school related to fear of encountering a spider.

▸ Exposure to the specific feared object or situation, which immediately provokes the onset of clinically significant levels of anxiety

▷ This anxiety may fit the criteria for cued panic attack.

▷ The level of anxiety is directly related to how physically close the object or situation is to the person and the degree to which escape from the object or situation is possible.

▸ Patient engages in avoidant behavior to prevent reaction to object or situation or endures object or situation with dread.

▷ Avoidant behavior is distressful and has implications for social, recreational, or occupational or school functioning.

► Assess for subtypes:

▸ There are five common subtypes: situational, natural environment, blood-injection-injury, animal, and other.

▸ A person can experience more than one subtype at a time.

▸ A phobia to one object or situation in a subclass predisposes a person to another phobia within the same subclass (e.g., fear of rats increases the risk for fear of spiders).

1. **Situational Type:** Cued by specific situations; examples include driving, enclosed spaces, tunnels or bridges, or flying

▷ Most common adult form

▷ In older adults, fear of closed-in situations most common

▷ Bimodal peak of onset

▸ First peak, childhood

▸ Second peak, mid-20s

2. **Natural Environment Type:** Fear cued by objects in the natural environment; examples include storms, lightning, water, or heights.

▷ Second most common adult form

▷ Onset usually during childhood

3. **Blood-Injection-Injury Type:** Cued by seeing blood or an injury or by receiving an injection or other invasive medical procedure.

▷ Third most common adult form

▷ Strong vasovagal component that can produce other somatic sensations

▸ May exacerbate underlying cardiac or respiratory disorders

▸ Person often presents with fainting as chief complaint

▸ Experiences paroxysmal tachycardia and hypertension followed by deceleration of heart rate and drop in blood pressure

▸ Clinical presentation and disease natural history similar to panic disorder with agoraphobia.

4. **Animal Type:** Fear cued by animals or insects; examples include rats, snakes, or spiders.

▷ Fourth most common adult form

▷ Onset usually during childhood.

5. **Other Type:** Fear cued by range of other stimuli; examples include fear of choking, vomiting, or fear of a specific illness.

▷ In children, often manifests as fear of loud sounds or costumed characters.

Physical Exam

▶ Nonspecific

Mental Status Exam

▶ Consistent with finding for anxiety

▶ Thought content consistent with criteria for phobia

Diagnostic Studies

▶ Nonspecific

Differential Diagnosis

▶ Avoidance behavior in PTSD, OCD, separation anxiety disorder, or psychotic disorders

Management

▶ Follow guidelines of general clinical management of anxiety disorders

Pharmacologic Treatment

▶ SSRIs

▶ TCAs

▶ Short-term use of BNZs

Nonpharmacologic Treatment

▶ CBT

▶ Biofeedback

▶ Desensitization therapy

SOCIAL ANXIETY (PHOBIA) DISORDER

Description

▶ Social anxiety disorder is a marked and persistent fear of social or performance situations in which embarrassment may occur.

▶ Anxiety levels often are sufficient to fit criteria for a situationally bound panic attack.

▶ The disorder has an estimated 3%–13% prevalence rate among the U.S. population.

▶ Rates are equal for the genders.

Assessment

History

▶ Assess for the following:

▷ Some degree of social anxiety is common and normative in adolescence.

▷ Social phobia should be diagnosed only if symptoms persist for longer than 6 months.

▷ Onset is in the mid-teens, often following stressful or humiliating experience and tends to remit with age.

▷ Differential diagnosis is assisted by awareness that people with social phobia do *not* feel better or experience decrease anxiety when accompanied by a trusted companion.

▷ Common descriptive features:

▷ Hypersensitivity to criticism

▷ Negative self-evaluations

▷ Sensitivity to rejection

▷ Low self-esteem

▷ Inferiority feelings

▷ Lack of assertiveness

- Protracted anticipatory anxiety may occur days or weeks before the feared social situation.
- Levels of subjective distress and impaired functioning can be significant and have been associated with suicidal ideation.

Physical Exam

- Findings for a patient who is acutely anxious
  - Sweating
  - Tremors
  - Palpitations
  - Muscle tension
  - Diarrhea
  - Blushing

Mental Status Exam

- Consistent for anxiety
- Thought content consistent with criteria for social anxiety

Diagnostic Studies

- Nonspecific

Management

- Follow guidelines of general clinical management of anxiety disorders

Pharmacologic Treatment

- SSRIs
- BNZs, for short-term use
- Beta-blockers
- Used for discrete episode relief
- Example, before having to attend a scheduled social function

Nonpharmacologic Treatment

- CBT
- Exposure therapy
- Relaxation therapy

OBSESSIVE–COMPULSIVE DISORDER (OCD)

Description

► OCD is the presence of anxiety-provoking obsessions or compulsions that function to reduce the person's subjective anxiety level.

  » Obsession

    ▷ Defined as experiencingrecurrent and persistent thought, impulse, or images that cause anxiety and distress

    ▷ Experienced as intrusive and inappropriate

    ▷ Ego-dystonic experience in which a person feels the content of obsession is alien to his or her belief structure and not the kind of common thought, impulse, or image he or she usually experiences.

  » Compulsion

    ▷ Defined as repetitive behaviors or mental actions that a person feels driven to perform in response to an obsession.

Incidence and Demographics

► Rates are equal in men and women.

► Onset is most common during adolescence or early adulthood.

  » Age of onset is earlier in men (usually age 15) than women (usually age 20).

Risk Factors

► Genetic loading

  » Familial transmission pattern

    ▷ Disease rates higher in persons with a first-degree relative who has OCD than in the general population.

    ▷ Rates are also higher in persons with a first-degree relative who has Tourette's syndrome than in the general population.

  » PANDAS (pediatric autoimmune neuropsychiatric disorders associated with streptococcal infections) should be considered in all children with sudden-onset OCD symptoms

Assessment

History

► Assess for the following:

  » Diagnostic criteria:

    ▷ Presence of *either* obsessions *or* compulsions

      » The patient recognizing that the obsession or compulsion is excessive or unreasonable

- The obsession or compulsion is causing marked distress, is time-consuming, or interferes with normal daily activity.

▷ Common obsessions include

- Repeated thoughts about contamination, dirt, or germs

- Repeated doubts, such as having hit someone with a car or having left an oven on, without evidence

- Need to have things in a specific order, with marked distress when that order is disturbed

- Aggressive or horrific thoughts

- Sexual imagery

  ▷ Obsessions usually do not involve real-world worries such as concern over finances.

- The person recognizes that the thought, impulse, or images are a product of his or her own mind.

- The person attempts to ignore or suppress thoughts, impulse, or images or to override them with other thoughts or actions.

- People often avoid situations in which content of obsession may be encountered (e.g., avoiding public restrooms to avoid contamination)

▷ Common compulsions include

- Repetitive actions, usually behavioral, and often called *rituals*

  ▷ Hand-washing

  ▷ Excessive cleaning

  ▷ Checking to see, for example, if the lights are turned off, the stove is turned off, or the doors are locked

  ▷ Needing to place objects in certain order

▷ Common mental actions include

  ▷ Counting

  ▷ Silently repeating words

  ▷ Praying

▷ Behaviors or mental acts are not experienced as pleasurable and are intended to prevent or reduce distress and subjective anxiety.

▷ If the person resists the compulsion, anxiety and subjective tension usually increase.

▷ Some people believe the compulsion can prevent some dreaded event or situation that is experienced as an obsession, such as sexual or horrific images.

Physical Exam

▶ Nonspecific

▶ Dermatitis often present related to excessive hand-washing or overuse of caustic cleaning agents.

▶ Hypochondriasis and somatic fixation common

Mental Status Exam

▶ Consistent with finding for anxiety

▶ Thought content dominated by obsessions

▶ Behavioral manifestations of rituals may be noted

Diagnostic Studies

▶ Nonspecific

Differential Diagnosis

▶ Body dysmorphic disorder

▶ Eating disorders

▶ Trichotillomania

▶ Hypochondriasis

▶ Obsessive–compulsive personality disorder

▶ Tic or stereotypic movement disorder

Management

▶ Follow guidelines of general clinical management of anxiety disorders

Pharmacologic Treatment

▶ SSRIs

▶ TCAs

Nonpharmacologic Treatment

▶ CBT

▶ Exposure therapy

Special Considerations

▶ Children

　▹ Common in childhood, usually with prepubertal onset

　▹ More common in boys than girls

　▹ Washing, checking, and ordering the most common behavioral manifestations

　▹ Common comorbidities in children:

> Learning disorders

> Disruptive behavioral disorders

> Tourette's syndrome

» Associated in children with Group A beta-hemolytic streptococcal infections (e.g., scarlet fever, strep throat)

▶ Older adults

» More obsessions than compulsions usually present

» Obsessive content characteristically about dying

» Compulsions characteristically about washing and cleaning

Common Comorbidities

▶ Major depression

▶ Eating disorders

▶ Other anxiety disorders

POSTTRAUMATIC STRESS DISORDER (PTSD)

Description

▶ PTSD is the re-experiencing of an extremely traumatic event accompanied by symptoms of increased arousal and avoidance of stimuli associated with the trauma.

▶ The traumatic event can be experienced directly or witnessed.

» Common *experienced* trauma includes

> Military combat

> Violent personal assault such as robbery or rape

> Kidnapping or hostage situation

> Terrorist attack

> Torture

> Prolonged sexual abuse

> Natural or human-made disasters

» Common *witnessed* trauma includes

> Observing the death of or significant injury to another

> Unexpectedly witnessing of any of the above traumas

> Learning of the sudden or unexpected death of or significant injury to family member or close friend

ANXIETY DISORDERS 237

▷ A relationship exists between the person's physical proximity to the traumatic event and the likelihood of symptom onset.

Risk Factors

▶ Experienced trauma or witnessed trauma

▶ Genetic loading

    ▸ Assumed to have strong genetic etiological component and tends to run in families

    ▸ History of major depression in first-degree relative related to increased risk of developing PTSD

Assessment

History

▶ Assess for the following:

    ▸ Symptoms cannot predate exposure to trauma

    ▸ Presenting symptoms and history can be delineated as one of *three subtypes:*

        ▷ *Acute:* Duration of symptoms less than 3 months

        ▷ *Chronic:* Symptoms lasting 3 months or longer

        ▷ *Delayed onset:* At least 6 months between traumatic event and the onset of symptoms

▶ Diagnostic criteria (symptoms for 1 month or longer):

    ▸ Exposure to a traumatic event

        ▷ The person experienced, witnessed, or was confronted with an event involving the actual or threatened death or serious injury, **and** the person's response involved intense fear, helplessness, or horror.

        ▷ The traumatic event is persistently re-experienced

    ▸ One or more re-experiencing symptoms

        ▷ Recurrent and intrusive distressing recollection of the event, including images, thoughts, and perceptions

        ▷ May be experienced as flashbacks

        ▷ Rare cases involve dissociative states lasting hours to days

        ▷ Recurrent distressing dreams about the event

        ▷ Acting or feeling as if the traumatic event were reoccurring

        ▷ Intense psychological distress at exposure to cues that symbolize or resemble aspects of the traumatic event

        ▷ Physiological reactivity on exposure to cues that symbolize or resemble aspects of the traumatic event

238 PSYCHIATRIC–MENTAL HEALTH NURSE PRACTITIONER REVIEW MANUAL, 3RD EDITION

- Three or more avoidance symptoms
  - Persistent avoidance of stimuli associated with the traumatic event and numbing of responsiveness
  - Efforts to avoid talking about or thinking about traumatic event
  - Avoidance of activities, places, or people that arouse recollections of traumatic event
  - Inability to recall important aspects of event
  - Marked decreased interest or participation in activities
  - Feelings of detachment or estrangement from others
  - Restricted range of affect
  - Sense of foreboding and of shortened future, premature death, or no expectation for success or happiness
- Two or more increased arousal symptoms
  - Persistent symptoms of increased arousal
  - Difficulty falling asleep
  - Irritability or outburst of anger
  - Difficulty concentrating
  - Hypervigilance
  - Exaggerated startle response
- Symptoms causing significant distress or impairment in activities of daily functioning
- Symptoms usually occur within 3 months of trauma
- Duration of symptoms highly variable
- Symptoms remit within 3 months in half of cases
- Common waxing and waning of symptoms related to internal and external cues that resemble the trauma

Physical Exam
- ▶ Nonspecific
- ▶ Increased rates of somatic complaints
- ▶ Insomnia frequently chief complaint on presentation for evaluation
- ▶ Distractibility in motor tasks
- ▶ Measurable increased autonomic functioning
  - Tachycardia
  - Diaphoresis
  - Increased respiratory rates
  - Pupilary dilation
  - Increased startle response

ANXIETY DISORDERS 239

Mental Status Exam

▶ Consistent with finding for anxiety

▶ Thought content consistent with criteria for PTSD and often dominated by traumatic experience

▶ May demonstrate some psychotic findings during flashback episodes

Diagnostic Studies

▶ Nonspecific.

Differential Diagnosis

▶ Adjustment disorder

▶ Brief psychotic disorder

▶ Acute stress disorder

▶ Intrusive thoughts in OCD

Management

▶ Follow guidelines of general clinical management of anxiety disorders.

Pharmacologic Treatment

▶ SSRIs

▶ TCAs

▶ BNZs

▶ Antipsychotics may be useful during episodes of flashbacks.

▶ Alpha antagonists (e.g., Prazosin) may be used for treating nightmare (off-label use).

Nonpharmacologic Treatment

▶ CBT

▶ Supportive group therapy

▶ Relaxation therapies

▶ Eye movement desensitization and reprocessing

Common Comorbidities

▶ Major depression

▶ Dysthymia

▶ Substance abuse or dependence

Special Considerations

▶ Can occur at any age, including childhood

▶ Children

  ▹ Expression of fear and horror occurs in disorganized or agitated behavior.

  ▹ Repetitive play behaviors show themes or aspects of trauma.

  ▹ Frightening dreams, but without recognized content, are common.

GENERALIZED ANXIETY DISORDER (GAD)

Description

▶ In GAD, excessive worry, apprehension, or anxiety about events or activities occurs more days than not for a period of at least 6 months.

  ▹ The person finds it hard to control the anxiety.

  ▹ No clear link exists between the anxiety and life events or stressors.

  ▹ Worry and anxiety interfere with activities of daily living.

  ▹ The nature and focus of worry shift frequently.

  ▹ Symptoms wax and wane

▶ Symptoms worsen as life events stress the person.

Incidence and Demographics

▶ Onset usually by age 20

▶ More frequent in women than in men

  ▹ Two-thirds of patients are female.

Risk Factors

▶ Genetic loading, with familial pattern of transmission

Assessment

History

▶ Assess for the following:

  ▹ In GAD, anxiety and worry are out of proportion to the actual likelihood or impact of the feared event.

    ▸ People report subjective distress caused by the constant worry but do not always describe the worry as excessive.

  ▹ Excessive anxiety and worry last for more days than not for at least 6 months.

  ▹ The person finds it difficult to control anxiety.

Physical Exam

► Nonspecific

► Associated with other health states

　► Irritable bowel syndrome

　► Migraine and other headache disorders

► Physical signs of anxiety

　► Muscle tension

　► Generalized muscle ache and soreness

　► Tremors

　► Twitching

　► Subjective complaints of shakiness

　► Shortness of breath

　► Autonomic hyperarousal signs

　► Tachycardia

　► Increased respiratory rates

　► Dizziness

　► Numbness

　► Easily fatigued, often experienced as activity intolerance

　► Muscle tension and increased tone

　► Sleep disturbance

Mental Status Exam

► Appearance

　► Psychomotor restlessness

► Mood

　► Anxious

　► Feeling keyed up or on edge

　► Irritability

► Concentration

　► Difficulty concentrating

► Thought content

　► Thematic for the anxiety and worry

　► Descriptive of the significant distress and impairment in daily functioning caused by GAD

Diagnostic Studies

▶ Nonspecific

Management

Pharmacologic Treatment

▶ SSRIs

▶ Buspar

▶ BNZs as p.r.n. agents

Nonpharmacologic Treatment

▶ Good candidates for therapy as single-treatment modality

▶ CBT

▶ Relaxation therapies

▶ Stress management

▶ Supportive counseling

Differential Diagnosis

▶ PTSD

▶ Adjustment disorder with anxiety

▶ Obsessions in OCD

▶ Anxiety associated with another disorder such as hypochondriasis or social phobia

Common Comorbidities

▶ Mood disorders

▶ Other anxiety disorders

▶ Substance-related disorders

Special Considerations

▶ Children

  » Anxiety is common in children, but it is important to assess normal vs. pathological levels.

  » Anxiety is manifested in excessive worry over competence or quality of performance in school or work, sports, or other activities.

  » Common worry often manifests as anxiety over punctuality or natural catastrophes such as earthquakes or war.

  » Often accompanied by

    ▷ Overly conforming behavior

ANXIETY DISORDERS 243

> ▷ Perfectionist self-expectations

> ▷ Excessive seeking of approval of others

> ▷ Need for frequent reassurance about performance

► In older adults, may result in significant social isolation

CASE STUDY

John, a 47-year-old teacher, has a long-standing history of GAD disorder. He had been doing well until about 4 weeks ago. At that time he was traveling overseas with his church group participating in a caring mission in South America. He began to feel more and more depressed and anxious as he saw the "poverty and despair" in developing countries. He has started not sleeping and having "bad dreams" whenever he did try to sleep. He is beginning to think he is physically sick, as his anxiety is now beginning to interfere with work, and he is worried that he may need to be in the hospital to find out "what's wrong with me."

One week ago he began to feel overwhelmingly anxious, was convinced he was dying, and had his first of 6 discrete episodes he calls "panic attacks." He went to the local ER and was diagnosed with anxiety and given Valium 5 mg #30 to use p.r.n. He at first felt like the Valium was helping, but now he is feeling "like nothing helps." He is increasingly despondent, sure he is dying and that no one will believe him, and has contemplated suicide. He says he would not do it but is bothered by thinking about suicide. He is having increased tremors with anxiety, headaches, and nausea, which the ER diagnosed as anxiety reaction. His wife agrees that all of his symptoms are anxiety, but she reports that he is sure he is dying of cancer and no one will tell him the truth.

Mental Status Exam

► Appearance: Well-nourished, well-dressed

► Motor: Some motor restlessness

► Speech: Some pressure

► Affect: Anxious

► Mood: Depressed

► Thought process/content: Thematic for fear of becoming sicker and of dying early and some vague suicidality without intent or plan; denies delusions or hallucinations.

► Abstractive on proverbs

► Memory: Impaired

► Concentration: Impaired

Social History

▶ Married and has 3 children

▶ Works as high school gym teacher

▶ Overweight at 280 lbs., with sedentary lifestyle

▶ Smokes 2 packs a day

▶ Does not drink alcohol for religious reasons

▶ Wife very concerned and supportive

Past Psychiatric History

▶ Hospitalized in 1998 for "nerves"

▶ At that time started on Paxil 20 mg/d

▶ After 3 months, dose raised to 40 mg/d; has been doing well until recently

▶ Has had no significant exacerbation of symptoms since initial treatment

Past Medical History

▶ History of seizure disorder since childhood; well controlled with levetiracetam (Keppra)

▶ Recent exposure to TB during international travel

Current Medications

▶ Paxil 40 mg

▶ Valium 5 mg p.o. p.r.n. q 4 hrs.

▶ Isoniazid for prophylaxis treatment for 6 months

Labs

▶ All labs within normal limits

Screening Tools

▶ BAI: Severe score range

In planning care for this patient, the PMHNP has many issues to consider:

▶ What is the most likely diagnosis?

▶ How will you separate comorbidity from complications of current diagnosis?

▶ What medication adjustments would you make?

▶ How will you address the family issues?

▶ How often will you plan to see the patient?

REFERENCES

American Nurses Association. (2000). *Scope and standards of psychiatric–mental health clinical nursing practice.* Washington, DC: American Nurses Association.

American Psychiatric Association. (2000). *Diagnostic and statistical manual of mental disorders* (4th ed., text rev.). Washington, DC: American Psychiatric Association.

Bremner, J. D. (2002). Neuroimaging studies in post-traumatic stress disorder. *Current Psychiatric Reports, 4,* 254–263.

Christensen, D. D. (2001). The challenge of obsessive–compulsive hoarding. *Primary Psychiatry, 6*(2), 79–84.

Davidson, J. R. (2000). Trauma: The impact of post-traumatic stress disorder. *Journal of Psychopharmacology, 14*(Suppl. 1), 5–12.

Fernandez-Lewis, R., Hinton, D., Laria A., Patterson, E., Hofmann, S., Craske, M. G., & Liao, B. (2010). Culture and the anxiety disorders: Recommendations for DSM-V. *Depression and Anxiety, 27, 212–229.*

Gold, P. W., & Chrousos, G. (1998). The endocrinology of melancholic and atypical depression: Relation to neurocircuitry and somatic consequences. *Proceedings of the Association of American Physicians, 111*(1), 22–34.

Goodman, W. K., Price, L. H., Rasmussen, S. A., Mazure, C., Fleischmann, R. L., Hill, S. A., & Chamey, D. S. (1989). The Yale-Brown obsessive-compulsive scale I: Development, use, and reliability. *Archives of General Psychiatry, 46,* 1006–1011.

Gould, E., Reeves, A. J., & Fallah, M. (1999). Hippocampal neurogenesis in adult Old World primates. *Proceedings of the National Academy of Sciences USA, 96,* 5263–5267.

Guess, K. (2006). Posttraumatic stress disorder: Early detection is key. *The Nurse Practitioner, 31*(3), 1–8.

Hamilton, M. (1959). The assessment of anxiety states by rating. *British Journal of Medical Psychology, 32*(1), 50–55.

Hembree, E. (2002). Psychosocial treatment of post-traumatic stress disorder. *Primary Psychiatry, 9*(2), 49–52.

Kessler, R. C., Chin ,W. T., Merikangas, K. R., Demler, O. M., & Walters, E. E. (2005). Prevalence, severity and comorbidity of 12-month DSM-IV disorders in the National Comorbidity Survey Replication. *Archives of General Psychiatry, 62,* 617–627.

Lopez, I., Rivera, F., Ramirez, R., Guarnaccia, P.. Canino, G., & Bird, H. (2009). Ataques de Nervios and their psychiatric correlates in Puerto Rican children from two different contexts. *Journal of Nervous and Mental Disease, 197*(12), 923–929.

Margolin, G., & Gordis, E. B. (2000). The effects of family and community violence on children. *Annual Review of Psychology, 51,* 445–479.

Mathew, J. (2002). Future pharmacotherapy for post-traumatic stress disorder: Prevention and treatment. *Psychiatric Clinics of North America, 25,* 427–441.

Meredith, P. V., & Horan, N. M. (2000). *Adult primary care.* Philadelphia: W. B. Saunders.

Narrow, W. E., Rae, D. S., & Regier, D. A. (1998). *NIMH epidemiology note: Prevalence of anxiety disorders. One-year prevalence best estimates calculated from ECA and NCS data.* Washington, DC: National Institute of Mental Health.

National Institute of Mental Health, Genetics Workgroup. (1998). *Genetics and mental disorders* (NIH Publication No. 98-4268). Rockville, MD: Author.

Regier, D. A., Rae, D. S., & Narrow, W. E. (1998). Prevalence of anxiety disorders and their comorbidity with mood and addictive disorders. *British Journal of Psychiatry(Suppl. 34), 24–28.*

Stuart, G. W., & Laraia, M. (2001). *Principles and practice of psychiatric nursing.* St. Louis, MO: Mosby.

Turner, S. (1999). Place of pharmacotherapy in PTSD. *Lancet, 354,* 1404–1407.

Yehuda, R. (1999). Biological factors associated with susceptibility to posttraumatic stress disorder. *Canadian Journal of Psychiatry, 44*(1), 34–39.

Yehuda, R. (2000). Biology of posttraumatic stress disorder. *Journal of Clinical Psychiatry, 61*(Suppl. 7), 14–21.

Zung, W. W. K. (1971). A rating instrument for anxiety disorders. *Psychometrics, 12,* 371–379.

CHAPTER 10

SCHIZOPHRENIA AND OTHER PSYCHOTIC DISORDERS

This chapter describes a category of disorders that represents some of the most debilitating severe mental illnesses. Schizophrenia, the prototypic disorder of this category of illnesses, is multifaceted and gravely affects a person's ability to function in many spheres of daily life. Of the psychotic disorders, schizophrenia is the illness that has been most heavily researched and the one we know the most about.

The other disorders that constitute this category of illnesses will be presented after the in-depth discussion of schizophrenia. Almost all of the information provided for schizophrenia and for the clinical management of this disorder will pertain to the other psychotic disorders presented in this chapter.

GENERAL DESCRIPTION OF PSYCHOTIC DISORDERS

▶ These brain-based psychiatric disorders are grouped together because of similarity in frequent psychotic symptoms. Each disorder has a different etiology.

▶ Psychotic disorders are some of the most debilitating classes of psychiatric illnesses, as determined by the degree of functional impairment and financial burden of this severe mental illness.

▶ *Psychotic* implies inability to test reality.

▶ Manifests in symptoms (see Table 10–1) such as:

  ▻ Hallucinations

  ▻ Delusions

  ▻ Disorganized thinking and speech

- ▹ Referential thinking
- ▹ Frequent illusional perceptions
- ► Psychotic disorders are generally known to have a strong genetic component.

TABLE 10-1. SYMPTOMS OF PSYCHOSIS

CLINICAL MANIFESTATION	DEFINITION	TYPE
Hallucinations	False sensory experience without stimuli being present	(Arranged in order of commonality) ► Auditory ► Visual ► Tactile ► Olfactory ► Gustatory **NOTE:** *Hypnogogic* and hypnopompic** are considered normative and do not fall under psychotic hallucinations, related to sleep
Delusions	A false belief firmly maintained despite evidence to the contrary	► Persecutory ► Religious ► Grandiosity ► Somatic ► Referential ► Jealous ► Erotomanic
Disorganized thinking (often referred to as *formal thought disturbance* or *disorder*)	Problems with information organization and interpretation that is best assessed in the speech patterns of patients	► Loose association ► Derailment ► Tangentially ► Word salad
Disorganized behavior	Unusual behavior ranging from childlike silliness to anger	► Silliness ► Unpredictable anger ► Difficulties with activities of daily living ► Disheveled ► Odd or unusual dress ► Inappropriate sexual activity ► Stereotypic motor activities
Referential thinking and delusions of control	Belief that events, actions, or situations in the environment hold special significance or meaning	► Thought insertion ► Thought withdrawal ► Thought control ► Thought broadcasting
Illusionals	Misperception of actual environmental stimuli	► Auditory ► Visual ► Tactile ► Olfactory ► Gustatory

Note. Hypnopompic hallucination = a false perception that occurs when one is waking up; *hypnogogic hallucination* = a false perception that occurs when one is falling asleep; neither is considered pathological.

SCHIZOPHRENIA

Description

► Schizophrenia causes significant disturbance in many areas of functioning:

- Cognition
- Perception
- Emotion
- Behavior
- Eye movement
- Socialization

Etiology

► Multiple theories exist, ranging from psychological to neurobiological.

► A probable multifactorial etiological profile exists.

► Neurobiological theory

- Implicates three areas of neurobiological functioning: genetics, neurodevelopment, and neurobiological defects

► Genetics

- Studies of twins have identified schizophrenia as having a strong genetic etiological component.

- Incidence increases from 1% risk of illness in general population to

  ▷ 50% risk in monozygotic twin of a person with schizophrenia

  ▷ 15% risk in dizygotic twin of a person with schizophrenia

  ▷ 40% risk in children if both parents have schizophrenia

- No one specific gene has yet been identified.

- A polygenic SNP defect is believed to exist.

- Chromosomes 5, 6, 8, 11, 18, 19, and 22 have been implicated (Gershon & Badner, 2001).

► Neurodevelopment

- Genetic defects are believed to cause abnormal neuronal cell development, connection, organization, and migration.

- These include inadequate synapse formation, excessive pruning of synapses, and excitotoxic death of neurons.

- Intrauterine insults may contribute to etiological picture:

  ▷ Prenatal exposure to toxins, including viral agents

  ▷ Oxygen deprivation

  ▷ Maternal malnutrition, substance use, or other illness

► Neurobiological defect

    ► Several abnormal brain structures have been identified in people with schizophrenia:

        ▷ Enlarged ventricles

        ▷ Smaller frontal and temporal lobes

        ▷ Cortical atrophy

        ▷ Decreased cerebral blood flow

        ▷ Hippocampal reduction (Lencz, Bilder, & Cornblatt, 2001)

    ► Abnormalities lead to suspected impaired neuronal communication:

        ▷ Suspected alterations in chemical neuronal signal transmission

            ► Excess dopamine in mesolimbic pathway

            ► Decreased dopamine in the mesocortical pathway

            ► Excess glutamate

            ► Decreased GABA

            ► Decreased serotonin

Incidence and Demographics

► Geographic and historical variations in incidence give insight into etiological factors:

    ► Higher rates in urban-born

    ► Higher rates in first-born

    ► Higher rates in lower socioeconomic status

► Schizophrenia is equally prevalent in men and women.

    ► *Men:* Onset ages 18–25 years

        ▷ Tend to have more negative symptoms than women

        ▷ Tend to have poorer prognosis, more hospitalizations, and less responsiveness to medications than women

    ► *Women:* Onset ages 25–35 years

        ▷ Usually have less premorbid dysfunction than men

        ▷ Usually experience more dysphoria than men

        ▷ Tend to have paranoid delusions and more hallucinations than men

    ► Age of onset has pathophysiological and prognostic significance:

    ► Earlier age of onset

        ▷ Tend to be men

        ▷ Have poorer premorbid functioning

        ▷ Have more evidence of structural brain abnormalities

- Have more prominent negative symptoms
- Have more cognitive impairment
- Have poorer prognosis
- Later age of onset
  - Tend to be women
  - Have less evidence of structural abnormalities
  - Have less cognitive impairment
  - Have better prognosis

Possible Risk Factors
- Genetic loading
  - First-order relative with schizophrenia
- Prenatal exposure to flu or virus
- Prenatal malnutrition
- Obstetrical complications
- Central nervous system (CNS) infection in early childhood

Prevention and Screening
- At-risk family education
- Community education
  - Stigma reduction
  - Signs and symptoms of illness
  - Treatment potential for control of symptoms
- Early recognition, intervention, and initiation of treatment
  - Significant and protracted prodromal symptom period usually noted before full onset of illness
  - Usually mild manifestations of criteria symptoms:
    - Odd or unusual beliefs but not to delusional proportion
    - Feel unliked or picked on but not to delusional proportion
    - Odd speech patterns but not illogical
      - Digressions
      - Tangentiality
  - Overly concrete or abstractive
  - Odd behavior but not disorganized

- ▷ Collects odd or worthless items

- ▷ Mumbles to self

- ▷ Isolates self and avoids interaction with others

Assessment

History

▶ Assess for the following:

- ▹ There exists no single pathognomonic symptom of schizophrenia, but rather a constellation of symptoms.

- ▹ Schizophrenia is a disease of information processing.

- ▹ The symptoms are behavioral and cognitive.

- ▹ The illness is associated with marked difficulty in social or occupational functioning.

- ▹ Prominent dysfunctions exists in many spheres of daily living.

  - ▷ Interpersonal relationships

    - ▹ 60%–70% of clients do not marry

- ▹ Social or occupational functioning

  - ▷ "Downdrift" functionality is noted over time.

    - ▹ Lower academic achievement compared to unaffected siblings

    - ▹ Difficulty holding a job

    - ▹ Underemployed relative to intellectual capacity

- ▹ Self-care deficits

  - ▷ Poor hygiene

  - ▷ Difficulty with financial management

  - ▷ Limited independent living skills.

- ▹ Characteristic symptom clusters for the illness (see Table 10–2) include

  - ▷ Positive symptom cluster

  - ▷ Negative symptom cluster

  - ▷ Associated symptoms

SCHIZOPHRENIA AND OTHER PSYCHOTIC DISORDERS **253**

TABLE 10-2. POSITIVE AND NEGATIVE SYMPTOM CLUSTERS OF SCHIZOPHRENIA

SYMPTOM CLUSTER	EXPLANATION	CLINICAL MANIFESTATIONS
Positive symptoms	► Symptoms that respond positively to and that can be controlled by typical antipsychotic medications ► Reflect excesses or distortions of normal brain functioning ► Caused by increased dopamine in the mesolimbic pathway	► Hallucinations ► Delusions ► Referential thinking ► Disorganized behavior ► Hostility ► Grandiosity ► Mania ► Suspiciousness
Negative symptoms	► Symptoms less responsive to typical antipsychotic medications but may respond to and be controlled by atypical antipsychotic medications ► Represent a decrease or loss of normal functioning ► Caused by decreased dopamine in the mesocortical pathway	► Affective flattening ► Alogia or poverty of speech ► Avolition ► Apathy ► Abstract-thinking problems ► Anhedonia ► Attention deficits
Associated symptoms	► Symptoms not required to be present to diagnose the disorder but often are present and a focus of treatment	► Inappropriate affect ► Dysphoric mood ► Depersonalization ► Derealization ► High anxiety

► *DSM-IV-TR* (American Psychiatric Association, 2000) diagnostic criteria for schizophrenia

  ► Two or more of the following frequently are present during a 1-month period (only 1 if delusions are bizarre or hallucinations consist of a voice that is running commentary or 2 or more voices conversing with each other):

    ▷ *Delusions:* Bizarre and unorganized type; examples include delusions that manifest as loss of control over mind or body:

      ► Thought withdrawal

      ► Thought insertion

    ▷ *Hallucinations:* Bizarre and unorganized type; examples include hallucinations that are improbable or readily apparent as not likely to have occurred

      ► Disorganized speech

      ► Grossly disorganized behavior

      ► Presence of negative symptoms

    ▷ Significant impairment usually is evident by social or occupational dysfunction.

    ▷ Duration of symptoms lasts for at least 6 months.

- Complete remission is uncommon.
- The course of illness is variable.
  - Many patients have a fairly stable illness course.
  - Some patients have clear episodic remissions and exacerbation periods.
  - Negative symptoms tend to appear first as the illness develops.
  - Positive symptoms appear to decrease over time, but negative symptoms persist.
- Factors predictive of good prognosis
  - High level of premorbid functioning
  - Acute onset
  - Later age of onset
  - Clear precipitating event
  - Married or partnered
  - Good support system
  - Positive symptoms
  - Short interval between treatment and onset of first symptoms
    - The sooner the patient is treated, the better the prognosis.
    - Longer untreated premorbid period is associated with a poorer prognosis.
  - Absence of structural brain abnormalities
  - Family history of mood disorders
  - No family history of schizophrenia

▶ Subtypes of schizophrenia
- Subtypes are defined by predominant patient symptomology (see Table 10–3).
  - Disorganized type: Most severe
  - Paranoid type: Least severe
  - Catatonic type
  - Undifferentiated type
  - Residual type
- Subtype identification is of limited clinical value, because illness course, response to treatment, and prognosis appear unrelated to subtype.

TABLE 10-3. SUBTYPES OF SCHIZOPHRENIA

SUBTYPE	CHARACTERISTIC
Paranoid	▶ Prominent delusions or auditory hallucinations ▶ Lack of prominence of disorganized speech or behavior
Disorganized	▶ Prominence of disorganized speech, behavior, and flat or inappropriate affect
Catatonic	▶ Prominence of motor symptoms, including immobility as evidenced by catalepsy or stupor, excessive motor movement that is purposeless and not influenced by environmental stimuli, extreme negativity, mutism, oddities of posturing, echolalia,* and echopraxia*
Undifferentiated	▶ Presence of symptoms consistent with schizophrenia but not a prominence of symptoms consistent with any of the other subtypes
Residual	▶ Absence of prominent delusions, hallucinations, disorganized speech, and disorganized or catatonic behavior, and the continued presence of disturbance as indicated by presence of negative symptoms

Note. Echolalia = repetition of the last-heard words of other speakers; *echopraxia* = imitation of observed behavior or movements.

Physical Exam

▶ Abnormal smooth-pursuit eye movements

▶ Abnormal saccadic eye movement

▶ Poor eye–hand coordination

  ▹ Patient identified as "clumsy" or "awkward"

▶ Presence of neurological nonlocalizing "soft signs":

  ▹ *Astereognosis*: Loss of ability to judge the form of an object by touch

  ▹ Twitches, tics, or rapid eye-blinking

  ▹ *Dysdiadochokinesia*: Impairment of the ability to perform rapidly alternating movements

  ▹ Impaired fine-motor movement

  ▹ Left–right confusion

  ▹ Mirroring

▶ Presence of neurological localizing "hard signs":

  ▹ Weakness

  ▹ Decreased reflexes

▶ Other abnormalities that may be noted:

  ▹ Highly arched palate

  ▹ Narrow or wide-set eyes

  ▹ Subtle malformations of the ears

Mental Status Exam

- ▶ Appearance
  - ‣ Odd
  - ‣ Unusual
  - ‣ Peculiar
- ▶ Speech
  - ‣ Bizarre content
  - ‣ Disorganized
  - ‣ Tangential
  - ‣ Loose association
- ▶ Affect
  - ‣ Blunted
  - ‣ Flat
  - ‣ Inappropriate
- ▶ Mood
  - ‣ Blandness
  - ‣ Impoverished
- ▶ Thought process
  - ‣ Psychotic
    - ▷ Hallucination
    - ▷ Delusion
    - ▷ Referential
    - ▷ Thought control, insertion, or withdrawal
- ▶ Thought content
  - ‣ Thematically matched to psychotic content
  - ‣ May be impoverished
- ▶ Cognition
  - ‣ Illogical
  - ‣ Disorganized
- ▶ Orientation
  - ‣ Usually intact
- ▶ Memory
  - ‣ May cause impaired short-term
- ▶ Concentration
  - ‣ Impaired during acute episodes

- ► Abstraction
  - ▻ Concrete on formal testing
- ► Judgment
  - ▻ Impaired for self-welfare

Diagnostic Studies
- ► No specific diagnostic lab findings exist.
- ► Abnormalities noted in structural studies
  - ▻ Enlargement of lateral ventricles
  - ▻ Widened cortical sulci
  - ▻ Diffuse decrease in volume of white and gray matter
  - ▻ Decreased volume of temporal lobe
  - ▻ Hypovolume in hippocampus, amygdala, and thalamus (Lencz, Bilder, & Cornblatt, 2001)
- ► Abnormalities noted in functional studies
  - ▻ Hypofrontality
  - ▻ Decreased cerebral blood flow and metabolism
  - ▻ Diffuse hypometabolic action in cortical–subcortical circuitry

Differential Diagnosis
- ► Nonpsychiatric disorders
  - ▻ Epilepsy
  - ▻ CNS neoplasm
  - ▻ AIDS
  - ▻ Acute intermittent porphyria
  - ▻ B_{12} deficiency
  - ▻ Heavy-metal poisoning
  - ▻ Huntington's disease
  - ▻ Neurosyphilis
  - ▻ Systemic lupus erythematosus
  - ▻ Wernicke–Korsakoff syndrome
  - ▻ Wilson's disease
- ► Psychiatric disorders
  - ▻ Bipolar affective disorder
  - ▻ Substance-induced psychotic disorder
    - ▹ Amphetamines
    - ▹ Hallucinogens

258 PSYCHIATRIC-MENTAL HEALTH NURSE PRACTITIONER REVIEW MANUAL, 3RD EDITION

▷ Alcoholic hallucinosis

▷ Barbiturate withdrawal

▷ Cocaine

▷ PCP

► Mood disorders with psychotic features (see Chapter 8)

► Schizoaffective disorder (see below)

► Schizophreniform disorder (see below)

► Brief psychotic disorder (see below)

► Delusional disorder (see below)

► Schizotypal personality disorder (see Chapter 13)

► Schizoid personality disorder (see Chapter 13)

► Paranoid personality disorder (see Chapter 13)

Management

▶ Assess for acuity level

► During acute psychotic episodes, client may require brief hospitalization to

▷ Ensure patient safety

▷ Rapidly stabilize patient's symptom level in a controlled environment

▷ Monitor treatment adherence with the goal of stabilization and recovery

► Clinical management during non-acute episodes occurs most often in community settings.

Pharmacologic Treatment

▶ Pharmacological therapy is the primary treatment modality, augmented by nonpharmacological treatments.

Pharmacologic Treatment

▶ Most patients will require lifelong medication

▶ Patient and family education is important for treatment adherence

▶ Adjunctive medications may be used to achieve full symptom control:

► Antidepressants

► Anxiolytics

► Anticonvulsants

Nonpharmacologic Treatment

▶ Individual therapy

► Usually supportive rather than insight-oriented

▷ Focuses on establishing reality testing

▷ Builds daily-life skills

▷ Assists patient in establishing and meeting life goals

▸ CBT for management of hallucinations and delusions.

▶ *Atypical antipsychotics* (see Table 10–4)

   ▸ Primary first-line treatment agents

   ▸ First introduced in the 1990s

   ▸ Have less significant neurological side effects

   ▸ Effectively treat positive *and* negative symptoms

   ▸ Function as serotonin–dopamine antagonists

      ▷ D_2 and 5HT2a blockade

   ▸ Expensive (some generics now available)

   ▸ Fewer clinically significant side effects

      ▷ Can cause extrapyramidal side effects (EPSE; see 5 common types in Table 10–5) but with lower risk compared to typical antipsychotics

      ▷ Lower incidence of tardive dyskinesia (TD; see below).

   ▸ Improved compliance

▶ *Mode of action:*

   ▸ In addition to the dopaminergic blockade found in first-generation antipsychotics, second-generation drugs capitalize on the interplay between dopamine and serotonin. Serotonin binds to 5HT2a heteroreceptors on DA neurons, thus further shutting off release of DA. By antagonizing (blocking) the 5HT2a heteroreceptors on DA neurons, DA release in the nigrostriatal, tuberoinfundibular, and mesocortical pathways is enhanced.

   ▸ *Dopamine pathways:* These explain both the therapeutic effects *and* the side effects of the atypical antipsychotics.

      ▷ *Mesolimbic pathway:* SDAs block dopamine in this pathway, causing decreased positive symptoms.

      ▷ *Mesocortical pathway:* SDAs increase dopamine in this pathway, causing decreased negative symptoms

      ▷ *Nigrostriatal pathway:* Dopamine has a reciprocal relationship with acetylcholine

      ▷ *Acetylcholine pathway:* When serotonin is blocked by the SDA, dopamine increases; therefore, ACh decreases, which causes decreased EPSE. (EPSE are caused by increased ACh.)

      ▷ *Tuberoinfundibular pathway:* Dopamine inhibits prolactin. The blockade of dopamine by SDAs causes prolactin to increase, causing galactorrhea and gynecomastia.

   ▸ Hyperprolactinemia associated with the antipsychotics may cause sexual problems, galactorrhea, amenorrhea, gynecomastia, and bone demineralization in postmenopausal women not on estrogen.

TABLE 10-4. ATYPICAL ANTIPSYCHOTICS

AGENT	BRAND NAME	DOSAGE FORMS & DAILY DOSAGE	SIDE EFFECTS	COMMENTS
Clozapine	Clozaril	Tablet or oral disintegrated Tablet, 25–900 mg/d	► *Common:* Tachycardia, drowsiness, dizziness, sialorrhea, weight gain, hyperlipidemia ► *Rare:* Agranulocytosis, myocarditis, neuroleptic malignant syndrome	► Only drug for treatment-resistant schizophrenia ► WBC with differential monitoring required due to risk of agranulocytosis ► During first 6 months: weekly; during second 6 months: every 2 weeks; then monthly if WBC/ANC normal ► Monitor for myocarditis ► Dose-related seizure risk ► Significant weight gain and risk of diabetes ► Rare hyperprolactemia ► Monitor weight, BMI, waist circumference ► Monitor serum lipids and glucose ► Assess family and personal history of cardiovascular disease
Quetiapine	Seroquel and Seroquel XR	Tablet, 50–800 mg/d	► *Common:* Sedation and hypotension (orthostatic hypotension), weight gain ► *Rare:* Cataract formation	► Transient and asymptomatic elevated LFTs ► Monitor for cataract development ► Divided doses: b.i.d. or t.i.d. ► No prolactin elevation ► Monitor weight, BMI, waist circumference ► Monitor serum lipids and glucose ► Assess family and personal history of cardiovascular disease
Olanzapine	Zyprexa, Zyprexa Zydis, Zyprexa Relprev	Tablet and intramuscular injection (acute), 5–20 mg/d; injection, 150–405 mg every 2–4 weeks	► Sedation, weight gain, hyperlipidemia, elevated glucose, elevated LFTs, ► Mild prolactin elevation ► Long-acting Preparation (Zyprexa Relprev) requires that patients be monitored for 3 hours postinjection due to risk of postinjection delirium sedation syndrome	► Significant weight gain ► Monitor weight, BMI, waist circumference ► Monitor serum lipids and glucose ► Assess family and personal history of cardiovascular disease

CONTINUED ▶

TABLE 10-4. ATYPICAL ANTIPSYCHOTICS CONTINUED ▶

AGENT	BRAND NAME	DOSAGE FORMS & DAILY DOSAGE	SIDE EFFECTS	COMMENTS
Risperidone	Risperdal, Risperdal Consta	Tablet, liquid, orally disintegrated tablets; 2–8 mg, injectable (25–50 mg IM) every 2 weeks	▶ Hypotension, galactorrhea nausea, insomnia	▶ Doses > 6 mg associated with a higher incidence of extrapyramidal symptoms ▶ Less weight gain than with clozapine or olanzapine ▶ Greatest prolactin elevation among atypical psychotics ▶ Monitor weight, BMI, waist circumference ▶ Monitor serum lipids and glucose ▶ Assess family and personal history of cardiovascular disease
Ziprasidone	Geodon	Tablets, 40–200 mg/d; injectable, 10–20 mg IM (acute treatment)	▶ Hypotension, sedation, ▶ dizziness ▶ *Rare:* Prolongation of QTc interval	▶ Requires QTc monitoring ▶ Avoid co-administration with other drugs known to prolong QTc ▶ Taking with food increases absorption twofold ▶ Use caution when administering with patients at risk for hypokalemia, hypomagnesemia, after myocardial infarction, or with congestive heart failure ▶ Monitor weight, BMI, waist circumference ▶ Monitor serum lipids and glucose ▶ Assess family and personal history of cardiovascular disease
Paliperidone	Invega, Invega Sustenna	Tablets (3–12 mg/d) injection, 39 mg–234	▶ Orthostatic hypotension, hyperpro-lactinemia, GI upset, dizziness, headache	▶ Same as extended-release Risperidone
Aripiprizole	Abilify	Tablets, 5–30 mg/d; injection (acute agitation), 5.25–15 mg IM every 4 weeks; long-acting, 200 –400 mg IM monthly	▶ Headache, agitation, anxiety, insomnia, somnolence, akathisia, GI problems	▶ Is a partial agonist of D_2 receptors ▶ Monitor weight, BMI, waist circumference ▶ Monitor serum lipids and glucose ▶ Assess family and personal history of cardiovascular disease

CONTINUED ▶

TABLE 10-4. ATYPICAL ANTIPSYCHOTICS CONTINUED ▶

AGENT	BRAND NAME	DOSAGE FORMS & DAILY DOSAGE	SIDE EFFECTS	COMMENTS
Iloperidone	Fanapt	12–24 mg/ day in divided doses	▶ Orthostatic hypotension, sedation, dizziness	▶ Titrate slowly due to the alpha 1 antagonist properties ▶ Might be helpful for posttraumatic stress disorder hyperarousal symptoms due to alpha 1 blocking ▶ Monitor weight, BMI, waist circumference ▶ Monitor serum lipids and glucose ▶ Assess family and personal history of cardiovascular disease
Asenapine	Saphris	5–10 mg p.o. b.i.d., sublingual	▶ Akathisia, somnolence	▶ Monitor weight, BMI, waist circumference ▶ Monitor serum lipids and glucose ▶ Assess family and personal history of cardiovascular disease
Lurasidone	Latuda	40–160 mg/d	▶ Akathisia, sedation, and nausea	▶ Should be taken with food to increase absorption ▶ Use with caution at lower doses in patients with renal and hepatic impairment ▶ Monitor weight, BMI, waist circumference ▶ Monitor serum lipids and glucose ▶ Assess family and personal history of cardiovascular disease

Note. All atypical antipsychotic medications have a warning: increase in mortality in elderly patients with dementia-related psychosis

TABLE 10-5. EXTRAPYRAMIDAL SIDE EFFECTS (EPSE)

SIDE EFFECT	DEFINITION
Akathisia	Motor restlessness; inability to remain still; rocking, pacing, or constant motion of unilateral limb—also can manifest as a subjective sense of restlessness without objective finding *Note:* Often mistaken for increasing anxiety
Akinesia	Absence of movement, difficulty initiating motion, subjective feeling of lack of motivation to move *Note:* Often mistaken for laziness or lack of interest
Dystonia	Muscle spasm; spasticity of muscle group, especially back or neck muscles; subjectively painful *Note:* Often mistaken for agitation or unusual, stereotypic movements characteristic of schizophrenia
Pseudo-Parkinson's	Presence of symptoms of Parkinson's disorder produced by D_2 blockade; includes shuffling gait, motor slowing, mask-like facial expression, pill-rolling, tremors, and muscle rigidity *Note:* Mask-like facial expression often confused as affective blunting or flattening
Tardive dyskinesia	Involuntary abnormal muscle movement of the mouth, tongue, face, and jaw that may progress to limbs; can be irreversible; can occur as an acute process at initiation of medications or as a chronic condition at any point in treatment

▶ *Typical antipsychotics* (first-generation; see Table 10–6)

    ▹ Cross-classified as neuroleptics because of significant side effects

    ▹ First introduced in the 1950s

    ▹ Useful for treating positive symptoms by blocking dopamine in the mesolimbic pathway

    ▹ Can make negative symptoms worse by blocking dopamine in the mesocortical pathway

    ▹ Therapeutic effect related primarily to D_2 receptor blockade

    ▹ Generic (inexpensive)

    ▹ Can be used as sustained-released injectable agents

        ▹ Decanoate long-acting injectable dose forms of typical antipsychotics:

            ▹ Prolixin-D (Limited availability due to low production)

            ▹ Haldol-D

▶ *High potency*: Have a greater risk of EPSE but less risk of sedation and anticholinergic symptoms

► *Low potency:* Have a greater risk of sedation and anticholinergic side effects but less risk of EPSE

► Caffeine and nicotine cause diminished antipsychotic effect; dose may need to be higher

► Because of multiple clinically significant side effects, are not considered first-line treatment agents

- Side effects leading to poor adherence

- High patient teaching needs

- EPSE most common side effect.

  ▷ Caused by D_2 receptor antagonism (when dopamine receptors are blocked, ACh increases, which causes EPSE; a reciprocal relationship exists between ACh and dopamine.)

  ▷ Treated by use of anti-Parkinsonian drugs (cross-classified; see Table 10–7)

  - Anticholinergics

  - Antihistamines

  - Dopamine agonists

  - Benzodiazepines (BNZs)

- Tardive dyskinesia (TD)

  ▷ TD is a potentially irreversible movement disorder that most commonly occurs after a person has been on an antipsychotic for a year or more.

  ▷ TD more commonly occurs with typical antipsychotic medication, but also can occur with atypical antipsychotic medication.

  ▷ Symptoms consist of abnormal, involuntary movements such as lip smacking, chewing, tongue protrusion, or twisting movements of the trunk or limbs.

  ▷ Perioral movements are most common.

  ▷ Treatment involves discontinuation of the offending agent and often, starting an atypical antipsychotic.

  ▷ Patients on typical antipsychotics should have routine abnormal involuntary muscle movement screening (AIMS or DISCUS) every 3–6 months.

  ▷ Patient and family education on the detection of early signs and symptoms of abnormal movements

  ▷ If abnormal movements are noted, consider reducing the dosage or switching to an atypical antipsychotic.

  ▷ Risk factors include

  - Long-term treatment with neuroleptics

  - Older age

  - Female gender

  - Presence of mood or cognitive disorder

- Assessment of abnormal movement rating scales
  - Abnormal Involuntary Movement Scale (AIMS)
  - Dyskinesia Identification System Condensed User Scale (DISCUS)
  - Simpson-Angus Scale (SAS)
- Neuroleptic malignant syndrome (NMS)
  - Rare but potentially life-threatening
  - Can occur at any point during treatment
  - Most common with typical but has been reported in atypical antipsychotics
  - Risk factors include
    - Rapid dose escalation
    - Use of high-potency typical antipsychotic
    - Parental administration of antipsychotics
  - Assess for the following abnormal labs:
    - Elevated CPK (creatine phosphokinase)
    - Elevated WBCs (white blood cell count)
    - Elevated LFTs (liver function tests)
  - Assess for symptoms known to occur first:
    - Altered sensorium
    - Hyperthermia
    - Hyperreflexia
  - Assess for symptoms of autonomic instability:
    - Hypotension
    - Extreme muscular rigidity
    - Hyperthermia
    - Tachycardia
    - Diaphoresis
    - Tachypnea
    - Coma and potentially death
  - Treatment
    - Seek immediate medical care for treatment
    - Discontinue antipsychotic medication(s)
    - Administration of Dantrium (dantrolene) or Parlodel (bromocriptine) for antipsychotic-induced dopamine receptor blockade
    - Antipyretic (acetaminophen) and cooling blanket for hyperthermia
    - Intravenous hydration
    - Benzodiazepine for muscular rigidity (catatonic symptoms)

TABLE 10-6. TYPICAL ANTIPSYCHOTICS

AGENT	BRAND NAME	FORMS & DAILY DOSAGE	SIDE EFFECTS	COMMENTS
Chlorpromazine	Thorazine	Tablet, SR, liquid, 50–2,000 mg/d	▸ *High:* Sedation, hypotension ▸ *Moderate:* EPS, anticholinergic	▸ Allergic dermatitis ▸ Photosensitivity ▸ EKG changes; QTc monitoring
Mesoridazine	Serentil	Tablet, liquid, injection, 100–400 mg/d	▸ *High:* Anticholinergic, sedation, hypotension ▸ *Low:* EPS	▸ EKG changes; QTc monitoring
Thioridazine	Mellaril	Tablet, liquid, 50–800 mg/d	▸ *High:* Anticholinergic, sedation, hypotension, prolonged QT interval ▸ *Low:* EPS	▸ EKG changes: QTc monitoring ▸ Irreversible retinal pigmentation at doses > 800 mg/d ▸ Decreased libido ▸ Retrograde ejaculation
Fluphenazine	Permitil Prolixin	Tablet, liquid, injection, 2–40 mg/d, 12.5–75 mg/IM every 2 weeks (decanoate)	▸ *Very high:* EPS ▸ *Low:* Anticholinergic, sedation, hypotension	
Perphenazine	Trilafon	Tablet, liquid, injection, 8–64 mg/d	▸ *High:* EPS ▸ *Low:* Anticholinergic, sedation, hypotension	
Trifluoperazine	Stelazine	Tablet, injection, 5–80 mg/d	▸ *High:* EPS ▸ *Low:* Anticholinergic, sedation, hypotension	
Haloperidol	Haldol	Tablet, liquid, injection, 2–40 mg/d, 50–300 mg IM, every month (decanoate)	▸ *Very high:* EPS ▸ *High:* Anticholinergic, sedation ▸ *Low:* hypotension	▸ In older adults, monitor for oculogyric crisis and pneumonia
Loxapine	Loxitane	Capsule, liquid/ 20–250/d	▸ *High:* EPS ▸ *Moderate:* Sedation, hypotension ▸ *Low:* Anticholinergic	
Molindone	Moban	Tablet, liquid, 50–225 mg/d	▸ *High:* EPS ▸ *Low:* Anticholinergic, hypotension ▸ *Very low:* sedation	▸ Less or no weight gain
Thiothixene	Navane	Capsule, liquid, injection/5–60 mg/d	▸ *High:* EPS ▸ *Low:* Anticholinergic, sedation, hypotension	

TABLE 10-7. MEDICATIONS USED TO TREAT EPSE SYMPTOMS

EFFECTIVE DRUG AND CROSS-CLASSIFICATION	AKINESIA	AKATHISIA	DYSTONIA	PSEUDO-PARKINSON'S	TARDIVE DYSKINESIA
Cogentin (benztropine) 0.5 mg-2 mg p.o. t.i.d. *Anticholinergic*	X	X	X	X	▶ Best treatment strategy is prevention through careful monitoring
Kemadrin (procyclidine) 2.5-0.5 mg p.o. b.i.d.-q.i.d. *Anticholinergic*	X	X	X	X	
Artane (trihexyphenidyl) 2-5 mg p.o. t.i.d. *Anticholinergic*	X	X	X	X	▶ If present, treat by reducing current dose, or change client to atypical agent
Benadryl (diphenhydramine) 25 mg p.o. q.i.d. *Antihistamine*	X		X	X	
Symmetrel (amantadine) 100-200 mg p.o. b.i.d.: *Dopamine agonist*	X			X	
Inderal (propranolol) 20-40 mg p.o. t.i.d. *Beta blocker*		X			
Catapres (clonidine) 0.1 mg p.o. t.i.d. *Alpha 2 agonist*		X			
Klonopin (clonazepam) 1 mg p.o. b.i.d. *Benzodiazepine*		X	X		
Ativan (lorazepam) 1 mg p.o. t.i.d. *Benzodiazepine*		X	X		

► Other common side effects related to effects on receptors other than dopamine:

  ▸ Alpha adrenergic blockade

    ▷ Cardiovascular side effects

    ▷ Orthostatic hypotension

  ▸ Muscarinic cholinergic blockade

    ▷ Dry mouth

    ▷ Blurred vision

    ▷ Constipation

    ▷ Urinary retention

  ▸ Endocrine side effects

    ▷ Weight gain

    ▷ Increased prolactin levels

  ▸ Neurological side effects

    ▷ Lowering of seizure threshold

  ▸ Other side effects

    ▷ Photosensitivity

    ▷ Agranulocytosis

► Group therapy

  ▸ Focuses on problem-solving

  ▸ Focuses on education

    ▷ Medication groups

    ▷ Life skills groups

► Proactive crisis management planning to deal with potential relapse needs

  ▸ Identify symptom triggers.

  ▸ Identify symptoms that indicate relapse.

  ▸ Identify past pattern of relapse to help predict future relapses.

  ▸ Identify self-care interventions.

  ▸ Identify point at which professional intervention is required.

  ▸ Identify support network of family and friends.

  ▸ Identify other resources to be mobilized when symptom level increases.

  ▸ Assertive community treatment (ACT)

    ▷ Evidence-based case management program

    ▷ Multidisciplinary treatment team

- Illness management recovery (IMR)
    - Evidence-based recovery program
- Education modules
    - Recovery strategies, information on mental illness, building supports, using medication, drugs and alcohol, coping, reducing relapse, mental health system, advocacy, and stress-vulnerability model (Whitley, Gingerick, Lutz, & Mueser, 2009).
- Milieu therapy
    - Provides for structure and safety needs
    - Provides socialization and interpersonal support
    - Encourages independency
- Patient and family education
    - Explain underlying pathology of illness.
    - Discuss signs and symptoms.
    - Assist in identifying strategies for living with illness.
    - Assist in understanding and making decisions about care options.
    - Develop relapse prevention plan.
    - Promote overall health.

Common Comorbidities

- Rates of substance abuse and dependency are high.
    - 20%–40% comorbidity
- Nicotine dependence is especially high.
    - 80%–90% comorbidity
    - Tend to use cigarettes with highest nicotine content
    - Drug interaction with antipsychotic medications
- May need to reduce doses when patient quits or cuts back.
- Other common psychiatric comorbidities are anxiety disorders (see Chapter 9), especially panic disorder and obsessive–compulsive disorder.

Special Considerations

- Schizophrenia is significantly associated with shorter-than-expected life span when compared to the general population.
- Persons with a severe mental illness (SMI) prematurely die 10–25 years earlier as compared to the general population.
    - Reasons are unclear but may include overall general lack of routine health care and high levels of comorbidity (see below).

▶ Suicide

  ▸ Suicide rates are high; assess for suicidal ideations at every visit.

  ▸ 10% commit suicide.

  ▸ 20%–40% attempt suicide.

  ▸ Known risk factors for suicide include

    ▷ Male gender

    ▷ Ages 45 or younger

    ▷ Presence of depressive symptoms

    ▷ Hopelessness

    ▷ Unemployed

    ▷ Noncompliance

    ▷ Recent hospitalization

    ▷ Postpsychotic period

    ▷ Comorbid substance abuse

▶ General medical illnesses

  ▸ Patients need access to ongoing primary care.

  ▸ Monitor patient for development of metabolic syndrome, diabetes, hypertension, hyperlipidemia, respiratory illnesses, and cardiac illnesses.

    ▷ Monitor weight gain, lipids, and blood glucose

    ▷ Provide weight management and nutritional assistance.

    ▷ Use body mass index (BMI) as the accepted standard for determining if a patient's weight places him or her at risk of developing serious health problems.

    ▷ BMI categories

      ▸ *Underweight:* less than BMI 18.5

      ▸ *Normal weight:* BMI 18.5–24.9

      ▸ *Overweight:* BMI 25.0–29.9

      ▸ *Obese:* BMI 30.0–39.9

      ▸ *Severely obese:* BMI 40 and higher

  ▸ Risks related to BMI

    ▷ Clients who are overweight to obese as determined by BMI have

      ▸ 2.9 times increased risk for diabetes

      ▸ 2.9 times increased risk for hypertension

      ▸ 2.1 times increased risk of coronary artery disease

      ▸ 3.0 times increased risk for endometrial cancer

      ▸ 2.7 times increased risk for colon cancer

Special Considerations

- ► Children
  - ▸ Hallucinatory and delusional content less rich, elaborate, and bizarre
  - ▸ Visual hallucinations more common than auditory
- ► Older adults
  - ▸ More women than men with rare late onset
  - ▸ Although exhibiting prodromal social isolation, are more often married
  - ▸ Prognosis usually better; more responsive to medications due to dominance of positive symptom cluster (see below)
  - ▸ All atypical antipsychotic medications have a black box warning: increase in mortality in elderly patients with dementia-related psychosis
  - ▸ Risk factors
    - ▹ Postmenopausal states
    - ▹ Presence of human leukocyte antigen
    - ▹ Positive family history
  - ▸ Symptoms
    - ▹ Predominance of positive symptoms
    - ▹ High levels of persecutory delusions and hallucinations
    - ▹ Lower levels of disorganized behavior
    - ▹ Preservation of social and occupational interest
    - ▹ Fewer negative symptoms.

Follow-up

- ► Chronic illness
  - ▸ Usually requires lifelong treatment
  - ▸ Case management necessary to coordinate aspects of care
- ► Relapse periods
  - ▸ Develop relapse plan with patient and family.
- ► Multiple health needs
  - ▸ Perform frequent assessment of general health status.
  - ▸ Address comorbid nicotine addiction.
- ► Preventative care
  - ▸ Monitor routine labs to screen for complications of treatment:

- ▶ Serum glucose and lipid panels
  - ▹ Weight, body mass index
  - ▹ Liver and kidney function (based on medication)
  - ▹ Complete blood count
  - ▹ American Diabetes Association, American Psychiatric Association, American Association of Clinical Endocrinologists, and North American Association for the Study of Obesity Guidelines (2004)
  - ▹ Perform annual eye exam if on typical antipsychotic agent or Seroquel
- ▶ Clinical outcome measures
  - ▹ Standardized rating scales include
    - ▷ Positive and Negative Syndrome Scale (PANNS; Kay & Fiszbein, 1987)
    - ▷ Brief Psychiatric Rating Scale (BPRS; Overall & Gorham, 1962)
    - ▷ Scale for Assessment of Positive Symptoms (SAPS; Andreason & Olsen 1982)
    - ▷ Scale for Assessment of Negative Symptoms (SANS; Andreason, 1982).

SCHIZOPHRENIFORM DISORDER

Description
- ▶ Closely resembles schizophrenia
- ▶ Two differences from schizophrenia:
  - ▹ Total duration of the illness is at least 1 month but less than 6 months, including prodromal, active illness period and residual symptom phase
  - ▹ Does not require for diagnosis that there be impaired social or occupational functioning, although may be present.

Etiology
- ▶ Similar to schizophrenia

Risk Factors
- ▶ Similar to schizophrenia

Assessment

History

▶ Assess for the following:

    ▸ Two or more of the following frequently present during a 1-month period

        ▷ Delusions

        ▷ Hallucinations

        ▷ Disorganized speech

        ▷ Grossly disorganized behavior

        ▷ Presence of negative symptoms

    ▸ Duration of symptoms for at least 1 month and for no longer than 6 months

    ▸ Almost all information provided for schizophrenia pertains to this disorder, except

        ▷ Occurs much less often than schizophrenia; incidence is 0.03% of general U.S. population

        ▷ Approximately one-third recover completely within 6 months

        ▷ Remaining two-thirds develop schizophrenia or schizoaffective disorder (see below).

Physical Exam

▶ Similar to schizophrenia

Mental Status Exam

▶ Similar to schizophrenia

Diagnostic Studies

▶ Similar to schizophrenia

Management

▶ Similar to schizophrenia

▶ Assess for acuity level

▶ During acute psychotic or affective episodes, patient may require brief hospitalization to

    ▸ Ensure patient safety

    ▸ Rapidly stabilize patient's symptom level in a controlled environment

    ▸ Ensure patient compliance with treatment to reach stabilization

        ▷ Clinical management during nonacute episodes occurs most often in community settings.

Pharmacologic Treatment

▶ Similar to schizophrenia

Nonpharmacologic Treatment

▶ Similar to schizophrenia

Follow-up

▶ Similar to schizophrenia

SCHIZOAFFECTIVE DISORDER

Description

▶ An uninterrupted period of illness in which the person experiences psychotic symptoms similar to those seen in schizophrenia as well as mood symptoms similar to major depressive disorder (MDD) or bipolar (BP) disorder (see Chapter 8).

Assessment

History

▶ Assess for the following:

- Symptoms of schizophrenia—two or more of the following frequently present during a 1-month period:
  - ▷ Delusions
  - ▷ Hallucinations
  - ▷ Disorganized speech
  - ▷ Grossly disorganized behavior
  - ▷ Presence of negative symptoms but usually less severe than those in schizophrenia
- Symptoms of one or more of mood disorders (see Chapter 8):
  - ▷ Major depressive episode
  - ▷ Manic episode
  - ▷ Mixed-mood episode
- Presence of delusions or hallucinations for at least 2 weeks in the absence of prominent mood symptoms.
- Subtypes
  - ▷ Two subtypes differentiated by type of mood-related symptoms:
    - *Depressive*: When prominent mood symptoms are of the depressive type only
    - *Bipolar*: When predominant mood symptoms are manic or mixed type

Physical Exam
▶ Similar to schizophrenia

Mental Status
▶ Similar to schizophrenia

Diagnostic Studies
▶ Similar to schizophrenia

Management

Pharmacologic Treatment
▶ Similar to schizophrenia

▶ Similar to MDD or BP disorder (see Chapter 8).

Nonpharmacologic Treatment
▶ Similar to schizophrenia

▶ Similar to MDD or BP disorder (see Chapter 8).

Follow-up
▶ Similar to schizophrenia

▶ Similar to MDD or BP disorder (see Chapter 8)

DELUSIONAL DISORDER

Description
▶ Presence of 1 or more nonbizarre delusions lasting for at least 1 month

▶ Psychosocial functioning and daily behavior not at all impaired except as they surround content of delusion

▶ Seldom any other symptoms; in rare cases may have hallucinations or mood disturbances.

Assessment

History
▶ Assess for the following

  ▹ Presence of delusions

    ▷ Well-organized and potentially believable

    ▷ Any unusual behavior is explainable if content of delusion understood

- Subtypes (categorized by thematic content of delusion)
  - Erotomanic
    - Delusional content focused on false belief that another person is in love with the patient
    - Usually focused on idealized or spiritual love and only infrequently has strong sexual content
    - Focus of love usually famous or powerful person who does not usually know the patient
    - In rare cases, the person may know patient
    - Leads to obsessive behaviors such as surveillance or stalking
  - Grandiose
    - Delusional content focuses on the patient having some great talent, skill, or knowledge
    - May have strong religious component, such as prophecy or deity connections (special connection to God)
  - Jealous
    - Delusional content focuses on false belief that patient's spouse or partner is being unfaithful with someone else
    - Belief has no connection with realistic evidence
    - Usually seen in men
    - Patient may try to control behavior of spouse or partner in an attempt to prevent imagined infidelities.
  - Persecutory
    - Delusional content focuses on patients' belief that others are out to harm them, spy on them, or otherwise do them harm
    - Often angry and hostile at perceived persecution
  - Somatic
    - Delusional content focuses on bodily functions and sensations
    - Often belief that a body part is infected, absent, omits a strange odor, or is misshapen or malformed
  - Mixed
    - No clear predominant theme for the delusional content
- Related symptoms that can be present but are not required for diagnosis include
  - May become depressed over protracted problems with thematic content
  - May become involved in legal difficulties related to behaviors based on delusional content
  - May be subjected to or request unnecessary medical tests and procedures.

Physical Exam
► Nonspecific

Mental Status Exam
► Normal except for delusions
   ▹ Abstraction
      ▹ May be concrete on proverbs during delusional episodes
   ▹ Thought process
      ▹ Presence of delusions
      ▹ Perseveration on topics related to delusion
   ▹ Thought content
      ▹ Thematic for type of delusion

Diagnostic Studies
► Nonspecific

Management

Pharmacologic Treatment
► Similar to schizophrenia

Nonpharmacologic Treatment
► Similar to schizophrenia

BRIEF PSYCHOTIC DISORDER

Description
► Disorder with sudden onset of psychotic symptoms lasting at least 1 day but less than a month

Assessment

History
► Assess for the following:
   ▹ Age of onset in adolescence or early adulthood
   ▹ Positive-type psychotic symptoms:
      ▹ Delusions
      ▹ Hallucinations

▷ Grossly disorganized behavior

▷ Disorganized speech

» Can occur with or without identified stressor

» Patient always returns to premorbid level of functioning

Physical Exam

► Nonspecific

Mental Status Exam

► Similar to schizophrenia

Diagnostic Studies

► Nonspecific

Management

Pharmacologic Treatment

► Similar to schizophrenia

Nonpharmacologic Treatment

► Similar to schizophrenia

► Acute episode requires frequent monitoring for safety needs because of the following:

» Confusion

» Rapid shifting in emotions

» Impaired judgment

» Inability to meet nutritional and hygiene needs.

SHARED PSYCHOTIC DISORDER (FOLIE Á DEUX)

Description

► Characterized by development of a delusion in a patient who has a close relationship with another person who already has a psychotic disorder with a prominent delusion

Assessment

History

▶ Assess for the following:

  ▶ Patient in close contact with an individual who already has a delusion and

   ▷ That a person usually has schizophrenia.

   ▷ That person usually is the dominant person in the relationship.

   ▷ That individual gradually imposes his or her delusion on the patient.

   ▷ Usually the relationship is long-term and very close.

  ▶ Aside from the delusional content, the patient's behavior is otherwise normal.

Physical Exam

▶ Nonspecific

Mental Status Exam

▶ Similar to schizophrenia

  ▶ Diagnostic and laboratory findings

▶ Nonspecific

Management

Pharmacologic Treatment

▶ Similar to schizophrenia

Nonpharmacologic Treatment

▶ Similar to schizophrenia

▶ Chronic disease course

▶ Poor prognosis if relationship continues, especially if person with delusion goes untreated.

▶ Good prognosis if the patient can be separated from the person with the delusion.

CASE STUDY

Jim is a 28-year-old patient newly diagnosed with schizophrenia. He initially experienced a psychotic episode while serving in the military and now is living at home with his parents. Jim is still reluctant to accept his diagnosis and continues to believe that he "got bad weed" in the service and that he will be fine once the weed is out of his body. He has not been adherent with treatment, and his parents are threatening to evict him from the house if he does not start accepting treatment.

Jim has a history of juvenile-onset diabetes and has struggled to maintain a diabetic diet and to control his weight. When asked to identify his current goals, Jim will state only that he wishes to find a good wife and settle down to a normal life. There are many issues to consider in planning care with this patient.

► What is the top priority for the psychiatric–mental health nurse practitioner (PMHNP)?

► What medications are reasonable to consider for the patient at this time?

► What is the relationship between his diabetes and schizophrenia?

► How will his comorbid illness affect your care planning?

► What routine ongoing monitoring will he require?

REFERENCES

American Diabetes Association, American Psychiatric Association, American Association of Clinical Endocrinologists, & North American Association for the Study of Obesity. (2004). Consensus development conference on antipsychotic drugs and obesity and diabetes. *Diabetes Care, 27(2)*, 596–601.

American Psychiatric Association. (2000). *Diagnostic and statistical manual of mental disorders* (4th ed., text rev.). Washington, DC: American Psychiatric Association.

Andreason, N. C. (1982). Negative symptoms in schizophrenia: Definition and reliability. *Archives of General Psychiatry, 39(7)*, 784–788.

Andreason, N. C., & Olsen, S. (1982). Negative vs. positive schizophrenia: Definition and validity. *Archives of General Psychiatry, 39(7)*, 789–794.

Brzustowicz, L. M., Hodgkinson, K. A., Chow, E. W. C., Honer, W. G., & Bassett, A. S. (2000). Location of a major susceptibility locus for familial schizophrenia on chromosome 1q21-q22. *Science, 288*, 678–682.

Dolder, C. R., Lacro, J., Dunn, L., & Jeste, D. (2002). Antipsychotic medication adherence: Is there a difference between typical and atypical agents? *American Journal of Psychiatry, 159*, 103–108.

Gershon, E. S., & Badner, J. A. (2001). Progress towards discovery of susceptibility genes for bipolar manic-depressive illness and schizophrenia. *CNS Spectrums, 6*, 965–977.

Guy, W. (n.d.). *ECDEU assessment manual for psychopharmacology* (rev. ed.). Washington, DC: U.S. Department of Health and Human Welfare.

Harkavy-Friedman, J., & Nelson, E. (1997). Management of the suicidal patient with schizophrenia. *Psychiatric Clinics of North America, 20*, 625–629.

Harrop, C. E. (2002). The development of schizophrenia for late-life adolescence. *Current Psychiatric Reports, 4*, 293–298.

Heinssen, R. K., Perkins, R., Appelbaum, P., & Fenton, W. (2001). Informed consent in early psychosis. *Schizophrenia Bulletin, 27*, 571–584.

Heresco-Levy, U., Javitt, D. C., Ermilov, M., Mordel, C., Silipo, G., & Liechtenstein, M. (1999). Efficacy of high-dose glycine in the treatment of enduring negative symptoms of schizophrenia. *Archives of General Psychiatry, 56*, 29–36.

Herz, M., Lamberti, S., Mintz, J., Scott, R., O'Dell, S., McCartan, L., & Nix, G. (2000). A program for relapse prevention in schizophrenia. *Archives of General Psychiatry, 57*, 277–283.

Kay, S. R., & Fiszbein, A. (1987). The positive and negative syndrome scale for schizophrenia. *Schizophrenia Bulletin, 13*, 261–275.

Lencz, T., Bilder, R. M., & Cornblatt, B. (2001). The timing of neurodevelopmental abnormality in schizophrenia: An integrative review of the neuroimaging literature. *CNS Spectrums, 6*, 233–253.

Lewis, D. A., & Lieberman, J. A. (2000). Catching up on schizophrenia: Natural history and neurobiology. *Neuron, 28*, 325–334.

Lindsay, H. (2000). Neurodevelopment of schizophrenia reveled. *Clinical Psychiatric News, 3*, 34–39.

Lyon, E. (1999). A review of the effects of nicotine on schizophrenia and antipsychotic medications. *Psychiatric Services, 50*, 1346–1349.

Mathalon, D. H., Sullivan, E., Lim, K. & Pfefferbaum, A. (2001). Progressive brain volume changes and the clinical course of schizophrenia in men. *Archives of General Psychiatry, 58*, 148–157.

Newcomer, J. W., Haupt, D., Fucetola, R., Melson, A., Schweiser, J., Cooper, B., & Selke, G. (2002). Abnormalities in glucose regulation during antipsychotic treatment of schizophrenia. *Archives of General Psychiatry, 59,* 337–345.

Overall, J. E., & Gorham, D. R. (1962). The brief psychiatric rating scale. *Psychological Reports, 10,* 790–812.

Rector, N. A., & Beck, A. (2002). A clinical review of cognitive therapy for schizophrenia. *Current Psychiatric Reports, 4,* 284–292.

Richardson, C., Faulkner, G., McDevitt, J., Skrinar, G., Hutchinson, D., & Piette, J. (2005). Integrating physical activity into mental health services for persons with serious mental illness. *Psychiatric Services, 56*(3), 324–331.

Sable, J. A. (2002). Antipsychotic treatment for late-life schizophrenia. *Current Psychiatric Reports, 4,* 299–306.

Staal, W. G., Hulshoff Pol, H., Schnack, G., van Haren, N.E., Seifert, N. & Kahn, R. (2001). Structural brain abnormalities in chronic schizophrenia at the extremes of the outcome spectrum. *American Journal of Psychiatry, 158,* 1140–1142.

Stahl, S. M. (2011). The prescriber's guide Stahl's essential psychopharmacology (4th ed.). New York: Cambridge University Press.

Tamminga, C. (2001). Treating schizophrenia now and developing strategies for the next decade. *CNS Spectrums, 6,* 987–991.

Tandon, R., & Jibson, M. D. (2001). Pharmacologic treatment of schizophrenia: What the future holds. *CNS Spectrums, 6,* 980–986.

U.S. Food and Drug Administration/Protecting and Promoting Your Health. (2013). *FDA Drug Safety Communication: FDA is investigating two deaths following injection of long-acting antipsychotic Zyprexa Relprevv (olanzapine pamoate).* Retrieved from www.fda.gov/Drugs/DrugSafety/ucm356971.htm

Walker, A. (2000). The family and schizophrenia. *Issues in Mental Health Nursing, 21,* 27–31.

Whitley, R., Gingerich, S., Lutz, W, & Mueser, K. (2009). Implementing the illness management and recovery program in community mental health settings: Facilitators and barriers. *Psychiatric Services, 60*(2), 202–209.

CHAPTER 11

DELIRIUM, DEMENTIA, AND OTHER COGNITIVE DISORDERS

Cognitive disorders often are thought of as disorders of older adults. Although most common in this population, cognitive disorders can occur at any age. Very young or very old people with cognitive disorders have multiple health needs. Older adult patients usually have more than one chronic illness, and psychiatric disorders can be accompanied by other comorbidities.

Psychiatric–mental health nurse practitioners (PMHNPs) must approach patients with cognitive disorders by conducting a multisystem assessment.

COGNITIVE DISORDERS

Description
▶ Cognitive disorders cause a clinically significant deficit in cognition that represents a major change from the person's previous baseline level of functioning.
▶ Two common disorders are
  ▹ Delirium
  ▹ Dementia

Etiology
▶ Cognitive disorders are a complex general medical condition resulting in changes in multiple domains, including memory, interpersonal relationships, and behavior. Cognitive disorders can result from substance use or abuse, a reaction to medications or other ingested agents, or a combination of some or all of these factors.

DELIRIUM

Description

▶ Delirium is a syndrome and not a disease, with an acute onset that causes short-term changes in cognition.

▶ The hallmark symptom is a disturbance of consciousness accompanied by changes in cognition.

▶ Delirium is not caused by current medical condition(s).

▶ Subtypes of delirium

  ▸ Hyperactive: Agitated, restless, hyperalert

  ▸ Hypoactive: Lethargic, slowed, apathetic

  ▸ Mixed: Cycles between hyperactive and hypoactive

Incidence and Demographics

▶ Common, especially in older adults

▶ Often overlooked and mistaken for other medical conditions or dementia

▶ In persons with psychiatric disorders, often mistaken for worsening of psychotic symptoms instead of a distinct condition

▶ Prevalence varies based on age, patient setting, and sample

  ▸ 0.4% in general U.S. population ages 18 years or older

  ▸ 1% to 2% in those ages 65 or older

  ▸ 14% to 56% of hospitalized patients

  ▸ 1.4% to 70.3% of patients in long-term care

  ▸ 25% in clients with cancer

  ▸ 40% in hospitalized patients with AIDS

  ▸ 80% in terminal patients nearing death

  ▸ Poor prognosis

    ▷ 1 year mortality rate of patients with delirium is up to 50%

Risk Factors

▶ Advancing age

▶ Multisystem medical illness

  ▸ The more physically ill the patient, the higher the risk.

▶ Substance abuse

▶ Visual or hearing impairment

▶ Past episode of delirium or preexisting brain disorder or cognitive impairment

Prevention and Screening

- ► At-risk family education
- ► Community education
    - ▸ Stigma reduction
    - ▸ Signs and symptoms of illness
    - ▸ Treatment potential for control of symptoms
- ► Use of the Confusion Assessment Method (CAM) instrument
- ► Early recognition, intervention, and initiation of treatment
    - ▸ Whenever a patient's clinical presentation changes rapidly from baseline, consider delirium as one possible differential diagnosis.

Assessment

History

- ► Assess for the following:
    - ▸ Key findings
        - ▷ Disturbance of consciousness develops over a short time, usually hours to days.
        - ▷ This disturbance tends to fluctuate during the day.
    - ▸ Sleep–rest cycle disturbances
        - ▷ Reversal of the sleep–wake cycle is common: patients are awake at night and sleep during the day.
    - ▸ Impaired recent and intermediate memory
    - ▸ Psychomotor agitation
        - ▷ The patient exhibits purposeless, random actions.
- ► Course of illness may resolve within hours to days
    - ▸ The more quickly the underlying physiological disturbance is recognized and treated, the more rapidly the delirium will resolve.
    - ▸ Symptoms, when unrecognized, may persist for months.
    - ▸ Most symptoms resolve within 3 to 6 months.

Physical Exam

- ► Evidence that significant clinical symptoms are a consequence of direct physiological processes, substance use or abuse, or general medical condition
- ► Usually nonspecific neurological abnormalities
    - ▸ Tremors
    - ▸ Incoordination

- Urinary incontinence
- Myoclonus
- Nystagmus
- Asterixis—a flapping motion of the wrists
- Increased muscle tone and reflex

Mental Status Exam

- ► General appearance
  - Unconcerned with appearance
  - Disheveled
  - Highly inattentive
- ► Speech
  - Impaired
  - Disorganized
  - Rambling
  - Incoherent
  - Slurred
- ► Affect
  - Rapid, unpredictable shifts in affective state without known precipitation
    - ▷ Lethargic
    - ▷ Agitated
- ► Mood
  - Difficult to elicit from patient
- ► Thought process
  - Disorganized
  - Distractible
  - Perceptual disturbances
    - ▷ Illusions most common
    - ▷ Hallucinations are typically visual and accompanied by illusions
- ► Thought process and content
  - Disorganized, distorted thought
  - Delusions and hallucinations are common.
- ► Orientation
  - Disorientation is usually the first symptom to appear
  - Patient usually disoriented to time and place

DELIRIUM, DEMENTIA, AND OTHER COGNITIVE DISORDERS **287**

► Memory

  ▸ Impaired recent and immediate memory

► Concentration

  ▸ Grossly impaired

► Abstraction

  ▸ Grossly impaired

► Judgment

  ▸ Grossly impaired

Diagnostic Studies

► Findings consistent with underlying physiological etiology

► Workup includes standard tests

  ▸ Blood chemistry

  ▸ Complete blood count

  ▸ Thyroid function tests

  ▸ Syphilis

  ▸ Human immunodeficiency antibody test

  ▸ Urinalysis

  ▸ Chest radiograph

  ▸ Serum or urine drug screen

► EEG abnormalities

  ▸ Generalized slowing

  ▸ Generalized increased activity if delirium is related to alcohol withdrawal

Differential Diagnosis

► Dementia (see below)

► Substance intoxication or withdrawal (see Chapter 12)

► Schizophrenia (see Chapter 10)

► Schizophreniform disorder (see Chapter 10)

► Mood disorders with psychotic features (see Chapter 8)

Management

► Undertake treatment of underlying condition or disorder.

► Avoid the use of new medications whenever possible, because using them can cloud the diagnostic picture.

Pharmacologic Treatment

► Symptomatic treatment

► Agitation and psychotic symptoms

  ▹ Antipsychotic agents

    ▷ Haloperidol (Haldol)

    ▷ Atypical antipsychotic agents

    ▷ Anxiolytic agents for insomnia

Nonpharmacologic Treatment

► Monitor for safety needs.

► Determine reality orientation frequently.

► Pay attention to basic needs:

  ▹ Hydration

  ▹ Nutrition

► Patient should be neither sensory-deprived nor overstimulated.

► It is helpful to have in the patient's room familiar people, familiar pictures or decorations, and a clock or calendar; regular orientation to person, place, or time.

Special Considerations

► Delirium is associated with high morbidity and mortality.

► High morbidity results from injury or is associated problems related to inactivity:

  ▹ Pneumonia

  ▹ Hydration and nutritional deficits

► Safety concerns exist

► Mnemonic DELIRIUM (Dick & Morency, 2011)

  ▹ **D**rugs

  ▹ **E**lectrolyte abnormality

  ▹ **L**ow oxygen saturation

  ▹ **I**nfection

  ▹ **R**educed sensory input

  ▹ **I**ntracranial

  ▹ **U**rinary or renal retention

  ▹ **M**yocardial

DELIRIUM, DEMENTIA, AND OTHER COGNITIVE DISORDERS **289**

► Children

  ▸ Especially susceptible

  ▸ Related to immature brain development

  ▸ Often mistaken for uncooperative behavior

    ▷ If a child is not soothed by common methods (e.g., parental presence), delirium is suspected.

      ▸ Most common in febrile states

      ▸ Medications known to affect cognition

  ▸ Especially common with anticholinergic medications

► Older adults

  ▸ Susceptibility related to physiological changes of aging

  ▸ Older men more prone than older women for unknown reasons

DEMENTIA

Description

► Dementia is a group of disorders characterized by gradual development of multiple cognitive deficits:

  ▸ Impaired executive functioning

  ▸ Impaired global intellect with preservation of level of consciousness

  ▸ Impaired problem-solving

  ▸ Impaired organizational skills

  ▸ Altered memory

► Various forms of dementia share common symptoms but have different underlying pathology.

► Dementia of Alzheimer's type (DAT)

  ▸ Most common type

  ▸ Gradual onset and progressive decline without focal neurological deficits

  ▸ Hallmark amyloid deposits and neurofibrillary tangles.

► Vascular dementia (VD)

  ▸ Second most common type

  ▸ Formerly called *multi-infarct dementia*

  ▸ Primarily caused by cardiovascular disease and characterized by step-type declines

  ▸ Most common in men with preexisting high blood pressure and cardiovascular risk factors

290 PSYCHIATRIC–MENTAL HEALTH NURSE PRACTITIONER REVIEW MANUAL, 3RD EDITION

- Hallmarks carotid bruits, fundoscopic abnormalities, and enlarged cardiac chambers

▶ Dementia due to HIV disease

- Classified as a subcortical dementia
- Parenchymal abnormalities visualized on MRI scan
- HIV-associated neurocognitive disorder or HIV encephalopathy are less severe forms
- HIV can cause many psychiatric symptoms
- Manifests by progressive cognitive decline, motor abnormalities, and behavioral abnormalities
- Co-occurs with obsessive–compulsive disorder, posttraumatic stress disorder, generalized anxiety disorder, depression, and mania
- Development of dementia in patient with HIV is an indicator of poor prognosis; death usually occurs within 6 months
- Psychotic symptoms usually occur in late-stage infection
- Clinical signs of late-stage HIV-related dementia include cognitive, motor, behavioral, and affective impairment:
  ▷ Global cognitive impairment
  ▷ Mutism
  ▷ Seizures
  ▷ Hallucinations
  ▷ Delusions
  ▷ Apathy
  ▷ Mania
- Antiretrovirals and protease inhibitors can interact with psychotropic medications, because many are metabolized by the P450 system or are CYP3A4 inhibitors. Therefore, prescribing psychotropic medications in this patient population should be done with caution while monitoring for drug interactions.

▶ Pick's disease

- Also known as *frontotemporal dementia*
- Neuronal loss, gliosis, and Pick's bodies present
- More common in men
- Personality and behavioral changes in early stage
- Cognitive changes in later stages
- Kluver–Bucy syndrome: hypersexuality, hyperorality, and placidity

▶ Creutzfeldt–Jakob disease

- Fatal and rapidly progressive disorder

- Occurs mainly in adults in middle age or older
- Initially manifests with fatigue, flulike symptoms, and cognitive impairment
- Later manifests with aphasia, apraxia, emotional lability, depression, mania, psychosis, marked personality changes, and dementia
- Death usually occurs within 6 months.

▶ Huntington's disease
- Subcortical type of dementia
- Characterized mostly by motor abnormalities (e.g., choreoathetoid movements)
- Psychomotor slowing and difficulty with complex tasks
- Memory, language, and insight usually intact until late stages
- High incidence of depression and psychosis

▶ Lewy body disease
- Caused by Lewy inclusion bodies in the cortex
- Presents with recurrent visual hallucinations
- Parkinson features (bradykinesia, cogwheel rigidity, tremor)
- Adversely react to antipsychotics

Etiology
▶ Multiple theories ranging from psychological to neurobiological
- Probable multifactorial etiological profile

▶ Primary causes mostly unknown

▶ General medical condition, result of substance use or abuse, reaction to medications or other ingested agents, or combination of some or all of these factors

▶ Diffuse cerebral atrophy and enlarged ventricles in DAT

▶ Decreased acetylcholine (Ach) and norepinephrine in DAT

▶ Genetic loading
- Genes on chromosomes 1, 14, and 21 have been identified in families with a history of DAT
- Autosomal dominant trait
- Inherited alleles for apolipoprotein E4 (APOE4) on chromosome 19 are suspected to be related to late-onset dementia.

Incidence and Demographics

▶ Often misdiagnosed or unrecognized, especially in early stages and in young patients

▶ Prevalence of 1.6% for people in the United States ages 65 or older

  ▸ 16% to 25% in people ages 85 or older

▶ DAT the most common

  ▸ Affects an estimated 4 million in the United States

  ▸ Duration of illness averages 8 to 10 years

Risk Factors

▶ Age

▶ Multisystem medical illnesses

▶ Genetic loading

  ▸ Family history of dementia in first-order relative

▶ History of substance use or abuse

Prevention and Screening

▶ At-risk family education

▶ Community education

  ▸ Stigma reduction

  ▸ Signs and symptoms of illness

  ▸ Treatment potential for control of symptoms

▶ Early recognition, intervention, and initiation of treatment

  ▸ Allows for ruling out age-related memory changes or unidentified conditions

  ▸ Cognitive and functional evaluation at least every 3 years for people ages 65 or older

  ▸ Baseline and regular cognitive evaluation to monitor cognitive decline and treatment response to medications in persons diagnosed with dementia

▶ Routine screening in primary care not recommended (USPSTF, 2003).

Assessment

History

▶ Assess for the following:

  ▸ Detailed history of present illness, including time frame, progression, and associated symptoms

  ▸ Past medical history of hypertension, strokes, head trauma, and psychiatric illness

  ▸ Psychiatric history of depression, anxiety, and schizophrenia

DELIRIUM, DEMENTIA, AND OTHER COGNITIVE DISORDERS 293

- Social history, including present living situation; marital status; occupation; education; and alcohol, tobacco, or illicit drug use

- Medications, including prescription, over-the-counter, herbals, supplements, and home remedies

- Initial and periodic functional history and assessment

- Validate history with family or caregiver

► Memory impairment immediate and intermediate

- Most prominent feature of disorder

- Usually earliest symptom

- Produces multiple deficits in daily functioning

  ▷ Unable to learn new information

  ▷ Forgets past information

  ▷ Loses valuables

  ▷ Forgets daily activities like eating and dressing

  ▷ Becomes easily lost

  ▷ Has other cognitive deficits such as impaired executive functioning

► Instruments for assessing level of impairment

- Mini-Mental State Examination (MMSE, not in public domain; Crum, Anthony, Bassett, & Folstein, 1993)

- Montreal Cognitive Assessment (MoCA)

  ▷ In public domain

- Mini-Cog

► Remember to always consider visual, sensory, language, physical disabilities, and education when administering mental status tests.

Physical Exam

► *Amaurosis fugax*: Unilateral transient vision loss, described as "curtain over eye"

► Unilateral focal–motor weakness

► Asymmetrical reflexes

Mental Status Exam

► General appearance

- Apraxia

- Decreased self-care activities of daily living.

► Speech

- Deterioration of language skills

- Aphasia
- Circumlocutory phrases
- Indefinite object recognition (such as calling items "things" and being unable to find discrete name)
- In advanced stages are
  - Mutism
  - Echolalia

▶ Affect
- Lability

▶ Mood
- Depressed
- Often difficult to elicit from patient

▶ Thought process
- Agnosia

▶ Thought content
- Difficult to elicit from patient

▶ Orientation
- Disoriented to time and place
- Disoriented to person in late stages of disorder.

▶ Memory
- Impaired in many dimensions of memory:
  - Word registration
  - Recall
  - Retention
  - Recognition

▶ Concentration
- Distractible

▶ Abstraction
- Concrete on proverb testing.

▶ Judgment
- Grossly impaired for self- and social judgment.

Diagnostic Studies

▶ CBC, chemistry profile, thyroid function tests, B_{12} level, and folate level to rule out metabolic causes or unidentified conditions

▶ Drug toxicity screening if indicated

▶ Alcohol and illicit drug screen if suspected or indicated

▶ Urinalysis if urinary tract infection suspected

▶ Arterial oxygen or pulse oximetry if hypoxemia suspected

▶ CT or MRI not routinely used

▶ EEG not useful

▶ Neuropsychological testing recommended to complete diagnostic assessment

Differential Diagnosis

▶ Nonpsychiatric

    ▸ Parkinson's disease

    ▸ Hearing loss

    ▸ B_{12} and folate deficiencies

    ▸ Trauma, especially with history of falls

    ▸ Hypothyroidism

    ▸ Infection

    ▸ Cerebrovascular accident

    ▸ Polypharmacy

    ▸ Alcohol intoxication

▶ Psychiatric

    ▸ Mood disorders (see Chapter 8)

    ▸ Delirium (see above)

    ▸ Anxiety disorders (see Chapter 9)

Management

▶ General considerations

    ▸ Rule out or treat any conditions that may contribute to cognitive impairment.

    ▸ Discontinue unnecessary medications, especially sedatives and hypnotics.

Pharmacologic Treatment

▶ Cognitive symptoms

    ▸ N-methyl D-aspartate glutamate receptor antagonists

    ▸ Prevent overexcitation of glutamate receptors and stabilize the neurodegenerative process

    ▸ Memantine (Namenda; 10 to 20 mg b.i.d.)

- ▷ May slow the degenerative process
- ▷ Promotes synaptic plasticity
- ▷ May be used in combination with cholinesterase inhibitors
- ► Cholinesterase inhibitors
  - ▷ May be initiated for mild to moderate Alzheimer's disease
  - ▷ Can lead to modest clinical improvement in some patients, with studies showing 2- to 3-point improvement in MSE testing
  - ▷ Treat only symptoms, slow loss of function, and may improve agitated behaviors
  - ▷ Do not prevent pathological progression of disease
  - ▷ Not effective in severe, end-stage disease
  - ▷ Should stop if side effects develop, usually nausea and vomiting
  - ▷ Commonly used agents:
    - ► Donepezil (Aricept; 5 to 10 mg/day; Stahl, 2011)
      - ▷ Approved for mild, moderate, and severe Alzheimer's disease
    - ► Nausea, diarrhea, vomiting, appetite and weight loss, abnormal dreams, insomnia, dizziness common
  - ▷ Rivastigmine tartrate (Exelon; 1.5 to 6 mg twice a day; increase gradually to avoid nausea)
    - ► Indicated for mild to moderate Alzheimer's disease and Parkinson's disease dementia (Stahl, 2011)
  - ▷ Transdermal: 9.5 mg once a day
    - ► Retitrate if a lapse in treatment occurs
- ► Psychosis and agitation
  - ► Try nonpharmacological therapies first.
  - ► Use antipsychotic agents for agitation or psychotic symptoms regularly.
  - ► Use lowest effective dose and attempt to wean periodically.
  - ► Antipsychotics may cause many side effects of significance in the older adult:
    - ▷ Extrapyramidal symptoms
    - ▷ Sedation
    - ▷ Postural hypotension
    - ▷ Anticholinergic side effects
  - ► Benzodiazepines may be used for treating anxiety or infrequent agitation.
    - ▷ Are not as effective as antipsychotics for severe symptoms (Jervis, 2002).

- ▶ Depression
  - ▹ Treat patients with depressive symptoms:
    - ▹ Depressed mood
    - ▹ Insomnia
    - ▹ Fatigue
    - ▹ Irritability
    - ▹ Appetite loss
- ▶ Use lowest effective dose
- ▶ Treat for 6 to 12 months, then attempt to taper; depression may reoccur and need to be treated as a chronic condition.
- ▶ Patients may have less depression as the dementia progresses and they become less aware of their circumstances.

Nonpharmacologic Management

- ▶ Educate patient and family about the illness, treatment, and community resources.
- ▶ Assist with long-term planning, including financial, legal, and advanced directives.
- ▶ Assess home and driving safety.
- ▶ Use behavioral therapy to identify causes of problem behaviors and changes to the environment to reduce the behavior.
- ▶ Use recreational therapy, art, and pet therapy to reduce agitation and promote normalized behavior.
- ▶ Use reminiscence therapy or life review to process through any unresolved issues and recollect the past.
- ▶ Maintain a simple daily routine for bathing, dressing, eating, toileting, and bedtime.
- ▶ Integrate cultural beliefs into the management of all patients with dementia (Cummings & Jeste, 1999).
- ▶ Psychotherapeutic approaches for HIV-related dementia
  - ▹ Major psychodynamic themes for people with HIV-related dementia are issues of guilt, self-esteem, and fear of dying.
  - ▹ Because the patient may not be able to give a complete and accurate history, family or friends should be questioned about any unusual behavior or mental status changes.
  - ▹ Changes in the level of activity, in interest in other people, or in personality are clues to an acute central nervous system disturbance.
  - ▹ Some changes are directly due to brain dysfunction, while other changes are due to psychological distress of a systemic problem—anxiety that the person is dying.
  - ▹ The spectrum of neuropsychiatric and neurological manifestations depends on the severity of immunosuppression.

298 PSYCHIATRIC–MENTAL HEALTH NURSE PRACTITIONER REVIEW MANUAL, 3RD EDITION

- Psychiatric disorders may preexist or result from HIV.
- Even subtle neurocognitive impairment can affect psychological coping.
- Neuropsychiatric disorders are much more prevalent in late-stage illness.

Special Considerations

▶ Primarily a disease of older adults but can occur in children

▶ Diagnosis based on impaired cognition; diagnoses not applicable until ages 4 to 6 years, when cognition can be fully assessed

- Dementia in children usually presents as deterioration in functioning, such as school performance or delay in normal development.

TRAUMATIC BRAIN INJURY (TBI) ASSOCIATED WITH MILITARY ACTION

Description

▶ May be described as mild, moderate, or severe

▶ Severity depends on length of loss of consciousness, degree of verbal and motor skills after injury, and duration of posttraumatic amnesia

▶ May result in a lifetime of impairments in behavioral, emotional, cognitive, and physical functioning

Etiology

▶ Brain injury resulting when the head is hit or violently shaken, such as from a blast or explosion.

Incidence and Demographics

▶ Estimated that 30% of returning soldiers have mild TBI

Risk Factors

▶ Combat duty exposing personnel to improvised explosive devices (IEDs) used by opposing factions

Prevention and Screening

▶ Mandatory postdeployment screening for all veterans returning from combat assignment

▶ The physically and emotionally traumatic environment in which they occur

▶ The potentially repetitive and cumulative nature of concussions sustained over a tour (or multiple tours) of combat duty

▶ The high incidence of comorbid mental health conditions

DELIRIUM, DEMENTIA, AND OTHER COGNITIVE DISORDERS 299

► The difficulty in following typical recommendations for postconcussion care (such as rest; Jaffee, Helmick, Girard, Meyer, Dinegar, & George, 2009)

Assessment

History

► Exposure to events (such as blasts, vehicle accidents, falls) that may have caused brain injury

► Immediate symptoms (such as loss of consciousness, feeling dazed, head injury, amnesia of event)

► Onset or worsening of problems (such as with memory, balance, headaches, dizziness, irritability, sensitivity to bright light, sleep problems) that may indicate brain injury

► Presence of symptoms in past week

► Four factors complicate recovery from combat-related concussions compared with mild TBI acquired in civilian settings.

Physical and Mental Status Exams

► Symptoms of TBI. See Table 11–1.

TABLE 11–1. SYMPTOMS OF TRAUMATIC BRAIN INJURY

MILD TBI	MODERATE TO SEVERE TBI
Mental status changes: ► Poor concentration ► Memory difficulty ► Intellectual impairment ► Irritability ► Depression ► Anxiety Physical findings: ► Dizziness ► Balance problems ► Headaches ► Tinnitus (ringing in the ears) ► Numbness and tingling ► Vision changes ► Sensitivity to light ► Sensitivity to sound ► Extreme fatigue ► Sleep problems Acute symptoms: ► Dazed and confused	Symptoms in first column plus: ► Chronic, worsening headaches ► Repeated nausea and vomiting ► Seizures ► Difficult to arouse from sleep ► Slurred speech ► Unequal pupils ► Confusion ► Restlessness and agitation ► Extreme weakness or numbness ► Loss of coordination

- ▶ Risk for suicide
  - ▹ Factors increasing risk for suicide attempt with TBI (Simpson & Tate, 2005):
    - ▷ Males
    - ▷ Ages 18 and 19
    - ▷ Psychiatric disorder
    - ▷ Aggressive behavior
    - ▷ Substance use

Diagnostic Studies

- ▶ No current diagnostic test can retrospectively diagnose mild TBI or determine that current symptoms or problems are due to a past mild TBI. Conventional structural neuroimaging studies are typically normal in mild TBI.

Differential Diagnosis

- ▶ Posttraumatic stress disorder (PTSD)
- ▶ Depression
- ▶ Anxiety
- ▶ Other mental health diagnosis

Management

Pharmacologic Treatment

- ▶ No specific medications for TBI
- ▶ Treat related symptoms according to current evidence-based standards
- ▶ Increased sensitivity to side effects of medication (secondary to head injury)
- ▶ Sedation
- ▶ Anticholinergic side effects ($\downarrow$ memory)
- ▶ Seizures with tricyclic antidepressants (TCAs), buproprion, and amantadine ($\downarrow$ seizure threshold)
- ▶ Extrapyramidal symptoms, neuroleptic malignant syndrome, tardive dyskinesia
- ▶ Neuroleptics: $\downarrow$ neuronal recovery
- ▶ Benzodiazepines: $\downarrow$ memory, $\uparrow$ confusion, $\downarrow$ coordination, abuse potential (Warden et al., 2006)
- ▶ Cognitive disorders recommendations
  - ▹ Methyphenidate: $\uparrow$ attention, processing speed, general cognitive function, learning and memory

- Dextroamphetamine: ↑ attention, processing speed
  - Bromocriptine (off label, possibly helpful): ↑ executive function
  - Amantadine (off label, possibly helpful): ↑ general cognitive function, attention and concentration (Warden et al., 2006)
- When using medications, start low and go slow

Nonpharmacologic Treatment

- Treat comorbidities (military personnel with TBI frequently have PTSD, which makes treatment of TBI more difficult)
- Safety plan for suicide risk; limit availability of means
- Teach family to identify signs of risk for suicide
- Follow up for 1 year after anyone with TBI makes a suicide attempt
- Treat vestibular dysfunction with physical therapy to reduce dizziness
- Treat traumatic vision syndrome with occupational therapy; scanning and accommodation difficulties lead to headaches, irritability, and fatigue
- Treat memory impairment with occupational therapy to teach memory improvement skills
- Teach about symptoms and implications for relationships, employment, etc.
- Avoid alcohol
- Neuropsychological testing
- Psychotherapy
  - Supportive
  - CBT
    - Increase understanding of relationships between cognition and emotion
    - Target adjustment or development of new beliefs and assumptions

- ▶ Behavioral
- ▶ Family
  - ▹ Behavioral, affective, and personality changes are most difficult for families to adjust to
  - ▹ Tips for families:
    - ▷ If concentration is an issue, ask the TBI survivor for one thing at a time. Use of white noise machines may reduce distractions. May take longer to complete tasks.
    - ▷ If memory is an issue, keep notepads near the phone for messages and in other places throughout the house. Keep a "memory book." Make a calendar and keep in a central location.
    - ▷ If anger or irritability is an issue, leave the situation if possible and wait for TBI survivor to calm down. Use a soft, calm voice. Keep your distance and give the TBI survivor space.
    - ▷ Resources
      - ▹ Defense and Veterans Brain Injury Center: http://www.DVBIC.org
      - ▹ Brain Injury Association of America: http://www.biausa.org
      - ▹ U.S. Dept. of Veteran Affairs: www.VA.gov
      - ▹ Texas Brain Injury Alliance: www.texasbia.org
  - ▹ Tips for the PMHNP for therapy with the patient with TBI
    - ▷ Determine what having a TBI means to the patient
    - ▷ Focus on "real life" difficulties in the here-and-now
    - ▷ Monitor speed and complexity of comments
    - ▷ Adjust session length according to level of attention and fatigue
    - ▷ Reestablish an acceptable sense of self
    - ▷ Instill hope without making predictions of a successful rehabilitation outcome

Special Considerations
- ▶ Mild TBI
  - ▹ Most patients achieve full recovery within 3 months; if residual symptoms continue, 80%–85% will clear within 6 months

Follow-up
- ▶ Symptoms may occur immediately but may also appear much later, which underscores the importance of screening for TBI; see Deployment Health Clinical Center (www.pdhealth.mil) for guidelines

CASE STUDY

Mrs. Dean, a 59-year-old homemaker with a positive family history for Alzheimer's disease, has been very worried lately over her belief that she is losing her memory. She has hesitated to go for an evaluation because of her concern and is very upset as she shares her beliefs with the PMHNP. She gives a social history of being happily married for the past 35 years and of having several children and two new grandchildren. She has had no recent stressors and has felt a slow decline in her memory for the past 2 years. She believes no one else has noticed, but recently it is harder to hide her deficit from her family.

She has been employed as a nurse for the past 25 years at the local hospital but has begun to notice a decline in her ability to keep track of all of the information needed to do her job well. She has a history of asthma and periodically uses a rescue inhaler and steroids to manage her asthma. She routinely takes one ASA a day and uses over-the-counter kava kava when she feels stressed. She has been taking pravastatin (Pravachol) 20 mg/day for her cholesterol level for the past 2 years. She has no significant physical findings but does show mild impairment in short-term memory testing during the MSE. There are many issues to consider in planning care with this patient:

- ▶ What is the probable diagnosis at this time?
- ▶ What further assessment is needed?
- ▶ What role does the medication taken by the patient play in decision-making?
- ▶ Would you include the family in care planning at this time?
- ▶ Are medications indicated at this time?
- ▶ What steps would you take to reduce the patient's discomfort as she discusses her concerns?

REFERENCES

American Geriatric Society. (1999). *Geriatric review syllabus.* New York: Kendall/Hunt.

American Psychiatric Association. (2000). *Diagnostic and statistical manual of mental disorders* (4th ed., text rev.). Washington, DC: Author.

Bickley, L. S. (2007). *Bates' guide to physical examination and history taking* (9th ed.). Philadelphia: Lippincott Williams & Wilkins.

Blessed, G., Tominson, B. E., & Roth, M. (1968). The association between quantitative measures of dementia and senile changes in cerebral gray matter of elderly subjects. *British Journal of Psychiatry, 114,* 797–811.

Borson, S., Scanlan, J., Brush, M., Vitaliano, P., & Dokmak, A. (2000). The mini-cog: a cognitive 'vital signs' measure for dementia screening in multilingual elderly. *International Journal of Geriatric Psychiatry,* 15, 1021–1027.

Burke, M., & Laramie, J. A. (2003). *Primary care of older adults* (2nd ed.). St. Louis, MO: Mosby.

Cummings, J., & Jeste, D. (1999). Alzheimer's disease and its management in the year 2010. *Psychiatric Services, 50,* 1173–1177.

de Lange, E., Verhaak, P. F., & van der Meer, K.. (2013). Prevalence, presentation and prognosis of delirium in older people in the population, at home and in long term care: A review. *International Journal of Geriatric Psychiatry, 28*(2), 127–134.

Desai, A., & Grossberg, G. (1999). Risk factors and protective factors for Alzheimer's disease. *Clinical Geriatrics, 7*(11), 43–47.

Dick, K., & Morency, C. R. (2011). Delirium. In K. Devereaux, & S. Crock (Eds.), *Geropsychiatric and mental health nursing* (2nd ed., p. 255–272). Sudbury, MA: Jones & Bartlett Learning.

Doornbos, M. M. (2002). Family caregivers and the mental health care system: Reality and dreams. *Archives of Psychiatric Nursing, 15*(4), 39–46.

Freidman, J. H. (1998). *Neurology in primary care.* Boston: Butterworth/Heinemann.

Jervis, L. L. (2002). Contending with problem behaviors in the nursing home. *Archives of Psychiatric Nursing, 15*(4), 32–38.

Melillo Devereaux, K., & Houde Crocker, S. (2011). *Geropsychiatric and mental health nursing* (2nd ed.). Sudbury, MA: Jones & Bartlett Learning.

Pfeiffer, E. (1975). A short portable mental status questionnaire for the assessment of organic brain deficit in elderly patients. *Journal of American Geriatric Society, 23,* 433–441.

Roalf, D., Mobergy, P., Xie, S., Wolk, D., Moelter, S, & Arnold, S. (in press). Comparative accuracies of two common screening instruments for classification of Alzheimer's disease, mild cognitive impairment, and healthy aging. *Alzheimer's & Dementia.*

Uphold, C. R. (2003). *Clinical guidelines in family practice* (4th ed.). Gainesville, FL: Barmarrae Books.

U.S. Preventive Services Task Force. (2003). *Screening for dementia recommendations and rationale.* Retrieved from http://www.uspreventiveservicestaskforce.org/3rduspstf/dementia/dementrr.htm

CHAPTER 12

SUBSTANCE-RELATED DISORDERS

One of the most common but least well-addressed classes of disorders is substance use, abuse, and dependence. Psychiatric–mental health nurse practitioners (PMHNPs) who work in primary psychiatric settings or integrated primary care settings commonly treat patients with substance-related disorders. These disorders can stand alone or be part of complex comorbid disorders with either general medical conditions or psychiatric disorders.

Many substances can be used and abused. No matter what the substance, two general categories of substance-related disorders exist: substance abuse and substance dependence. Although the specific drug of abuse will determine many of the physical, behavioral, and cognitive symptoms exhibited by the patient, some commonalities exist for all drugs.

This chapter focuses on the PMHNP role in determining the presence of either substance abuse or substance dependence, and the available clinical management and treatments. It also emphasizes alcohol abuse and dependency as the primary example of these two disorders. Alcohol is discussed because it is the most commonly abused substance; it is well researched and PMHNPs will most often encounter people in clinical settings with an alcohol-related disorder. Much of what is known about abuse of and dependence on alcohol is believed to be transferable to other substances.

SUBSTANCE-RELATED DISORDERS

Description
▶ *Substance-related disorders* are a cluster of disorders in which cognitive, behavioral, and physical symptoms indicate that a person is experiencing the effects of a drug of abuse.

- ▶ Psychiatric symptom clusters may be related to substance use, discontinuation of substance use, or withdrawal from habitual substance use.

- ▶ The word *substance* can describe a drug of abuse, a medication, or a toxin that produces psychoactivation and alters cognitive, behavioral, and affective perceptions.

- ▶ *Addiction* historically has been conceptualized as a disease, yet little is known about its underlying pathophysiology.

Etiology

- ▶ Multiple theories ranging from psychological to neurobiological

- ▶ Probable multifactorial etiological profile

  - ▸ Two common types of theories: psychodynamic and biological

  - ▸ Psychodynamic theory

    - ▷ Behaviors of abuse are seated in oral-stage fixation.

    - ▷ A person seeks gratification through oral behaviors.

    - ▷ Maladaptive regressive behaviors can become overlearned, fixed, and reinforced through dysfunctional family patterns.

    - ▷ Sociocultural factors attempt to explain population-based differences in substance abuse rates.

  - ▸ Biological theory

    - ▷ Genetic loading

  - ▸ People with a strong genetic vulnerability to addiction are thought to have defects in the working of the reward center of the brain, which predisposes them to stronger-than-normal positive rewards that draw them to substance use.

    - ▷ Gender differences

    - ▷ Ethnic differences

    - ▷ A person is predisposed to stronger-than-normal negative rewards, making it more difficult to stop abuse once it has begun.

- ▶ Involves two neurobiological processes:

  1. Reinforcement

     - ▷ Brain-based changes in structure and function can lead to addictive behavior.

     - ▷ The process of positive and negative rewards is physiologically linked to memory function.

     - ▷ Changes appear to occur with any drug of abuse.

     - ▷ Reinforcement results in "feel good" sensations when a drug of abuse is used and in "feel bad" sensations when the drug exits the body.

     - ▷ Positive rewards of reinforcement result in the social rewards commonly associated with drug use, such as disinhibition, euphoric mood, and anxiety reduction.

       - ▸ Mediated by dopamine (DA) pathways

- Negative rewards are aversive, such as increased anxiety and dysphoria.
  - Mediated by the gamma amino butyric acid (GABA) pathways
- Reinforcement occurs in the ventral tegmental area and the nucleus accumbens of the brain, collectively called the *reward center*.
- DA release within the reward center is enhanced further by the release of natural morphine-like neurotransmitters called *neuropeptides* (enkephalins, beta-endorphins).
- Neuropeptides further enhance the reinforcing pleasure experienced by the person.
- With repeated drug use, the DA system becomes increasingly sensitized.
- Eventually, associated drug use stimuli (e.g., pictures of drug paraphernalia) can cause DA release, leading to reinforcement of use and often to increased drug use.

2. Neuroadaptation
- Brain-based changes in structure and function can lead to *tolerance* and *withdrawal*.
- Drug-specific alterations in the normal level and function of neurotransmitters occur as the body adapts to the chronic presence of the substance of abuse.
- Neuroadaptive processes become very significant when the person stops substance use.
  - These processes become the basis for withdrawal symptoms, because adaptive responses are unopposed when the substance is no longer present.
- Neuroadaptive changes may be more enduring in some persons, possibly lasting for years, thus increasing their potential for relapse.
- This concept helps to explain why, after a long period of sobriety, a person who returns to substance abuse often picks up at the same level of tolerance and physical impact as experienced before sobriety.

Incidence and Demographics
- ▶ The United States has higher rates of substance abuse than any other developed country.
- ▶ More than 50% of U.S. patients with a psychiatric disorder have a comorbid substance abuse or dependence disorder.
  - Persons with schizophrenia are 4 times more likely to have a substance dependence comorbidity than the general population.
  - Persons with bipolar affective disorder are 5 times more likely to have a substance dependence comorbidity than the general population.
- ▶ More than 2 million admissions annually are made to inpatient substance abuse treatment facilities.
  - Though now legal in some states, marijuana is the most commonly abused illegal substance.
  - Alcohol is the most commonly abused legal substance.

- Rates are higher in men than in women.
  - 90% of men have used alcohol.
  - 70% of women have used alcohol.
- Rates are highest in Blacks, Hispanic Americans, and Native Americans; rates are lowest in Asian Americans.
- 55% of fatal driving accidents in the United States occur with a driver under the influence of alcohol.
- 50% of crimes in the United Stated are committed under the influence of alcohol.
- The lifetime risk for alcohol dependence is 15% in the general U.S. population.

Risk Factors
- Genetic loading
  - Family history of substance abuse or major depressive disorder (MDD)
- Association with peer structure with heavy substance use or abuse
- Co-occurring psychiatric disorder
- Age and gender
- Existence of chronic pain
- Untreated chronic, pathological-level anxiety

Prevention and Screening
- At-risk family education
- Community education
  - Stigma reduction
  - Signs and symptoms of illness
  - Treatment potential for control of symptoms
- Early recognition, intervention, and initiation of treatment to prevent disease and development of complications of disorder
- Implications of alcohol and other drugs of abuse during pregnancy:
  - Fetal alcohol syndrome (FAS)
  - Birth defects
- Acute alcohol intoxication in nontolerant persons such as teenagers:
  - Coma
  - Respiratory depression
  - Death
- CAGE screening test most commonly used screening tool for alcohol abuse (see Table 12–1)

TABLE 12-1. CAGE SCREENING TEST

C	Have you ever felt you ought to **cut down** on your drinking?
A	Have people **annoyed** you by mentioning your drinking?
G	Have you ever felt bad or **guilty** about your drinking?
E	Have you ever had a drink first thing in the morning to steady your nerves or get rid of a hangover (**eye-opener**)?

Adapted from "The CAGE Questionnaire: Validation of a New Alcoholism Instrument," by Mayfield, McLeod, Hall, 1974, *American Journal of Psychiatry, 131,* 1121–1123. Adapted with permission.

- Administered by asking the patient four questions

- Each positive answer scored as 1 point; negative answers receive no score

- The more positive answers, the greater the likelihood of an alcohol abuse disorder.

- Clients scoring 2 or greater are at mild to moderate risk for alcohol dependency, and the score is considered clinically significant

- Clients scoring 3 to 4 are considered at high risk for alcohol dependency

► Other screening

- AUDIT: Alcohol Use Disorders Identification Test

- S-MAST: Short Michigan Alcoholism Screening Test (or Geriatric Version)

- CRAFFT: Children under 21 years of age

- COWS: The Clinical Opiate Withdrawal Scale

Assessment

History

► Assess for the following:

- Detailed history of present illness, including time frame, progression, and associated symptoms

- Social history, including present living situation; marital status; occupation; education; and alcohol, tobacco, or illicit drug use

- Medication use, including prescription, over-the-counter, alternative, supplements, and home remedies

- Initial and periodic functional history and assessment

- Validate history with a family member

- Identify the category of drug abused by the patient

  ▷ Knowing category allows for anticipation of physical impact of drug and to predict potential symptoms of withdrawal

  ▷ Patients often abuse drugs from categories with similar pharmacological properties.

▷ Categories of abused agents:

- ► Alcohol
- ► Amphetamines or similar sympathomimetics
- ► Caffeine
- ► Cannabis
- ► Cocaine
- ► Hallucinogens
- ► Inhalants
- ► Nicotine
- ► Opioids
- ► Phencyclidine (PCP) or similar arylcyclohexylamines
- ► Sedatives
- ► Hypnotics
- ► Anxiolytics

► Assess for presence of substance abuse

- ► Maladaptive pattern of substance use manifested by recurrent and significant adverse consequences related to repeated use of a substance
- ► Is *not* synonymous with *use, misuse,* or *hazardous use*
- ► Specific criteria needed to identify substance use as abuse:
  - ▷ Maladaptive pattern of use occurring for at least a 12-month period of sustained abuse
  - ▷ Must be accompanied by repeated failure to fulfill major role obligation
  - ▷ Must be accompanied by use in situation that presents as physically hazardous, such as drinking and driving
  - ▷ Abuse continues despite multiple problems related to substance use patterns, such as legal, interpersonal, or social problems

► Assess for presence of substance dependence

- ► Cluster of cognitive, behavioral, and physiological symptoms indicating that the person continues use of a substance despite significant substance-related problems
- ► Synonymous with *addiction*
- ► Pattern of repeated use that leads to clinically significant impairment or distress with 3 or more of the following symptoms within a 12-month period:
  - ▷ Tolerance
  - ▷ Withdrawal
  - ▷ Using larger amounts than intended

SUBSTANCE-RELATED DISORDERS **311**

▷ Persistent craving or unsuccessful attempts to cut down

▷ Large amount of time spent obtaining substance, using substance, or recovering from its effects

▷ Activities decreased or given up because of use

▷ Using despite consequences

▸ Specify "with physiological dependence" or "without physiological dependence"

▸ Physiological dependence implies tolerance and withdrawal

▸ Symptoms of tolerance or withdrawal not needed to be present to meet criteria for substance dependence

▸ Degree of tolerance and withdrawal symptoms are substance-specific.

▷ *Tolerance:* The need for markedly increasing amounts of a substance to achieve desired effect

▷ *Withdrawal:* Maladaptive behavioral change with physiological and cognitive symptoms, occurring after blood or tissue concentrations of the substance declines in a person who has had prolonged heavy substance use

▸ Can be physical, psychological, or both, depending on the substance

▸ Withdrawal symptoms almost always the opposite of the acute action of the substance

▸ Categories of abused substances with pronounced, obvious withdrawal symptoms:

▷ Alcohol

▷ Opioids

▷ Sedatives

▷ Hypnotics

▷ Anxiolytics

▸ Categories of abused substances with less pronounced, less obvious withdrawal symptoms:

▷ Stimulants

▷ Nicotine

▷ Cannabis

▸ Categories of abused substances with little to no pronounced, obvious withdrawal symptoms:

▷ Hallucinogens

▷ PCP

▸ Course modifiers for substance dependence

▷ *Early partial remission:* One or more criteria (but not full criteria) have been met for substance dependence for at least 1 month but less than 12 months

- *Sustained partial remission:* One or more criteria (but not full criteria) have been met for substance dependence for 12 months or longer

- *Early full remission:* No criteria met for abuse or dependence for at least 1 month but less than 12 months

- *Sustained full remission:* No criteria met for abuse or dependence for 12 months or longer

▶ Assess for the presence of substance withdrawal or intoxication

- Patients abusing substances present for assessment either under the influence of the drug (intoxication) or experiencing problems related to cessation of substance use (withdrawal)

  - *Intoxication:* Reversible substance-specific syndrome due to recent ingestion of a psychoactivating substance

  - *Withdrawal:* Potentially nonreversible substance-specific syndrome due to cessation or significant reduction in heavy prolonged use of a substance.

- Blood alcohol levels determine presence of alcohol

  - Tolerant persons often have higher blood levels with less impairment than nontolerant persons

  - Must interpret blood alcohol levels of a patient based on his or her degree of tolerance

- Diagnostic criteria for substance withdrawal:

  - Cessation or reduction in alcohol use that has been heavy or prolonged

  - Two or more of the following symptoms within several hours or days of reduction or cessation:

    - Hand tremor

    - Insomnia

    - Autonomic hyperactivity (sweating, increased heart rate, and increased blood pressure)

    - Nausea or vomiting

    - Hallucinations or illusions

    - Psychomotor agitation

    - Anxiety

    - Seizures

    - Structured interview (see Table 12–2) allows for assessment of the use patterns and consequences of a person's substance use

- Assess for all dimensions of the impact of substance abuse and dependence in the person

TABLE 12–2. STRUCTURED INTERVIEW

DATA SET	POTENTIAL ASSESSMENT QUESTION
Current drug use	▸ Please tell me about your use of [substance]. ▸ What prescribed and self-prescribed drugs do you take regularly? ▸ Do you think you have a drug problem? ▸ Does anyone important to you think you have a drug problem?
Patterns of use	▸ Type and amount of [drug] consumption ▸ What is the longest period recently that you have gone without drug use? ▸ What happens when you go this long without [drug]? ▸ When was your last [drug] use? ▸ Have you had blackouts or memory loss during [drug] use? ▸ Is your [drug] use different now than it was 1 year ago? Five years ago?
Social consequences	▸ Have you ever been arrested related to your [drug] use (such as DUI)? ▸ Have you ever gotten into trouble at work or school because of your [drug] use? ▸ Have you ever behaved in a way you have regretted when using [drug]?
Relational aspects	▸ Have you ever gotten into arguments with your partner or spouse because of your [drug] use? ▸ Have you ever behaved toward your partner or spouse in a way you have regretted when using [drug] (such as being abusive)?
Sequelae of dependency	▸ Has your physical health suffered because of your [drug] use? ▸ Have you suffered any injury or trauma related to your [drug] use? ▸ Have you ever not complied with recommended medical care because it would mean you had to be [drug] free?

From *Practice Guideline for the Advanced Practice Nurse: Alcohol Withdrawal in the Acute Care Setting* by the Society of Psychiatric Mental Health Nurses, 2001, Philadelphia: International Society of Psychiatric Mental Health Nurses. Reprinted with permission.

Physical Exam

▶ Substance abuse or dependence produces many physical symptoms

▶ Usually a result of sequelae of use or abuse rather than findings specific to abuse or dependence

▶ Generally nonspecific when viewed in isolation

▶ Must be considered as a cluster of symptoms that raise an index of suspicion of addiction potential

  ▹ Abdominal pain and tenderness

  ▹ Nausea

  ▹ Weight loss

  ▹ Gastrointestinal bleeding

  ▹ Hypertension

  ▹ Anxiety

  ▹ First episode seizure in adult

▶ Physical findings (see Table 12–3) are drug-specific; alcohol-induced physical findings are the most well known.

TABLE 12-3. PHYSICAL FINDINGS SUGGESTIVE OF ALCOHOL DEPENDENCY

ORGAN SYSTEM	FINDING
Gastrointestinal	► Abdominal tenderness ► Splenomegaly ► Hepatomegaly (in some cases, size decreases)
Dermatological	► Diaphoresis ► Alopecia (especially distal extremity) ► Unexplained bruises ► Spider nevi, telangiectases, or angioma ► Palmer erythema ► Rosacea ► Superficial infections
Cardiovascular	► Tachycardia ► Cardiomyopathy ► Arrhythmia ► Hypertension
Respiratory	► Alcohol odor on breath ► Aspiration pneumonia ► Chronic upper respiratory infection
Neuropsychiatric	► Depression ► Anxiety ► Nystagmus ► Ataxia ► Emotional lability ► Irritability ► Peripheral neuropathy ► Hallucinations (especially tactile)
Endocrine	► Testicular atrophy ► Gynecomastia ► Sexual dysfunction

Adapted from *Alcohol's Effect on Organ Function, 21(1)*, 5–93. Copyright 1997 by the National Institute on Alcohol Abuse and Alcoholism (NIAAA). Adapted with permission.

Mental Status Exam (MSE)

► Nature of findings (see Table 12–4) depends heavily on whether the patient is experiencing substance intoxication or withdrawal, or is substance-free at the time of assessment.

► Index of suspicion for substance-related disorder should be raised if patient presents differently during different periods of assessment.

SUBSTANCE-RELATED DISORDERS **315**

TABLE 12–4. MSE FINDINGS CONSISTENT WITH SUBSTANCE ABUSE

CATEGORY OF ABUSED SUBSTANCE	CLINICAL FINDINGS	
Stimulant agents	► Anxiety ► Agitation ► Restlessness ► Aggression ► Panic episodes ► Grandiosity ► Elated mood	► Irritability ► Mood swings ► Hallucinations ► Impotence ► Dilated pupils ► Chest pain
Depressant agents	► Dysphoria ► Mood swings ► Ataxia ► Aggression ► Lack of impulse control ► Disinhibition ► Impaired attention ► Impaired memory	► Impaired judgment ► Hallucinations ► Paranoia ► Psychomotor retardation ► Slurred speech ► Drowsiness ► Myalgia
Hallucinogens	► Mood swings ► Ataxia ► Severe anxiety ► Panic episodes ► Aggression ► Hallucinations ► Paranoia ► Flashbacks	► Tremors ► Impaired concentration ► Impaired memory ► Impaired judgment ► Inability to make decisions ► Dilated pupils ► Nystagmus
Cannabis	► Paranoia ► Confusion	► Time distortion ► Hallucinations
Inhalants	► Ataxia ► Agitation ► Irritability ► Delirium	► Confusion ► Stupor ► Hallucinations ► Illusions

From *Medical Consequences of Drug Abuse/Mental Health Effects.* Copyright 2005 by the National Institute on Drug Abuse. Retrieved from www.drugabuse.gov/consequences/mortality.

Diagnostic Studies

► CBC, chemistry profile, thyroid function tests, and B_{12} level to rule out metabolic causes or unidentified conditions

► Drug toxicity screening, if indicated by history

► Alcohol dependence and abuse produce characteristic laboratory findings (see Table 12–5).

TABLE 12-5. LABORATORY FINDINGS SUGGESTIVE OF ALCOHOL DEPENDENCY

TEST	ABNORMALITY SUGGESTIVE OF ALCOHOL DEPENDENCY
Blood alcohol level (BAL)	> 100 mg/dL at the time of routine examination > 150 mg/dL without gross evidence of intoxication > 300 mg/dL at any time
Mean corpuscular volume (MCV)	Elevated (present in 60% of patients with alcohol dependency)
Gamma-glutamyltransferase (GGT)	Elevated 20% or more (present in 80% of patients with alcohol dependency)
Aspartate aminotransferase (AST)	Elevated 40% or more
Alanine aminotransferase (ALT)	Elevated 20% or more
Prothrombin time (PT)	Increased
Amylase	Elevated
White blood cell (WBC)	Low
Sodium (Na⁺)	Hyponatremia
Potassium (K⁺)	Hypokalemia
Serum lipids	Hyperlipidemia
Uric acid	Elevated
Triglycerides	Elevated

Adapted from *Principles of Addiction Medicine* (3rd ed.), by A. W. Graham, & T. K. Schultz, 2007, Baltimore: American Society of Addiction Medicine. Copyright 2007 by the American Society of Addiction Medicine. Adapted with permission.

Differential Diagnosis

▶ Endocrine disorders

　▸ Cushing's disease

▶ Neurological disorders

　▸ Seizure disorders

▶ Cardiovascular disorders

　▸ Myocardial infarction

▶ Mood disorders

　▸ MDD

　▸ Bipolar (BP) disorder

▶ Anxiety disorders

▶ Personality disorders

▶ Differential diagnostic consideration for acute alcohol withdrawal:

- Many acute general health conditions can mimic symptoms of alcohol withdrawal.
- In patients with a history of alcohol dependency, the PMHNP needs to consider not only withdrawal as a possible explanation for findings, but also the possibility of a general medical condition that can mimic alcohol withdrawal, such as hepatic encephalopathy or hypoglycemia.

Management

- ▶ Rule out or treat any conditions that may contribute to clinical findings.
- ▶ *Note:* 80% to 90% of people who require alcohol treatment do not get it.
  - Common reasons for failure to receive needed treatment:
    - ▷ Lack of diagnosis
    - ▷ Lack of referral
    - ▷ Lack of access to services
    - ▷ Resistance to treatment
  - The genetics of addiction vulnerability is becoming better known, which allows for preventative and early intervention treatments.
  - The knowledge base of pathophysiology of dependence has promoted new somatic interventions.
    - ▷ Psychopharmacology offers the promise of a new era in the treatment of addictions.
- ▶ Clinical management differs depending on the substance-related syndrome exhibited by the person.
  - Acute withdrawal
  - Acute intoxication
  - Long-term sobriety maintenance
  - Relapse prevention
- ▶ Alcohol withdrawal carries a high risk of mortality.
- ▶ Clinical management of alcohol withdrawal is a specialized treatment that requires specific experience in this type of care.
- ▶ Some clinical findings may assist in identification of patients at risk for severe alcohol withdrawal
  - Agitation
  - Decreased short-term memory
  - Disorientation
  - Hallucinations
  - Irregular pulse
  - Ophthalmoplegia

► Clinical Institute Withdrawal Assessment for Alcohol (CIWA–Ar; Sullivan, Sykora, Schneiderman, Naranjo, & Sellers, 1989)

▸ Used to determine likelihood of withdrawal and delirium tremens (DTs), which usually occur within the first 24 to 72 hours after cessation of alcohol

▹ Assesses 10 common withdrawal symptoms:

▸ Nausea and vomiting

▸ Tremors

▸ Paroxysmal sweats

▸ Anxiety

▸ Agitation

▸ Tactile disturbances

▸ Auditory disturbances

▸ Visual disturbances

▸ Headaches

▸ Altered sensorium

▸ Each symptom is graded on a 0- to 7-point scale, with the exception of orientation and sensorium, which is graded on a 0- to 4-point scale. The higher the total score (maximum = 67), the more likely the person will experience severe withdrawal and DTs: 0–8 = mild withdrawal, 9–15 = moderate withdrawal, > 15 = severe withdrawal and possible DTs

Pharmacological Treatment

► Pharmacological treatments are symptom-specific.

► Clinical management of acute withdrawal

▸ Detoxification (detox) agents substitute uncontrolled use of substance with slow tapering of controlled substance for uncontrolled use of substance to minimize neuroadaptive rebound.

▹ Multiple daily doses of benzodiazepines are used according to a fixed schedule and gradually tapered down over several days.

▹ Examples include:

▸ Lorazepam (Ativan)

▸ Chlordiazepoxide (Librium)

▸ Diazepam (Valium)

▸ Oxazepam (Serax)

▸ Polytherapy is a newer approach that matches drugs required for safe and effective withdrawal with neurotransmitter deficits created by substance use.

▹ Selected serotonin reuptake inhibitors

▷ Opioid antagonists nalmefene hydrochloride (Revex), naltrexone (Revia), or naltrexone for extended-release injectable suspension (Vivitrol)

▷ N-methyl-D-aspartate (NMDA) agonists

▸ Antiseizure medications such as carbamazepine (Tegretol) and valproic acid (Depakene) are sometimes used to decrease the potential of seizures

▸ Adrenergic medications are sometimes used to decrease high blood pressure and pulse associated with withdrawal.

► Clinical management of craving (see Table 12–6)

▸ Use anticraving medication such as naltrexone (Revia), acamprosate (Campral), ondansetron (Zofran), or buprenorphine (Buprenex).

▸ Use behavior treatment to help patient learn substitute behaviors.

▷ Clinical management and maintenance of sobriety (see Table 12–6)

▷ Patient may require ongoing treatment for comorbid psychiatric disorder.

▷ May use *aversion treatment* to avoid alcohol in persons with alcohol dependence.

▸ Disulfiram (Antabuse)

▷ Do not administer until the person has been alcohol-free for at least 12 hours.

▷ Advise patient to refrain from using anything that contains alcohol (e.g., vinegar, aftershave lotion, perfumes, mouthwash, cough medication) while taking disulfiram and up to 2 weeks after discontinuing disulfiram.

▷ Disulfiram can elevate liver function tests, so monitor.

▸ Antabuse may potentially induce mania in people with BP disorder.

TABLE 12-6. PHARMACOLOGICAL AGENTS USEFUL IN TREATING CRAVING AND MAINTAINING SOBRIETY FROM ABUSIVE SUBSTANCES

PHARMACOLOGICAL AGENT	CHEMICAL CATEGORY	ACTION	EFFECT
Celexa (celexa)	Selective serotonin reuptake inhibitor	Augment central serotonergic function	▸ Decreased desire and "liking"
Antabuse (disulfram)	Aldehyde dehydrogenase inhibitor	Aversive therapy; inhibits enzyme aldehyde dehydrogenase	▸ Causes symptoms of headache, nausea, vomiting, flushing if alcohol ingested
Narcan (naloxone)	Opioid antagonist, antidote	Blocks effects of opioids	▸ Used as an antidote for opioid overdose
Buprenex (buprenorphine)	Opioid partial agonist, opioid antagonist	Binds to opiate receptors in central nervous system (CNS), causing an analgesic effect; has agonist and antagonist activity	▸ Decreases heroin craving and use of opiates
Suboxone (buprenorphine and naloxone)	Narcotic analgesic, opioid agonist, opioid antagonist	Binds to opiate receptor, causing an analgesic effect; acts as an opioid antagonist	▸ Used in treatment of opioid dependence; ▸ Must meet qualification criteria to prescribe
Dolophine (methadone)	Narcotic analgesic	Binds to opiate receptors in the CNS, producing an analgesic effect, thus decreasing withdrawal symptoms	▸ Suppresses withdrawal symptoms from opiates; used as detox and maintenance treatment of narcotic addiction ▸ Must be part of FDA-approved program
Revex (nalmefene)	Opioid antagonist	Blocks ethanol-induced release of dopamine	▸ Increases abstinence; ▸ Decreases memory of drinking days
Revia; Vivitrol (naltrexone; extended release injectable)	Opioid antagonist	Blocks opioid receptors involved in rewarding effects of alcohol	▸ Increases abstinence; ▸ Decreases history of drinking days ▸ Assists with cravings
Campral (acamprosate)	Homotaurine	Agonist activity at GABA receptors and inhibitory activity at glutamate receptors	▸ Increases abstinence through decreased alcohol craving ▸ Thought to alter development of tolerance
Zofran (onadesteron)	Selective inhibitor of serotonin (5-HT_3)	Selective inhibition of Type 3 serotonin (5-HT_3) receptors that exhibit anti-emetic activity	▸ Increases abstinence; decreases craving

Adapted from *Principles of Addiction Medicine* (3rd ed.), by A. W. Graham, & T. K. Schultz, 2007, Baltimore: American Society of Addiction Medicine. Copyright 2007 by the American Society of Addiction Medicine. Adapted with permission.

► General health maintenance medication to treat vitamin deficiencies in persons with alcohol dependence include thiamine, folic acid, and B-complex vitamins.

Nonpharmacologic Treatment

► Multimodality treatment needed

► Lifetime treatment often required

► Inpatient treatment usually needed for safe and effective withdrawal from alcohol.

► Indications for inpatient alcohol detoxification include history of severe withdrawal symptoms, seizures, or delirium tremens; multiple past detoxifications; additional medical or psychiatric illness; recent significant alcohol consumption; lack of reliable support system; and pregnancy (Myrick & Anton, 1998).

► Reduce central nervous system stimulation by maintaining a quiet environment; put patient in room close to the nurses' station to facilitate frequent observation and monitoring; minimize abrupt changes in environment; decrease bright light and sharp, sudden noises; decrease room clutter; and do not restrain.

► Maintain hydration by monitoring intake and anticholinergic effects of benzodiazepines. Frequently offer fluids.

► Before discharge from acute-care setting, have a definite plan for follow-up treatment.

► Connect patient and family with support groups.

  ▸ 12-step groups in community

  ▸ Concrete plan for first week of support group attendance (may need daily)

► Connect patient with counseling or psychotherapy.

► Identify a primary healthcare provider.

► Note medical problems that will require further evaluation and potential treatment:

  ▸ Neurological sequelae of chronic alcohol consumption

  ▸ Nutritional deficiencies

  ▸ Cardiomyopathy, hypertension, arrhythmias, ischemic heart disease

  ▸ Blood dyscrasias

  ▸ Gastrointestinal inflammations

  ▸ Esophageal, liver, nasopharyngeal, and laryngeal cancers

► Individual care needs

  ▸ Substance abuse education classes

  ▸ Substance abuse counseling program

  ▸ Continued 12-step program involvement (e.g., Alcoholics Anonymous, Narcotics Anonymous)

  ▸ Halfway housing

  ▸ Cognitive–behavioral therapy.

► Family care needs

- Current and understandable information about condition, progress, and treatment plan

- Connect family to community support groups such as Al-Anon and Alateen

- Management of feelings such as guilt and anger

- Referrals to community resources

- Specific considerations: Relationship with treatment team; role strain; financial stresses; social isolation and "code of silence"; family support systems; family violence or marital and family strife; family members' work and school functioning; and history of mental disorders, including substance-related disorders

- Assist family in coping with difficulties incorporating drinking member back into routines; encourage further counseling to resolve these difficulties

- Refer for further treatment if family members report symptom clusters from anxiety and mood disorders, eating disorders, and addiction

Special Considerations

▶ Children and adolescents

- Most common period for starting drug use

- Significant impact of peer pressure on substance use patterns

- 30% to 40% of adolescents report drinking frequently

- 15% report binge drinking patterns

- Approximately 50% of high school–age students report at least a one-time use of illicit drugs.

▶ Older adults

- Referral to specialized treatment program that emphasizes interventions to deal with losses

- Large-print psychoeducation materials

- Transportation to service locations

- Treatment with same-age peer group

- Adaptations to home environment to cope with physical disabilities

- Close collaboration with primary-care physician for follow-up

CASE STUDY

Mrs. Day is a 61-year-old widow who has multiple health problems. She had been diagnosed with essential hypertension and chronic bronchitis and has non–insulin-dependent diabetes. She has been coming to your primary care clinic for 6 months, and before that she had been receiving her care from multiple other providers in the community, spending an average of 8 months with a practice group, then changing her care to another provider. She has Tricare as her insurance and receives Social Security Disability Insurance.

Mrs. Day's chief complaint for the past few months has been stasis ulcers on her lower left leg, which have not healed well despite multiple approaches to care. She also complains of problems with her "nerves." She currently is taking

- ▶ Multivitamin daily
- ▶ Ranitidine (Zantac) 150 mg q 12 hrs
- ▶ Alprazolam (Xanax) 1 mg b.i.d.
- ▶ Glipizide (Glucotrol) 20 mg b.i.d.

Mrs. Day is in today, and this is the first time you see her. On initial approach, she is hostile and difficult to get information from, stating, "You should know all this; you have my chart right there in your hand." She states that today she wants a refill of all of her prescriptions, and she wants you to write a letter to her landlord to "stop harassing me." She reports that her landlord is insisting that she place her garbage in the containers in the parking lot of the complex. She feels that is too far for her to walk, and she wants a letter supporting her current practice of leaving her garbage bags in the hallway outside her apartment door.

She also is reporting that her nerves are worse, and the pain in her legs is worse as well. She also believes that she has had a return of "chronic bronchitis," and she is requesting an antibiotic. She is requesting that you increase her alprazolam and add codeine or morphine or "any other thing like that" for her "constant pain." She states, "Just do this and get me out of here. I know what I need."

MSE

- ▶ *Appearance:* Moderately obese, well-dressed with appropriate hygiene, poor eye contact
- ▶ *Motor:* Mild psychomotor restlessness, slightly ataxic gait, tremulous
- ▶ *Speech:* Loud and pressured
- ▶ *Affect:* Angry
- ▶ *Mood:* Self-described as "cranky"; assessed as irritable
- ▶ *Thought processes:* Goal-directed and organized without evidence of psychotic processing but does show some mild thought-blocking and tangentiality

- *Thought content:* Thematic for mistrust of healthcare providers and of fear of pain continuing

- *Memory:* One-third of objects after 15 minutes

- *Concentration:* Refuses to do numbers testing, stating "I was never good with book work or numbers"

- *Abstraction:* Is abstract on proverbs; asks, "You got any more dumb questions?"

- *Judgment:* Intact for self-welfare

- *Education:* Completed 12th grade and went to 2-year secretarial/business school

- *Employment history:* Was a medical claims clerk for 32 years at the VA Medical Center

- *Social history:* No children; lives by herself; history of 2-pack-a-day smoker and "I drink a six-pack or so at night to relax myself—wouldn't you?"

Her physical exam is overall unremarkable. Her vital signs are within her documented baseline, with B/P 132/88, P 96, RR 26, temp 99 F, weight 209 lbs. Her lungs are overall clear. On her left leg she has a stasis ulcer, which is circular and approximately 6 cm in circumference. It is open and oozing white–yellow liquid drainage, with redness around the borders. She reports it is painful to touch and increasingly painful when weight-bearing. She was ordered silver sulfadiazene treatments with cling wrap and hot soaks q 6 hours. She refuses to cover it because "it hurts when I remove the bandage" and is not very clear about whether or not she is doing the hot soaks. Recent labs are all within normal limits, including TSH, electrolytes, and CBC.

- What is the primary health care concern of this patient?

- Is her use of potentially addictive prescription drugs warranted?

- What further assessment should be considered?

- If the patient is unwilling to participate in further assessment, how will you deal with her health needs?

REFERENCES

Barker, L. R., Burton, J. R., & Zieve, P. D. (2006). *Principles of ambulatory medicine* (7th ed.). Philadelphia: Lippincott Williams & Wilkins.

Bayard, M., McIntyre, J., Hill, K., & Woodside, J. (2004). Alcohol withdrawal syndrome. *American Family Physician, 69,* 1443–1450.

Brown, V. B., Ridgely, M. S., Pepper, B., Levine, I. S., & Ryglewicz, M. N. (1989). The dual crisis: Mental illness and substance abuse. *American Psychologist, 44,* 565–560.

DePetrillo, P., & McDonough, M. (1999). *Alcohol withdrawal treatment manual.* Glen Echo, MD: Focused Treatment Systems.

DiClemente, C., Bellino, L., & Neavins, T. (1999). Motivation for change and alcoholism treatment. *Alcohol Research and Health, 23*(2), 86–92.

Evans, K., & Sullivan, J. M. (2001). *Dual diagnosis: Counseling the mentally ill substance abuser* (2nd ed.). New York: Guilford Press.

Fuller, R., & Hiller-Sturmhofel, S. (1999). Alcoholism treatment in the United States: An overview. *Alcohol Research and Health, 23*(2), 69–77.

Graham, A. W., & Schultz, T. K. (2007). *Principles of addiction medicine* (3rd ed.). Baltimore: American Society of Addiction Medicine.

Hasin, D. S. (2001). The epidemiology of alcohol use and abuse in the United States: A review. *Economics of Neuroscience, 3*(12), 38–46.

Humphreys, K. (1999). Professional interventions that facilitate 12-step self-help group involvement. *Alcohol Research and Health, 23*(2), 93–98.

International Society of Psychiatric Mental Health Nurses. (2001). *Practice guideline for the advanced practice nurse: Alcohol withdrawal in the acute care setting.* Philadelphia: International Society of Psychiatric Mental Health Nurses.

Johnson, B., & Ait-Daoud, N. (1999). Medications to treat alcoholism. *Alcohol Research and Health, 23*(2), 99–106.

Kasper, D. (2005). *Harrison's principles of internal medicine* (16th ed.). New York: McGraw-Hill.

Lawson, A., & Lawson, G. (2004). *Alcoholism and the family: A guide to treatment and prevention* (2nd ed.). Gaithersburg, MD: Aspen.

Mayfield, D., McLeod, G., & Hall, P. (1974). The CAGE questionnaire: Validation of a new alcoholism instrument. *American Journal of Psychiatry, 131,* 1121–1123.

Miller, N., Gold, M., & Smith, D. (1997). *Manual of therapeutics for addictions.* New York: Wiley-Liss.

McCabe, S. (2000). Rapid detox: Understanding new treatment approaches for the addicted patient. *Perspectives in Psychiatric Care, 36,* 113–120.

McCabe, S., & Laraia, M. (2002). The neurobiology of medications to treat addictions. *APNA News, 14*(1), 12–14.

Minkoff, K., & Drake, R. (Eds.). (1991). *Dual diagnosis of major mental illness and substance disorder: New directions for mental health services.* San Francisco: Jossey-Bass.

Myrick, H., & Anton, R. (1998). Treatment of alcohol withdrawal. *Alcohol, Health, and Research World, 22(1),* 38–43.

Murray, C. J. L., & Lopez, A. D. (1996). *The global burden of disease: A comprehensive assessment of mortality and disability from diseases, injuries, and risk factors in 1990 and projected to 2020.* Cambridge, MA: World Health Organization & Harvard University School of Public Health.

Naegle, M. A., & D'Avanzo, C. E. (2001). *Addictions and substance abuse: Strategies for advanced practice nursing.* Upper Saddle River, NJ: Prentice Hall Health.

National Institute on Alcohol Abuse and Alcoholism. (1997a). *Alcohol and health* (DHHS Publication No. 97-4017). Rockville, MD: Author.

National Institute on Alcohol Abuse and Alcoholism. (1997b). Alcohol's effect on organ function. *DHHS Publication 21*(1), 5–93.

National Institute on Drug Abuse. (2005). *Medical consequences of drug abuse/mental health effects.* Bethesda, MD: National Institutes of Health. Retrieved from http://www.drugabuse.gov/consequences/mortality

Sciacca, K. (1987). New initiative in the treatment of the chronic patient with alcohol/substance abuse–use problems. *Tie-Lines, 3,* 5–6.

Sullivan, J. T., Sykora, K., Schniederman, J., Naranjo, C. A., & Sellers, E. M. (1989). The clinical institute withdrawal assessment for alcoholism. *British Journal of Addictions, 84*(11), 1353–1357.

Swift, R. M. (2001). The pharmacotherapy of alcohol dependence: Clinical and economic aspects. *Economics of Neuroscience, 3*(12), 62–66.

Vogel-Sprott, M. (1992). *Alcohol tolerance and social drinking: Learning the consequences.* New York: Guilford Press.

West, S., Garbutt, J. C., & Carey, T. S. (1999). *Pharmacotherapy for alcohol dependence: Evidence report/technology assessment* (AHCPR Publication No. 99-E0004). Rockville, MD: Agency for Health Care Policy and Research.

CHAPTER 13

PERSONALITY DISORDERS

This chapter reviews a category of illnesses called personality disorders, common disorders that can affect the quality of the general health care that a person receives. Although these disorders can create great difficulty for the given person, he or she remains able to perform routine daily functions. Often the person does not recognize a problem or seek treatment.

This chapter briefly reviews the concept of *personality* and then its disorders. Assessment and clinical management features of personality disorders are discussed.

PERSONALITY

Description

- ▶ *Personality* is the sum total of all emotional, cognitive, and behavioral attributes of a person.
- ▶ Personality involves an enduring pattern of perceiving, relating to, and thinking about the environment and one's self that are exhibited in a wide array of social and personal contexts.
- ▶ When healthy, personality structures allow for realistic, happy, and satisfying self-perceptions and interpersonal interactions.
- ▶ Characteristics
  - ▹ Personality is organized early in life and is dynamic and deeply ingrained; however, it can be altered.
  - ▹ Patterns of behavior based on personality can be perceived by the person as comfortable *(ego-syntonic)* or uncomfortable *(ego-dystonic):*
  - ▹ Ego-syntonic
    - ▹ Behavior consistent with personality

▷ Causes little concern to the person

▷ Person generally fails to recognize problem

▷ Person does not seek treatment

- Ego-dystonic

▷ Behavior inconsistent with personality

▷ Causes discomfort and concern to the person

▷ Person generally recognizes problem

▷ Person often seeks treatment

- Personality is reflected in behavioral traits habitually displayed by the person:

▷ Coping

▷ Interpersonal or interactive style

▷ Perceptions

▷ Cognitive beliefs about events, people, and situations

PERSONALITY DISORDERS

Description

▶ Personality disorders are chronically maladaptive patterns of behavior that cause functional impairment in work, school, or relationships.

▶ These disorders manifest as maladaptive patterns in four areas of functionality:

- Maladaptive *affective* traits, such as overly affectual patterns of response

- Maladaptive *behavioral* traits, such as poor impulse control patterns of response

- Maladaptive *cognitive* traits, such as unrealistic perceptual patterns of response

- Maladaptive *social* traits, such as maladaptive unsatisfying interpersonal patterns of response

▶ These disorders can cause *subjective distress.*

▶ A person is unlikely to recognize the problem or seek help if maladaptive patterns of behavior are ego-syntonic.

▶ A person is more likely to recognize problem and seek help if maladaptive patterns of behavior are ego-dystonic.

▶ Maladaptive patterns are *inflexible* and *pervasive* across most personal and social situations.

▶ These disorders are coded in the *DSM-IV-TR* (American Psychiatric Association, 2000) as Axis II disorders (see Table 13–1).

► Patients seldom fit neatly into one personality disorder diagnosis; rather, they often exhibit features of several similar disorders.

► For this reason, personality disorders often are referred to by the category of commonly manifesting symptom clusters (A, B, or C).

TABLE 13-1. CATEGORIES OF PERSONALITY DISORDERS

CATEGORY	CHARACTERISTIC BEHAVIOR	DISORDERS
Cluster A	Odd, unusual, eccentric, asocial	► Paranoid personality disorder ► Schizoid personality disorder ► Schizotypal personality disorder
Cluster B	Dramatic, affective instability	► Antisocial personality disorder ► Borderline personality disorder ► Histrionic personality disorder ► Narcissistic personality disorder
Cluster C	Anxious	► Avoidant personality disorder ► Dependent personality disorder ► Obsessive–compulsive personality disorder

Etiology

► Multiple theories ranging from psychological to neurobiological

► Probable multifactorial etiological profile

► Less empirical data available on neurobiological etiological factors

► Borderline personality disorder the most well researched

► Two common types of theories of personality disorders

1. Psychodynamic theory (primarily borderline personality disorder)—based on two etiological factors:

   ▷ Early separation problems

     ► Object relations theory

       ▷ Internalized intrapsychic experiences of interpersonal relationships

       ▷ Mental representation of the self in relation to others

       ▷ Stability and depth of a person's relationships

       ▷ During development, child must accomplish two tasks: *separation* and *individuation.*

         ► *Separation:* Develop intrapsychic self-representation distinct and separate from mother

         ► *Individuation:* Form distinct identity with characteristics unique to the person

     ▷ Four stages to the process of separation–individuation (Mahler, Pine, & Bergman, 1975)

- Differentiation

- Practicing

- Rapprochement

- Object constancy

  - Failure in separation–individuation is etiologically linked to development of personality disorders.

  - Different personality disorders linked to problems with different stages of the separation–individuation process.

- Disturbed parental interaction

  - Family background assumed to be dysfunctional:

    - Enmeshed family patterns

    - Role-reversal patterns of child–parent interaction

    - Restricted involvement of family with the rest of the environment

    - Social isolation

    - Confusion of parental authority and nurturing roles

    - Blurred family boundaries

  - Dysfunctional family patterns block separation–individuation processes; family rejection occurs if person attempts individuation.

2. Biological theory

   - Genetic factors

     - Familial tendency

     - Genetic overlap between loading for some Axis I disorders and personality disorders

   - Structural abnormalities

     - Reduced gray matter volume in prefrontal cortex

     - Limbic system deregulation

   - Neurotransmitter dysfunction

     - Decreased levels of serotonin

     - Elevated levels of norepinephrine

     - Dysregulation of dopamine receptors

   - Neurobiological impact of trauma

     - Most studied in borderline personality disorder

     - Assumes early childhood trauma alters basic brain patterns of response

     - In genetically susceptible people, may function as the environmental vulnerability that causes expression of genetic load.

Incidence and Demographics

▶ Difficult to estimate, because people with personality disorders are rarely hospitalized and often receive no treatment

▶ Incidence varies with disorder

▶ Generally assumed to be 0.5% to 5.4% in the general U.S. population

Risk Factors

▶ Genetic loading

▶ Dysfunctional family of origin

Prevention and Screening

▶ At-risk family education

▶ Community education

    ▸ Stigma reduction

    ▸ Signs and symptoms of illness

    ▸ Treatment potential for control of symptoms

▶ Early recognition, intervention, and initiation of treatment

▶ Preventative work with young children in identified dysfunctional family settings

Assessment

▶ Symptoms of personality disorder are enduring maladaptive patterns of behavior, generally seen as problems with living.

▶ Often several interviews are needed to clarify the diagnostic picture.

History

▶ Assess for the following:

    ▸ Detailed history of present illness, including time frame, progression, and associated symptoms

    ▸ Social history, including present living situation; marital status; occupation; education; and alcohol, tobacco, and illicit drug use

    ▸ Medication use, including prescription, over-the-counter, alternative, supplements, and home remedies

    ▸ Initial and periodic functional history and assessment

    ▸ Validate history with family member

        ▹ Long-term patterns of functioning

    ▸ Stability of traits over time and across situations

        ▹ Cultural issues vs. maladaptive personality traits

332 PSYCHIATRIC–MENTAL HEALTH NURSE PRACTITIONER REVIEW MANUAL, 3RD EDITION

- Issues of acculturation in new immigrants
- Cultural expression of habitual behavior
- Custom or religious practices

Assessment for Cluster A Disorders

▶ Patterns of pervasive distrust and suspiciousness, with odd and unusual behavior

- Present in a variety of contexts, even without supportive evidence

▶ Distrust usually not at psychotic level but can display brief psychotic episodes under stress

▶ Significant history includes the following:

- Limited social network
- Poor interpersonal relationships
- Limited disclosure or revealing of self to others, often refusing to answer personal questions
- Compliments often misinterpreted
- Pathological jealousy common
- Difficult to get along with
- Appearing cold and lacking in feelings
- High control needs
- Rigid and critical of others
- Often highly litigious
- Negatively perceive others; often biased and prone to stereotypes

▶ Differences in Cluster A disorders are in degree of suspiciousness and mistrust and in behavioral manifestations of those traits (see Table 13–2).

TABLE 13-2. CHARACTERISTICS OF CLUSTER A PERSONALITY DISORDERS

DISORDER	CHARACTERISTIC
Schizoid personality disorder	▶ Neither desires nor enjoys close relationships ▶ Chooses solitary activities ▶ Shows little to no interest in sexual activity with another person ▶ Derives no pleasure in social activities ▶ Lacks close friends or social supports ▶ Is indifferent of opinion of others ▶ Appears cold and detached ▶ Exhibits affective flattening
Schizotypal personality disorder	▶ Ideas of reference ▶ Odd beliefs ▶ Magical thinking ▶ Unusual perceptual experiences ▶ Paranoid ideation ▶ Inappropriate or constricted affect ▶ Behavior overtly odd, eccentric, or peculiar ▶ Few or no close friends ▶ Excessive social anxiety

Assessment for Cluster B Disorders

- ▶ Patterns of pervasive affective and interpersonal disruption

    - ▹ Present in a variety of contexts, even without supportive evidence

- ▶ Disturbance usually not at psychotic level but can display brief psychotic episodes under stress

- ▶ Disorders of Cluster B type may require hospitalization during period of active symptom expression and when patient under significant levels of stress

- ▶ Significant history includes the following:

    - ▹ Fluctuating emotional states

    - ▹ Dramatic qualities to how the person lives his or her life.

- ▶ Antisocial personality disorder

    - ▹ Usually diagnosed by age 18

    - ▹ More common in men

    - ▹ High substance abuse comorbidity

    - ▹ High impulsivity

    - ▹ Often diagnosed with conduct disorder as children.

- ▶ Borderline personality disorder

    - ▹ Predominantly in women

    - ▹ Often with positive history of significant childhood physical abuse, sexual abuse, neglect, or early parental separation or loss

- ▶ Differences in Cluster B disorders are in degree of affective instability, type of interpersonal disruption, and behavioral manifestations of those traits (see Table 13–3).

TABLE 13-3. CHARACTERISTICS OF CLUSTER B PERSONALITY DISORDERS

DISORDER	CHARACTERISTIC
Antisocial personality disorder	▶ Failure to conform to social norms ▶ Repeated acts that are grounds for arrest ▶ Deceitfulness, lying, and use of aliases for profit or pleasure ▶ Impulsivity and failure of future planning ▶ Reckless disregard for the welfare of others ▶ Consistent irresponsibility ▶ Lack of remorse; indifference to the feelings of others
Borderline personality disorder	▶ Frantic efforts to avoid real or imagined abandonment ▶ Pattern of unstable, intense interpersonal relationships ▶ Identity disturbances ▶ Impulsivity, often with self-damaging behavior ▶ Recurrent suicidal behavior ▶ Chronic feelings of emptiness ▶ Inappropriate, intensified affective anger responses ▶ Transient psychotic symptoms of paranoia and dissociation
Histrionic personality disorder	▶ Uncomfortable in situations in which he or she not center of attention ▶ Interactions with others characterized by inappropriate seductive or sexualized or provocative behavior, rapid shifting, and shallow emotional responses ▶ Consistent use of physical appearance to draw attention to self ▶ Speech excessively impressionistic and lacking in detail ▶ Suggestible and easily influenced ▶ Relationships considered more intimate than they are
Narcissistic personality disorder	▶ Grandiose sense of self-importance ▶ Preoccupation with fantasies of power, success, brilliance, and beauty ▶ Belief of self-importance and being special and unique ▶ Excessive admiration required ▶ Unreasonable expectations or sense of entitlement ▶ Interpersonally exploitative ▶ Empathy lacking ▶ Envy of others and belief that others envy him or her ▶ Arrogant and haughty behaviors

Assessment for Cluster C Disorders

▶ Patterns of pervasive anxiety and fear

- Present in a variety of contexts, even without supportive evidence

▶ Disturbance usually not at psychotic level but can display brief psychotic episodes under stress

▶ Significant history includes the following:

- Avoidant behavior

- Procrastination

- Difficulty in following through

- Fearful of rejection and criticism

- Difficulty relaxing
- ► Avoidant personality disorder
  - Must consider cultural variable when looking at avoidant behavior
  - Disorder equal for both genders
- ► Dependent personality disorder
  - Most frequently diagnosed personality disorder
  - Rates higher in women than in men
  - Commonly diagnosed in people with history of chronic physical illnesses
- ► Obsessive–compulsive personality disorder
  - Predominantly in men
  - Symptoms similar to but less severe than obsessive–compulsive disorder
- ► Differences in Cluster C disorders are in the degree of anxiety and fear and in behavioral manifestations of those traits (see Table 13–4).

Physical Exam
- ► Nonspecific

Diagnostic Studies
- ► CBC, chemistry profile, and thyroid function tests to rule out metabolic causes or unidentified conditions
- ► Drug toxicity screening if indicated by history

TABLE 13-4. CHARACTERISTICS OF CLUSTER C PERSONALITY DISORDERS

DISORDER	CHARACTERISTIC
Avoidant personality disorder	► Avoidance of activities involving significant interpersonal contact ► Fear of criticism, disapproval, or rejection ► Unwillingness to be involved with people unless sure of being liked ► Restraint in intimate relationships for fear of being shamed ► Preoccupation with being criticized or rejected in social settings ► View of self as socially inept, personally unappealing, or inferior ► Unusual reluctance to take personal risks or engage in new activities
Dependent personality disorder	► Difficulty making everyday decisions without excessive advice ► Needing others to assume responsibility for most areas of life ► Difficulty expressing disagreement ► Difficulty initiating projects by himself or herself ► Going to excessive lengths to obtain nurturing and support from others ► Urgent seeking of another relationship if a close relationship ends ► Unrealistic preoccupation with fears of being left alone
Obsessive-compulsive personality disorder	► Preoccupation with details, rules, order, and organization ► Perfectionism that interferes with task completion ► Excessive devotion to work and productivity ► Overly conscientious, scrupulous, and inflexible on issues of morality ► Inability to discard worn-out or worthless objects ► Reluctance to delegate tasks or work with others ► Adoption of a miserly spending style toward self and others ► Rigidity and stubbornness

Differential Diagnosis

► Comorbidity is common

► Mood disorders (see Chapter 8)

  » Affective instability of borderline personality disorder often mistaken for bipolar affective disorder

► Substance-induced disorders (see Chapter 12)

Management

► Rule out or treat any conditions that may contribute to cognitive impairment.

► Personality disorders are generally managed in a community setting.

► In some cases, hospitalization may be required (Clarkin, Foelsch, Levy, Hull, Delaney, & Kernberg, 2001).

Pharmacologic Treatment

► No specific class of pharmacological agents used to treat personality disorders

► Individualized symptom control

  » Impulsivity

PERSONALITY DISORDERS 337

 ▷ Selected serotonin reuptake inhibitors (SSRIs)

 ▷ Anticonvulsant mood stabilizers

 ▸ Affective instability

 ▷ SSRIs

 ▷ Anticonvulsant mood stabilizers

 ▸ Anxiety

 ▷ Nonbenzodiazepine (BNZ) anxiolytics

 ▷ SSRIs

 ▷ BNZs (use with caution)

Nonpharmacologic Treatment

▶ Most common form of treatment for personality disorders

▶ Focus on issues of limit-setting, protection from self-harm, improved coping, and enhanced interpersonal functioning

▶ Multiple therapeutic interventions may be used, such as

 ▸ Case management

 ▸ Psychotherapy

 ▷ Focus on the person gaining control

 ▷ Improvement of interpersonal skill level

 ▷ Enhanced coping

 ▷ Alteration of problematic patterns of behavior

 ▷ Forms of therapy:

 ▸ Dialectical–behavioral therapy

 ▸ Interpersonal therapy

 ▸ Behavioral therapy

 ▸ Cognitive–behavioral therapy (CBT)

 ▸ Milieu therapy

▶ Assist with realistic expectation formation.

▶ Structure environment.

▶ Improve realistic self-appraisal ability.

Special Considerations

▶ Children

- ▸ Before diagnosis is determined, sufficient life experiences must occur so that chronicity of maladaptive patterns can be observed.

- ▸ Features of personality disorder usually become apparent during adolescence to early adulthood.

- ▸ It is unusual for person to be given personality disorder diagnosis before ages 16 to 18 (an exception is antisocial personality disorder, which often is observable by onset of puberty; however, diagnosis of antisocial personality disorder is not made until age 18).

- ▸ Separation anxiety and chronic physical illness often precede and predict onset of dependent personality disorder.

Follow-up

▶ These are chronic disorders, and patients may be resistant to change.

▶ Relapse is common and frequent.

▶ How long to treat and success rates vary with individual characteristics and motivation.

▶ Prognosis is poor without treatment.

▶ Prognosis improves if treatment is started as early in life as possible.

CASE STUDY

Mr. Jevers is 42-year-old new patient who seeks health care for a general physical exam. The family nurse practitioner who examines Mr. Jevers asks the psychiatric–mental health nurse practitioner (PMHNP) to speak with him because of his odd presentation. The patient discusses with the PMHNP an unusual, recurrent experience he has been having.

Mr. Jevers lives in an apartment building downtown and works as a bartender in the late evening. He tells the PMHNP that every night as he walks home from work he watches to see if the wind "blows north to south or south to north." He relates that, on the occasions that wind goes north to south, he takes that as a sign that a woman will visit him. He tells of a woman who rides a bicycle down the road and, as she passes him, he receives a blessing from her that protects him from those who wish him harm. He believes the woman is a "spirit from the other side" and that no one but he can see the woman.

As Mr. Jevers tells his story, his affect is inappropriate, his mood pleasant and happy, and he exhibits some paranoid ideation as he worries that others will try to take away the spirit. His mental status examination (MSE) shows ideas of reference and some magical thinking as he shares his "blessing" with customers in the bar, and he describes odd, eccentric, and peculiar behaviors. Mr. Jevers is not at all bothered by his unusual experience and seems to enjoy telling it to others. He considers himself lucky to have "special powers" and to see and understand things that other do not. Mr. Jevers denies the presence of any typical manifestations of hallucinations or delusions, any mood disturbance or anxiety, and alcohol or other drug use. He reports having several close friends, a strong support network, and is in general good health but does experience significant social anxiety. He does not believe his unusual experience is a symptom of an illness and wishes no intervention or assistance at this time.

▶ What is the most probable diagnosis for this patient?

▶ What further assessment should occur?

▶ If the patient desires no treatment, should the PMHNP attempt to follow up with him?

▶ What treatment should be suggested at this time?

REFERENCES

Alper, G., & Peterson, S. J. (2001). Dialectical behavior therapy for patients with borderline personality disorder. *Journal of Psychosocial Nursing and Mental Health Services, 39*(10), 38–45.

American Psychiatric Association. (2000). *Diagnostic and statistical manual of mental disorders* (4th ed., text rev.). Washington, DC: American Psychiatric Association.

Burke, M., & Laramie, J. A. (2003). *Primary care of older adults* (2nd ed.). St. Louis, MO: Mosby.

Clarkin, J. F., Foelsch, P. A., Levy, K. N., Hull, J. W., Delaney, J. C., & Kernberg, O. F. (2001). The development of a psychodynamic treatment for patients with borderline personality disorder: A preliminary study of behavioral change. *Journal of Personality Disorders, 15,* 487–495.

Daghestani, A. N., Dinwiddie, M. D., & Hardy, D. W. (2001). Antisocial personality disorder in and out of correctional and forensic settings. *Psychiatric Annuals, 31,* 441–446.

Feinstein, R. E. (2000). Personality disorders in the primary care setting: Diagnosis, management, and intervention. *Resident and Staff Physician, 11,* 47–56.

Freidman, J. H. (1998). *Neurology in primary care.* Boston: Butterworth/Heinemann.

Keltner, N., Schwecke, L. H., & Bostrom, C. E. (2006). *Psychiatric nursing* (5th ed.). St. Louis, MO: Mosby.

Linehan, M,Comtois, K., Murray, A., Brown, M., Gallop, R., … Lindenboim, N. (2006). Two-year randomized controlled trial and follow-up of dialectical behavior therapy vs therapy by experts for suicidal behaviors and borderline personality disorder. *JAMA, 63*(7), 757–766.

Mahler, M., Pine, F., & Bergman, A. (1975). *The psychological birth of the human infant: Symbiosis and individuation.* New York: Basic Books.

Parker, L. (2001). Dialectical behavioral therapy: A working perspective. *Nursing Times, 9*(4), 38–39.

Schmahl, C. G., McGlashan, T. & Bremner, J. D. (2002). Neurobiological correlates of borderline personality disorder. *Psychopharmacology Bulletin, 36*(2), 69–78.

Stone, M. H. (2000). Clinical guidelines for psychotherapy for patients with borderline personality disorder. *Psychiatric Clinics of North America, 23,* 193–210.

Stuart, G. W., & Laraia, M. (2004). *Principles and practice of psychiatric nursing* (8th ed.). St. Louis, MO: Mosby.

Uphold, C. R. (2003). *Clinical guidelines in family practice* (4th ed.). Gainesville, FL: Barmarrae Books.

CHAPTER 14

DISORDERS OF CHILDHOOD AND ADOLESCENCE

Disorders first diagnosed in infancy, childhood, or adolescence, such as conduct disorder, oppositional defiant disorder, attention-deficit hyperactivity disorder, Asperger syndrome, Rett syndrome, autism spectrum disorder, eating disorders, and mental retardation, are considered brain-based illnesses and have many similarities to disorders diagnosed more commonly in adulthood. In addition, these disorders often are missed during childhood and adolescent years and are therefore not identified until early adulthood.

The disorders in this category differ in presentation, in developmental age of common onset, and in gender factors. Assessment, treatment planning, and therapeutic interventions for these disorders must always occur within the context of the family and assume a multimodal, systems-oriented approach to care. In addition, assessment of children is different from assessment of adults. Therefore, psychiatric–mental health nurse practitioners (PMHNPs) must apply principles of child assessment to care effectively for the patient and family experiencing or at risk for these disorders.

ASSESSMENT AND CARE PLANNING FOR CHILDREN AND ADOLESCENTS

▶ Requires alteration in assessment process

- ▹ Generally takes more time
- ▹ Nurse must develop trusting relationship with the child to put him or her at ease
- ▹ Interview the child and parent separately; child can provide information on internal symptoms and providers information on external signs (Hamrin & Gray Deering, 2012).

- Must attend to developmental needs and interests of the child

- Must attend to the cognitive and language abilities of the child.

▶ Mental status examination

- Modified to reflect developmental and other age-related issues in children

- Often requires establishment of a play environment to open communication with the child.

- Appearance

  ▷ Conclusions must consider age and developmental processes (e.g., physical appearance and dress for weather and age group)

  ▷ Gait and motor skills are assessed on expected normative behaviors for age.

▶ Speech

- Assessed on expected normative behaviors for age in comprehension, word selection, and range of vocabulary.

▶ Thought process

- Assessed on expected normative behaviors for age in degree of organization, goal orientation, and ability to focus

  ▷ Abstraction

    - Assessed on expected normative behaviors for age

    - Children ages 12 or younger not expected to have abstractive thought abilities (young children have concrete thinking)

    - Proverb testing and similarity testing require prior exposure to concept, word choices, and ability to think abstractly.

▶ Therapeutic care planning

- Variety of effective treatments commonly used with children and adolescents:

  ▷ Play therapy

  ▷ Game therapy

  ▷ Art therapy

  ▷ Bibliotherapy

  ▷ Orative therapy (such as storytelling, family narrative therapy)

  ▷ Behavioral therapy

  ▷ Milieu therapy

  ▷ Pharmacotherapy

OPPOSITIONAL DEFIANT DISORDER (ODD)

Description

▶ *Oppositional defiant disorder (ODD)* is an enduring pattern of negativistic, defiant, disobedient, hostile, and defiant behaviors, usually directed at an authority figure.

Etiology

▶ No single factor accounts for presentation.

▶ Etiology is largely unknown.

▶ Many biopsychosocial factors contribute to the development.

Incidence and Demographics

▶ ODD is more common in children of parents with a history of ODD, conduct disorder, ADHD, antisocial personality disorder, mood disorders, or substance abuse disorder.

▶ It affects 2% to 16% of the general U.S. population.

▶ Before puberty, boys with the disorder are more prevalent than girls; after puberty, the boy-to-girl ratio is equal.

▶ About 30% of children with ODD develop conduct disorder

Risk Factors

▶ Genetic loading

Prevention and Screening

▶ At-risk family education

▶ Community education

  ▹ Stigma reduction

  ▹ Signs and symptoms of illness

  ▹ Treatment potential for control of symptoms

▶ Well-child visit screening

▶ Mental health screening

▶ Early recognition, intervention, and initiation of treatment

  ▹ Secondary prevention important in younger patients

Assessment

▶ Detailed history of present illness, including time frame, progression, and associated symptoms

- Social history, including present living situation; education; and alcohol, tobacco, or illicit drug use
- Medication use, including prescription, over-the-counter, alternative, supplements, and home remedies
- Initial and periodic functional history and assessment
- Validate history with a family member.

History

- Assess for the following:
    - Criteria behaviors persisting for *at least 6 months* and including *at least 4* of the following:
        - Often loses temper
        - Often argues with adults
        - Often actively defies or refuses to comply with adults' requests or rules
        - Often deliberately annoys people
        - Often blames others for his or her mistakes or misbehavior
        - Often is touchy or easily annoyed by others
        - Often is angry and resentful
        - Often is spiteful or vindictive

Physical Exam

- Nonspecific

Mental Status Exam

- Mood
    - Liability: Low frustration tolerance, angry, argues and loses their temper
- Concentration
    - Impaired
- Thought content
    - Often blames others for mistakes

Diagnostic Studies

- No specific laboratory tests
- CBC, chemistry profile, thyroid function tests, and B_{12} level to rule out metabolic causes or unidentified conditions
- Drug toxicity screening, if indicated by history
    - Lead toxicity
    - Toxicology screen to rule out a substance abuse disorder

Differential Diagnosis

- ▶ ADHD (see below)
- ▶ Mood disorders (see Chapter 8)
- ▶ Substance abuse disorders (see Chapter 12)
- ▶ Mental retardation (see below)
- ▶ Conduct disorder (see below)
- ▶ Psychotic disorders (see Chapter 10)

Management

- ▶ Rule out or treat any conditions that may contribute to current symptom manifestation

Pharmacologic Treatment

- ▶ Nonspecific: Not first line
- ▶ Target symptoms: Mood or aggression

Nonpharmacologic Treatment

- ▶ Therapy is mainstay:
  - ▹ Individual therapy
  - ▹ Family therapy, with emphasis on child management skills
  - ▹ Evidence-based treatment: Child & parent problem-solving skills training (American Academy of Child and Adolescent Psychiatry [AACAP], 2007).
  - ▹ Incredible years (group intervention)
  - ▹ Parent–child interactional therapy (individual and family intervention)
  - ▹ Adolescent transitions program (ATP; individual and family and group intervention)

CONDUCT DISORDER

Description

- ▶ *Conduct disorder* is a persistent pattern of behavior in which the rights of others or societal norms or rules are violated.

Etiology

- ▶ No single factor accounts for presentation.
- ▶ Etiology is largely unknown.
- ▶ Many biopsychosocial factors contribute to the development

Incidence and Demographics

▶ Conduct disorder is more common in children of parents with antisocial personality disorder, alcohol dependence, mood disorders, or schizophrenia than in the general population.

▶ It affects 1% to 10% of general U.S. population, 6% to 16% of boys and 2% to 9% of girls.

▶ Onset is earlier for boys (10 to 12 years) than for girls (16 years).

Risk Factors

▶ Genetic loading

▶ Dysfunctional family patterns

▶ Substance abuse

Prevention and Screening

▶ At-risk family education

▶ Community education

- ▸ Stigma reduction

- ▸ Signs and symptoms of illness

- ▸ Treatment potential for control of symptoms

▶ Early recognition, intervention, and initiation of treatment

- ▸ Secondary prevention is important in younger patients

Assessment

▶ Detailed history of present illness, including time frame, progression, and associated symptoms

▶ Social history, including present living situation; education; and alcohol, tobacco, or illicit drug use

▶ Medication use, including prescription, over-the-counter, alternative, supplements, and home remedies

- ▸ Initial and periodic functional history and assessment

- ▸ Developmental history

- ▸ Validate history with a family member

History

▶ Assess for the following:

- ▸ Four categories of behaviors:

  1. Aggression toward people and animals

  2. Destruction of property

  3. Deceitfulness or theft

  4. Serious violation of rules

DISORDERS OF CHILDHOOD AND ADOLESCENCE **347**

▶ Must have 3 or more symptoms of the disorder in the past year and at least 1 symptom in the past 6 months

▶ Significant impairment in social, academic, and occupational functioning

  ▸ Childhood onset

    ▷ At least one criterion characteristic present before age 10 years

  ▸ Adolescent onset

    ▷ No criteria characteristic present before age 10 years

Physical Exam

▶ Nonspecific

Mental Status Exam

▶ Affect

  ▸ Irritable

  ▸ Angry

  ▸ Uncooperative

▶ Mood

  ▸ Anger

▶ Thought content

  ▸ Lack of empathy or concern for others

▶ Concentration

  ▸ Distractible

▶ Insight

  ▸ Poor

Diagnostic Studies

▶ No specific laboratory tests

▶ Drug screening to rule out possible substance abuse

▶ CBC, chemistry profile, thyroid function tests, and B_{12} level to rule out metabolic causes or unidentified conditions

Differential Diagnosis

▶ Attention-deficit hyperactivity disorder (ADHD; see below)

▶ Oppositional defiant disorder (ODD; see above)

▶ Mood disorders (see Chapter 8)

▶ Posttraumatic stress disorder (see Chapter 9)

348 PSYCHIATRIC–MENTAL HEALTH NURSE PRACTITIONER REVIEW MANUAL, 3RD EDITION

▶ Substance abuse disorders (see Chapter 10)

▶ Developmental disorders (see below)

Management

▶ Rule out or treat any conditions that may contribute to current symptom manifestation

Pharmacologic Treatment

▶ No specific pharmacological interventions

▶ Aggression and agitation treated with antipsychotics, mood stabilizers, selective serotonin reuptake inhibitors (SSRIs), and alpha agonists

Nonpharmacologic Treatment

▶ Multimodality treatment programs that use all available family and community resources

▶ Behavioral therapy is mainstay:

  » Individual therapy

  » Family therapy

Special Considerations

▶ May be diagnosed in patients ages 18 years or older if criteria for antisocial personality disorder are not met.

ATTENTION-DEFICIT HYPERACTIVITY DISORDER (ADHD)

Description

▶ *Attention-deficit hyperactivity disorder (ADHD)* is a persistent pattern of inattention or hyperactivity and impulsivity, or both, that is more frequent and more severe than that typically observed in people of the same developmental level.

Etiology

▶ Many biopsychosocial factors contribute to the development.

▶ Polygenic neurobiological deficits are associated with ADHD.

  » Problems with executive functioning

  » Abnormalities of fronto–subcortical pathways

    ▷ Frontal cortex

    ▷ Basal ganglia

  » Abnormalities of reticular activating system

> Structural abnormalities producing neurotransmitter abnormalities

  ▷ Dopamine dysfunction

  ▷ Norepinephrine dysfunction

Incidence and Demographics

► 3% to 5% of U.S. children have ADHD.

► Boys are more likely to be diagnosed (13.2%) than girls (5.6%; CDC, 2010).

► Average age of onset is 3 years; mean age of diagnosis is 9 years.

► Approximately 60% of clients have symptoms persisting into adulthood.

  ▸ Inattention symptoms are more persistent than hyperactivity/impulsivity symptoms.

Risk Factors

► Genetic loading

► Pregnancy and perinatal complications

► Family conflict

Prevention and Screening

► At-risk family education

► Community education

  ▸ Stigma reduction

  ▸ Signs and symptoms of illness

  ▸ Treatment potential for control of symptoms

► Early recognition, intervention, and initiation of treatment

  ▸ Secondary prevention is important in young patients.

Assessment

History

► Assess for the following:

  ▸ History of attention and impulse problems in patient's parents and grandparents because of high genetic load

  ▸ History of criteria symptoms in client

    ▷ Inattention

    ▷ Inattention to details

    ▷ Careless mistakes

    ▷ Difficulty sustaining attention

    ▷ Seeming not to listen

- Failure to finish tasks
- Difficulty with organizing
- Avoidance of tasks requiring sustained attention
- Loss of things
- Distractibility
- Forgetfulness

► Hyperactivity and impulsivity

- Blurting out answers before question is finished
- Difficulty awaiting his or her turn
- Interrupting or intruding on others
- Fidgeting
- Inability to stay seated
- Inappropriate running or climbing
- General restlessness
- Difficulty engaging in leisure activities
- Always "on the go"
- Excessive talking
- Variations in pervasiveness, frequency, and degree of impairment
- Subtypes:
  - ADHD, inattentive type
    - Inattentive symptoms dominate
    - Lack of criterion symptoms for hyperactivity and impulsivity
  - ADHD, hyperactive type
    - Hyperactivity and impulsivity symptoms dominate
    - Lack of criterion symptoms for inattention
  - ADHD, combined type
    - Criterion symptoms met for both inattention and hyperactivity and impulsivity

Physical Exam

► Nonspecific

► Minor physical anomalies at higher rates in people with ADHD than in general population:

- Hypertelorism
- Highly arched palate
- Low-set ears

► Higher-than-average accidental injury rates

Mental Status Exam

▶ Restlessness

▶ Inattention

▶ Distractible speech patterns

▶ Overproductive speech patterns

▶ Affective lability

▶ Poor memory

▶ Poor concentration

Diagnostic Studies

▶ Nonspecific

Differential Diagnosis

▶ Understimulated home environment

▶ Substance abuse

▶ MDD

▶ BP disorder

▶ Stereotypic movement disorder

Management

Pharmacologic Treatment

▸ Most commonly used agents (see Table 14–1) are stimulants (Schedule II)—controlled substances carry risk for abuse.

TABLE 14-1. MOST COMMONLY USED AGENTS FOR ADHD

DRUG	DOSAGE
Ritalin (methyphenidate hydrochloride), Schedule II	5–40 mg/day
Ritalin LA/Ritalin SR (methylphenidate hydrochloride), Schedule II	10–60 mg/day
Metadate CD (methylphenidate hydrochloride), Schedule II	10–60 mg/day
Metadate ER (methylphenidate hydrochloride), Schedule II	10–60 mg/day
Concerta (methylphenidate hydrochloride), Schedule II	18–72 mg/day
Methylin (methylphenidate hydrochloride), Schedule II	5–60 mg/day
Methylin ER (methylphenidate hydrochloride), Schedule II	10–60 mg/day
Daytrana (methylphenidate transdermal patch), Schedule II	10 mg–30 mg/day (9 hours)
Dexedrine (dextroamphetamine), Schedule II	2.5–20 mg/day
Adderall (amphetamine, dextroamphetamine), Schedule II	5–40 mg/d
Adderall XR (amphetamine, dextroamphetamine), Schedule II	5–60 mg/d
Focalin/Focalin XR (dexmethylphenidate), Schedule II	2.5–20 mg/d
Vyvanse (lisdexamfetamine dimesylate), Schedule II	30–70 mg/d
Strattera (atomoxetine hydrochloride), not a controlled substance	10–100 mg/day
Intuniv (guanfacine), alpha agonist; not a controlled substance; FDA approved	1–4 mg / day
Catapres (Clonidine), alpha agonist; not a controlled substance; not FDA approved	0.1–0.4 mg / day
Wellbutrin SR/XL (bupropion), norepinephrine dopamine reuptake inhibitor; not FDA approved	100–450 mg/day

- Monitor for side effects and adverse effects of stimulants:
  - GI upset
  - Cramps
  - Anorexia
  - Weight loss
  - Blood pressure
  - Growth suppression
  - Headache dizziness
  - Irritability
  - Psychosis (rare)

Nonpharmacologic Treatment

- Behavioral therapy
- Patient and parent cognitive-behavioral training program
- Psychoeducation
- Treatment of learning disorders
- Family therapy and education

▶ Parents of children with ADHD have many difficult emotions:
- Stress
- Self-blame
- Social isolation
- Embarrassment
- Depressive reaction
- Marital discord

▶ Typical family concerns:
- Stigma
- Anger
- Concerns over treatment options
- Presence of controversial information in media
  - Claims of dietary causes of disorder
  - Belief in family etiological factors

▶ Family educational needs:
- Environmental structuring
- Psychiatric comorbidities

- School issues and concerns
- Peer relationship-building
- Smoking and substance abuse rates
- Stress management

Common Comorbidities

- Major depressive disorder (MDD; see Chapter 8)
- Bipolar (BP) disorder (see Chapter 8)
- Anxiety disorders (see Chapter 9)
- Oppositional defiant disorder (see above)
- Substance abuse disorders (see Chapter 12)
- Tic disorder
- Learning disorders

Follow-up

- Monitor clinical progress over time.
- Use standardized rating scales such as:
  - Conners' Parent and Teacher Rating Scales (copyrighted; Conners, 1969)
  - Vanderbilt ADHD Diagnostic Parent and Teacher Rating Scales (public domain)
- Monitor attainment of growth and development milestones.
- Symptoms may persist into adulthood.
  - Plan for long-term needs.

ASPERGER SYNDROME

Description

- *Asperger syndrome* is severe, sustained impairment in social interaction and restricted, repetitive patterns of behavior, interests, and activities.
- Lacks language delays but is sometimes associated with motor delays

Etiology

- No single factor can account for presentation.
- Etiology is largely unknown.
- Many biopsychosocial factors contribute to the development.

Incidence and Demographics

▶ The disorder appears to be more common among family members who have the disorder or who have autism spectrum disorder (ASD).

▶ Prevalence is not known, but the disorder is more common in boys.

Risk Factors

▶ Genetic loading

Prevention and Screening

▶ At-risk family education

▶ Community education

  ▹ Stigma reduction

  ▹ Signs and symptoms of illness

  ▹ Treatment potential for control of symptoms

▶ Early recognition, intervention, and initiation of treatment

  ▹ Secondary prevention is important in young patients

Assessment

▶ Detailed history of present illness, including time frame, progression, and associated symptoms

▶ Social history, including present living situation; marital status; occupation; education; and alcohol, tobacco, or illicit drug use

▶ Medication use, including prescription, over-the-counter, alternative, supplements, and home remedies

▶ Initial and periodic functional history and assessment

▶ Validate history with a family member.

History

▶ Assess for the following:

  ▹ Qualitative impairment in social interaction

  ▹ Restricted, repetitive, and stereotyped patterns of behavior, interests, and activities

  ▹ Significant impairment in social, occupational, or other areas of functioning

  ▹ Diagnostic criteria very similar to autism, except no clinically significant delay in language, cognitive development, or adaptive behavior

Physical Exam

▶ Nonspecific

Mental Status Exam

- ▶ Appearance
    - ▹ Stereotyped or repetitive motor mannerisms
    - ▹ Poor eye contact
- ▶ Affect
    - ▹ Flat affect
- ▶ Reaction to interview
    - ▹ Lack of emotional reciprocity

Diagnostic Studies

- ▶ No laboratory tests
- ▶ CBC, chemistry profile, thyroid function tests, and B_{12} level to rule out metabolic causes or unidentified conditions
- ▶ Drug toxicity screening, if indicated by history

Differential Diagnosis

- ▶ ASD (see below)
- ▶ Rett syndrome (see below)
- ▶ Developmental disability
- ▶ Childhood disintegrative disorder (marked deterioration of functioning after a period of at least 2 years of normal functioning and development)
- ▶ Schizophrenia (see Chapter 10)
- ▶ Schizoid personality disorder (see Chapter 13)

Management

- ▶ Rule out or treat any conditions that may contribute to current symptom manifestation.

Pharmacologic Treatment

- ▶ Nonspecific
- ▶ Treat symptoms as indicated

Nonpharmacologic Treatment

- ▶ Multimodality treatment:
    - ▹ Behavioral therapy
    - ▹ Appropriate school placement
    - ▹ Occupational therapy
    - ▹ Physical therapy
    - ▹ Speech therapy

RETT SYNDROME

Description

▶ *Rett syndrome* is the development of specific deficits following a period of normal functioning after birth.

Etiology

▶ Etiology is unknown.

▶ There is a known, progressive, and deteriorating course after an initial period without apparent disability.

▶ It is compatible with probable metabolic disorder.

▶ Suspected genetic mutation exists.

Incidence and Demographics

▶ The disorder occurs primarily in girls.

▶ It is usually associated with severe or profound mental retardation (see below).

Risk Factors

▶ Mental retardation

▶ Seizure disorder

Prevention and Screening

▶ At-risk family education

▶ Community education

- Stigma reduction

- Signs and symptoms of illness

- Treatment potential for control of symptoms

▶ Screen for developmental delays at well-child visit (CDC, 2012).

- Modified Checklist for Autism in Toddlers (M-CHAT)

▶ Early recognition, intervention, and initiation of treatment

- Secondary prevention is important in young patients

Assessment

▶ Detailed history of present illness, including time frame, progression, and associated symptoms

▶ Social history, including present living situation

► Medication use, including prescription, over the counter, alternative, supplements, and home remedies

  ▹ Initial and periodic functional history and assessment

History

► Assess for the following:

  ▹ Normal prenatal and perinatal development

  ▹ Normal psychomotor development through the first 5 months after birth

  ▹ Normal head circumference at birth

  ▹ Onset of all of the following after the period of normal development:

    ▷ Deceleration of head growth between the ages 5 and 48 months

    ▷ Loss of previously acquired purposeful hand skills between ages 5 and 30 months, with the subsequent development of stereotyped hand movements

    ▷ Early loss of social engagement

    ▷ Appearance of poorly coordinated gait or trunk movements

    ▷ Severely impaired expressive and receptive language development with severe psychomotor retardation.

Physical Exam

► Associated features:

  ▹ Seizures

  ▹ Irregular respirations

  ▹ Scoliosis

  ▹ Loss of purposeful hand skills

  ▹ Stereotypic hand movements

Mental Status Exam

► Appearance

  ▹ Stereotyped hand movements

► Speech

  ▹ Expressive and receptive language impairment

► Affect

  ▹ Flat or blunted affect

Diagnostic Studies

► No specific laboratory or diagnostic findings

► CBC, chemistry profile, thyroid function tests, and B_{12} level to rule out metabolic causes or unidentified conditions

DISORDERS OF CHILDHOOD AND ADOLESCENCE **359**

► Drug toxicity screening, if indicated by history

► EEG and nonspecific abnormalities on brain imaging

Differential Diagnosis

- ASD (see below)

- Childhood disintegrative disorder

- Mental retardation (see below)

- Asperger syndrome (see above)

Management

► Rule out or treat any conditions that may contribute to current symptom manifestation.

Pharmacologic Treatment

► Nonspecific

Nonpharmacologic Treatment

► Multimodality treatment

► Treatment aimed at symptomatic intervention

AUTISM SPECTRUM DISORDER

Description

► *Autism spectrum disorder* involves the marked impairment of social and cognitive abilities.

Etiology

► Imbalances of glutamate, serotonin, and gamma-aminobutyric acid (GABA) are thought to be implicated in causation.

► Brain imaging studies (Gillberg, 1999) of children with autism reveal microscopic and macroscopic abnormalities of the amygdala, hippocampus, and cerebellum.

► Decreased numbers of Purkinje cells in the cerebellum are thought to play a role in the development.

Incidence and Demographics

► ASD is more common in children with a family history of pervasive developmental disorders.

► The concordant rate for an identical twin with autism is 60%.

► The incidence is 2 to 5 cases per 10,000 in the United States.

► The male-to-female ratio is 4:1.

360 PSYCHIATRIC-MENTAL HEALTH NURSE PRACTITIONER REVIEW MANUAL, 3RD EDITION

▶ Onset of symptoms is before age 3 years.

▶ About 10% of patients also have a genetic or chromosomal condition such as Down syndrome or fragile X syndrome (CDC, 2012).

Risk Factors

▶ Male

▶ Severe mental retardation

▶ Genetic loading

Prevention and Screening

▶ At-risk family education

▶ Community education

　▸ Stigma reduction

　▸ Signs and symptoms of illness

　▸ Treatment potential for control of symptoms

▶ Early recognition, intervention, and initiation of treatment

　▸ Secondary prevention is important in young patients.

Assessment

History

▶ Assess for the following:

　▸ Impairment with social interaction, communications, and behavior

　　▹ Impaired social interactions such as abnormal gaze, posture, and expression in social interactions

　▸ Lack of peer relationships, emotional reciprocity, and spontaneous seeking of enjoyment

　▸ Impaired communication, such as a delay or lack in the development of spoken language, impaired ability to initiate and sustain conversations, repetitive and stereotyped use of language, and inability to play with others

　▸ Restricted repetitive and stereotyped patterns of behavior, interests, and activities. such as inflexible adherence to specific nonfunctional routines and repetitive, stereotyped motor mannerisms (e.g., hand or finger flapping, rocking, swaying)

　▸ Parents may report any of the following symptoms:

　　▹ No cooing by age 1 year, no single words by age 16 months, no two-word phrases by age 24 months

　　▹ Loss of language skills at any time

　　▹ No imaginary play

　　▹ Little interest in playing with other children

> ▷ Extremely short attention span

> ▷ No response when called by name

> ▷ Little or no eye contact

> ▷ Intense tantrums

> ▷ Fixations on single objects

> ▷ Unusually strong resistance to changes in routines

> ▷ Oversensitivity to certain sounds, textures, or smells

> ▷ Appetite or sleep–rest disturbance, or both

> ▷ Self-injurious behavior

Physical Exam

▶ Nonspecific

Mental Status Exam

▶ Little or no eye contact

▶ Flat or blunted affect

▶ Lack of emotional reciprocity

▶ Stereotyped or repetitive motor mannerisms

> ▷ Expressive- and receptive-language impairment

Diagnostic Studies

▶ No specific laboratory tests

Differential Diagnosis

▶ Rett syndrome (see above)

▶ Asperger syndrome (see above)

▶ Childhood disintegrative disorder

▶ Mental retardation (see below)

▶ Hearing impairment

▶ Developmental language and speech disorders

▶ Tic disorders

▶ Stereotypic movement disorder

▶ Schizophrenia (see Chapter 10)

▶ Cluster A personality disorders (see Chapter 13)

Management

Pharmacologic Treatment

▶ No specific pharmacological interventions

▶ Antipsychotics effective for symptoms such as tantrums; aggressive behavior; self-injurious behavior; hyperactivity; and repetitive, stereotyped behaviors

▶ Antidepressants, naltrexone, clonidine, and stimulants used to diminish self-injurious and hyperactive and obsessive behaviors

Nonpharmacologic Treatment

▶ Behavioral therapy to improve cognitive functioning and reduce inappropriate behavior

▶ Occupational therapy to improve sensory integration and motor skills

▶ Speech therapy to address communication and language barriers

▶ Pivotal response training

▶ Appropriate school placement with a highly structured approach

EATING DISORDERS

Description

▶ *Eating disorders* are characterized by disordered patterns of eating, accompanied by distress, disparagement, preoccupation, and a distorted perception of one's body shape.

▶ Common forms of eating disorders:

- Anorexia nervosa

  ▷ Patients refuse to maintain a normal body weight

  ▷ Involves restricted caloric intake

  ▷ Patients have an intense fear of gaining weight because of a distorted body image

- Bulimia nervosa

  ▷ Patients engage in binge eating, combined with inappropriate ways of stopping weight gain

  ▷ Associated with efforts made to lose weight

- Binge eating disorder

  ▷ Recurrent episodes of binge eating with lack of control

  ▷ Bingeing occurs at least 2 days weekly for 6 months

  ▷ Not regularly associated with compensatory behaviors

DISORDERS OF CHILDHOOD AND ADOLESCENCE **363**

Etiology

▶ Etiology is multifactorial, with biological, social, and psychological factors implicated in causation.

▶ Neurobiological factors include decreased hypothalamic norepinephrine activation, dysfunction of lateral hypothalamus, and decreased serotonin.

Incidence and Demographics

▶ Incidence is more common in girls, with 85% to 95% of occurrences.

▶ Anorexia nervosa affects approximately 0.28% of the general U.S. population.

▶ Bulimia nervosa affects approximately 1.0% of the general U.S. population.

▶ Onset is typically between ages 14 and 18 years.

Risk Factors

▶ Genetic loading

▶ Increased risk of eating disorders among first-degree biological relatives of people with certain other psychiatric disorders:

  ▻ Eating disorders

  ▻ Mood disorders

  ▻ Substance abuse disorders

Prevention and Screening

▶ At-risk family education

▶ Community education

  ▻ Stigma reduction

  ▻ Signs and symptoms of illness

  ▻ Treatment potential for control of symptoms

▶ Early recognition, intervention, and initiation of treatment

  ▻ Secondary prevention is important in young patients

Assessment

▶ Detailed history of present illness, including time frame, progression, and associated symptoms

▶ Social history, including present living situation; marital status; occupation; education; and alcohol, tobacco, or illicit drug use

▶ Medication use, including prescription, over-the-counter, alternative, supplements, and homeremedies

▶ Initial and periodic functional history and assessment

▶ Validate history with a family member

History

▶ Anorexia nervosa

» Refusal to maintain a minimally normal body weight

» Weight less than 85% of expected weight

» Fear of gaining weight or becoming fat

» Distorted body image

▷ *Restricting type:* During the current episode, the patient has not regularly engaged in binge eating or purging behavior.

▷ *Binge eating/purging type:* During the current episode, the patient has regularly engaged in binge eating or purging behavior.

▶ Bulimia nervosa

» Recurrent, episodic binge eating

» Both binge eating and inappropriate compensatory behaviors occur at least twice weekly for 3 months

▶ Recurrent, inappropriate compensatory behaviors to prevent weight gain:

» Self-induced vomiting

» Laxatives

» Enemas

» Diuretics

» Stimulants

» Abuse of diet pills

» Fasting

» Excessive exercise

▶ Self-evaluation unduly influenced by body shape and weight

» *Purging type:* During the current episode, the patient regularly has engaged in purging or the misuse of laxatives, enemas, or diuretics.

» *Nonpurging type:* During the current episode, the patient has used other inappropriate compensatory behaviors, such as fasting or excessive exercise, but has not regularly engaged in purging or misuse of laxatives, enemas, or diuretics.

Physical Exam

▶ Anorexia nervosa:

» Low body mass index

» Amenorrhea

» Emaciation

» Bradycardia

- Hypotension
- ECG changes
  - ▷ Inversion of T-waves
  - ▷ ST segment depression
  - ▷ Prolonged QT interval
- Hypothermia
- Yellow skin secondary to carotenemia
- Dry skin
- Brittle hair and nails
- Lanugo growth on face, extremities, and trunk
- Peripheral edema
- Hypertrophy of the salivary glands
- Erosion of dental enamel
- Russell's sign—scarring or calluses on the dorsum of the hand secondary to self-induced vomiting.

▶ Bulimia nervosa
- Weight usually within normal range
- Erosion of dental enamel
- Russell's sign
- Hypertrophy of salivary glands
- Rectal prolapse

Mental Status Exam

▶ Appearance
- Emaciated appearance with anorexia nervosa

▶ Affect
- Lability
- Anxiety
- Constricted and sad

▶ Mood
- Dysphoric mood

- ► Thought content
  - ▸ Preoccupation with food and body weight
  - ▸ Suicidal ideation
  - ▸ Low self-esteem
- ► Concentration
  - ▸ Decreased concentration
- ► Judgment
  - ▸ Impaired for self-welfare
- ► Insight
  - ▸ Impaired

Diagnostic Studies

- ► CBC, chemistry profile, thyroid function tests, and B_{12} level to rule out metabolic causes or unidentified conditions
- ► Drug toxicity screening, if indicated by history
- ► Anorexia nervosa
  - ▸ No definitive laboratory test for diagnosis
  - ▸ Laboratory changes:
    - ▹ Normochromic, normocytic anemia
    - ▹ Leukopenia
    - ▹ Neutropenia
    - ▹ Anemia
    - ▹ Thrombocytopenia
    - ▹ Hypokalemia
    - ▹ Hypomagnesemia
    - ▹ Hypoglycemia
    - ▹ Decreased LH and FSH
- ► Bulimia nervosa
  - ▸ No definitive laboratory tests
  - ▸ Laboratory changes:
    - ▹ Hypotension
    - ▹ Bradycardia
    - ▹ Hypokalemia
    - ▹ Hyponatremia

DISORDERS OF CHILDHOOD AND ADOLESCENCE **367**

- ▷ Hypochloremia
- ▷ Hypomagnesemia
- ▷ Metabolic acidosis or alkalosis
- ▷ Elevated serum amylase

Differential Diagnosis

- ► General medical condition
- ► Mood disorders (see Chapter 8)
- ► Cluster B personality disorders (see Chapter 13)
- ► Obsessive–compulsive disorder (OCD; see Chapter 9)
- ► Schizophrenia (see Chapter 10)

Management

- ► Rule out or treat any conditions that may contribute to current symptom manifestation.

Pharmacologic Treatment

- ► Medication management as adjunctive therapy to psychotherapy
- ► No specific medication therapy for anorexia nervosa
- ► Fluoxetine is FDA-approved for bulimia nervosa
- ► SSRIs and tricylic antidepressants (TCAs) effective in reducing the frequency of bingeing and purging
- ► Treat associated symptoms, such as depression and anxiety, with appropriate pharmacological therapy

Nonpharmacologic Treatment

- ► Multimodal treatment
  - ▹ Medical and nutritional stabilization
    - ▷ Weight restoration
    - ▷ Correction of electrolyte disturbance
    - ▷ Vitamin supplementation
    - ▷ Nutrition counseling
  - ▹ Dental care
  - ▹ Psychotherapeutic interventions
    - ▷ Individual psychotherapy
    - ▷ Behavioral therapy
    - ▷ Cognitive–behavioral therapy

- ▷ Family therapy
- ▷ Group therapy
- ▸ Community resources
  - ▷ Eating disorder support groups
  - ▷ 12-step programs

MENTAL RETARDATION

Description

- ▶ *Mental retardation* is subaverage general intellectual functioning based on a standardized intelligence test.
- ▶ Onset must occur before age 18 years.
- ▶ IQ is below 70.
- ▶ Concurrent impairment exists in adaptive functioning in at least two of the following areas:
  - ▸ Communication
  - ▸ Self-care
  - ▸ Home living
  - ▸ Social or interpersonal skills

Etiology

- ▶ Heredity accounts for 5% of cases:
  - ▸ Inborn errors of metabolism errors (e.g., Tay–Sachs disease)
  - ▸ Single-gene abnormalities (e.g., tuberous sclerosis)
  - ▸ Chromosomal aberrations (e.g., translocation of chromosome 21 [Down syndrome] and X-linked gene of FMR-1 [fragile X syndrome])
- ▶ Early alterations of embryonic development account for 30% of cases.
  - ▸ Prenatal exposure to toxins (e.g., maternal alcohol consumption, infections)
- ▶ Pregnancy and perinatal problems account for 10% of cases:
  - ▸ Fetal malnutrition
  - ▸ Premature birth
  - ▸ Fetal hypoxia
  - ▸ Birth trauma

DISORDERS OF CHILDHOOD AND ADOLESCENCE **369**

► General medical conditions acquired during infancy or childhood contribute to approximately 5% of cases

  ► Infections

  ► Brain trauma

  ► Exposure to toxins (e.g., lead poisoning)

► No clear etiology can be found in 30% to 50% of cases.

► The most preventable cause of mental retardation is fetal alcohol syndrome.

► Characteristics of fetal alcohol syndrome include:

  ► Epicanthal skin folds

  ► Low nasal bridge

  ► Short nose

  ► Indistinct philtrum

  ► Small head circumference

  ► Small eye openings

  ► Wide-set eyes

  ► Thin upper lip

Risk Factors

► Genetic loading

► Adverse birth events

Incidence and Demographics

► Between 1% and 3% of the general population

Assessment

History

► Assess for the following:

  ► Mild mental retardation (IQ range 50–55 to 70)

    ▷ Accounts for 85% of cases

    ▷ Can develop social and communication skills

    ▷ Minimal sensorimotor abnormalities

    ▷ Can acquire academic skills up to approximately 6th-grade level

    ▷ Can achieve social and vocational skills adequate for minimum self-support

    ▷ Can live successfully in the community independently or in supervised settings

- Moderate mental retardation (IQ range 35–40 to 50–55)
  - Accounts for 10% of cases
  - Limited social awareness
  - Can acquire some communication skills
  - May benefit from vocational training
  - Seldom advances academically beyond the 2nd-grade level
  - Can be trained to care for most personal needs
  - Can perform unskilled or semiskilled work in sheltered job placements
  - Can live in the community but usually in a supervised setting such as a group home
- Severe mental retardation (IQ range 20–25 to 35–40)
  - Accounts for 4% of cases
  - Slow and poor motor development
  - Little or no communicative speech
  - May be able to learn to sight read some survival words such as *stop* and *exit*
  - May be able to perform simple tasks in tightly supervised settings
  - Can live in the community in group homes unless some other disability requires specialized nursing care
- Profound mental retardation (IQ below 20 to 25)
  - Accounts for 1% to 2% of cases
  - Minimal capacity for sensorimotor functioning
  - Poor cognitive and social capacities
  - Speech often absent
  - May develop minimal motor skills, self-care skills, and communication skills if appropriate training provided
  - May live in group homes or intermediate-care facilities
  - May be able to perform simple tasks in a closely supervised and sheltered setting

Physical Exam
- Oblique eye folds
- Small, flattened skull
- Large tongue
- Broad hands with stumpy fingers
- Single transverse palm crease
- High cheekbones
- Small height
- Brushfield spots on iris

- ► Abnormal finger and toe prints

- ► Cryptorchidism

- ► Congenital cardiac defects

- ► Early dementia

- ► Hypothyroidism

Mental Status Exam

- ► Communication deficits

- ► Dependency

- ► Passivity

- ► Poor self-esteem

- ► Low frustration tolerance

- ► Aggressiveness

- ► Stereotyped, repetitive motor movement

- ► Self-injurious behavior

Diagnostic Studies

- ► No specific laboratory findings

- ► Some laboratory findings associated with a variety of causes of mental retardation (e.g., metabolic disturbances)

Differential Diagnosis

- ► Borderline intellectual functioning

- ► Learning and communication disorders

- ► Pervasive developmental disorder (PDD)

   - ⯈ 75% of individuals with a PDD have comorbid mental retardation

- ► ADHD (see above)

- ► Stereotypic movement disorder

- ► General medical condition

Management

Pharmacologic Treatment

- ► Pharmacological treatment is symptom specific.

   - ⯈ Treat concomitant psychopathology (e.g., ADHD, depressive disorder, anxiety disorder, schizophrenia).

   - ⯈ Aggressive or self-injurious behavior may be controlled with antipsychotics and mood stabilizers.

372 PSYCHIATRIC–MENTAL HEALTH NURSE PRACTITIONER REVIEW MANUAL, 3RD EDITION

Nonpharmacologic Treatment

▶ Therapy

▶ Behavioral therapy

▶ Group therapy

▶ Family therapy

▶ Community resources

    ▹ Day care settings

    ▹ Sheltered workshops

    ▹ Group homes

▶ In *DSM-V*, "mental retardation" is replaced with the term "intellectual disabilities" and found in the chapter on Neurodevelopmental Disorders (*DSM-V*, 2013).

CASE STUDY

The parents of a child with attention-deficit hyperactivity disorder (ADHD) ask to speak to you privately after you complete your assessment of their child. They tell you they have several questions that they want answered, and they want to ask you to keep the answers to yourself and not tell their son what they ask. Their first question is about diet. They have read that ADHD can be managed by dietary therapy instead of medications, and they want your opinion about trying this strategy with their child. They also want to know how likely it is that he will "outgrow" the disorder. You have many issues to consider before answering the parents' questions.

▶ What is the most accepted theory of etiology regarding ADHD?

▶ What is the empirical database for dietary treatment in ADHD patients?

▶ What is the natural course of this illness? Is it likely that the son's symptoms will improve as he ages?

▶ What are the other issues to consider regarding the parents' request to keep confidential the concerns that they are expressing?

REFERENCES

American Academy of Child and Adolescent Psychiatry. (1997). Practice parameter for the treatment of children and adolescents with conduct disorder. *Journal of the American Academy of Child and Adolescent Psychiatry, 36*(10), 122S–139S.

American Academy of Child and Adolescent Psychiatry. (2007a). Practice parameter for the assessment and treatment of children and adolescents with attention-deficit/hyperactivity disorder. *Journal of the American Academy of Child and Adolescent Psychiatry, 46*(7), 894–921.

American Academy of Child and Adolescent Psychiatry. (2007b). Practice parameter for the assessment and treatment of children and adolescents with oppositional defiant disorder. *Journal of the American Academy of Child and Adolescent Psychiatry, 46*(1), 126–141.

American Psychiatric Association. (2000). *Diagnostic and statistical manual of mental disorders* (4th ed., text rev.).Washington, DC: American Psychiatric Association.

American Psychiatric Association. (2001). Practice parameters for the assessment and treatment of children and adolescents with suicidal behavior. *Journal of the American Academy of Child and Adolescent Psychiatry, 4*(Suppl. 7), 245–478.

American Psychiatric Association. (2013). *Diagnostic and statistical manual of mental disorders* (5th ed.).Washington, DC: Author.

Barlow, D. A., & Durand, V. M. (2004). *Abnormal psychology* (4th ed.). Pacific Grove, CA: Brooks/Cole.

Barkley, R. (2005). *Attention deficit hyperactivity disorder: A handbook for diagnosis and treatment* (3rd ed.). New York: Guilford Press.

Bernstein, G. A., & Shaw, K. (1997). Practice parameters for the assessment and treatment of children and adolescents with anxiety disorders. *Journal of the American Academy of Child and Adolescent Psychiatry, 36*(Suppl. 69), 80S–84S.

Blazer, D. G., & Kaplar, B. H. (2000). Controversies in community-based psychiatric epidemiology: Let the data speak for themselves. *Archives of General Psychiatry, 57,* 227.

Bremner, J. D. (1999). Devastating effects and clinical implications of childhood abuse. *Directions in Psychiatry, 19,* 147–160.

Centers for Disease Control and Prevention. (2010). Morbidity and mortality weekly report: Increasing prevalence of parent reported attention-deficit/hyperactivity disorder among children – United States, 2003 and 2007. *Morbidity and Mortality Weekly Report, 59*(44), 1–40.

Centers for Disease Control and Prevention. (2012). *Autism spectrum disorders.* Retrieved from http://www.cdc.gov/ncbddd/autism/facts.html

Conners, C. K. (1969). A teacher rating scale for use in drug studies with children. *American Journal of Psychiatry, 126,* 884–888.

Cyranowski, J. M., Frank, E., Young, E., & Shear, M. K. (2000). Adolescent onset of the gender difference in lifetime rates of major depression. *Archives of General Psychiatry, 57,* 21–27.

DelCarmen-Wiggins, R., & Carter, A. S. (2001). Assessment of infant and toddler mental health: Advances and challenges. *Journal of the American Academy of Child and Adolescent Psychiatry, 40*(1), 8–10.

Dohenwend, B. P. (1998). A psychosocial perspective on the past and future of psychiatric epidemiology. *American Journal of Epidemiology, 147,* 222–231.

Frances, A. (1998). Problems in defining clinical significance in epidemiologic studies. *Archive of General Psychiatry, 55,* 119.

Frankel, F. D. (2001). Common peer relationship problems in childhood. *Primary Psychiatry, 8*(12), 25–31.

Gadow, K., Sprafkin, J., & Nolan, E. (2001). DSM-IV symptoms in community and clinic preschool children. *Journal of the American Academy of Child and Adolescent Psychiatry, 40,* 1383–1392.

Gillberg, C. (1999). Neurodevelopmental processes and psychological functioning in autism. *Developmental and Psychopathology, 11,* 567–587.

Halmi, K. A., & Romano, S. J. (2001). Anorexia nervosa: An overview. *Primary Psychiatry, 6*(2), 35–56.

Hamrin, V. & Gray Deering, C. (2012). Mental health assessment of children and adolescents. In M. Boyd (Ed.), *Psychiatric nursing contemporary practice* (5th ed., pp. 661–678). Philadelphia: Lippincott Williams & Wilkins.

Harrison, P. L. (1999). Assessment and treatment of children with autism in the schools. *School Psychology Review, 28,* 533–693.

House, A. E. (2002). *DSM-IV diagnosis in the schools* (rev. ed.). New York: Guilford Press.

Kashani, J. H., & Orvaschel, H. (1990). A community study of anxiety in children and adolescents. *American Journal of Psychiatry, 147,* 313–318.

Kazdin, A. E. (2000). Developing a research agenda for child and adolescent psychotherapy. *Archives of General Psychiatry, 57,* 829–835.

McClellan, J., & Werry, J. S. (1997). Practice parameters for the assessment and treatment of children and adolescents with bipolar disorder. *Journal of the American Academy of Child and Adolescent Psychiatry, 36*(Suppl.), 157S–176S.

Nolan, E., Gadow, K., & Sprafkin, J. (2001). Teacher reports of DSM-IV ADHD, ODD, and CD symptoms in school children. *Journal of the American Academy of Child and Adolescent Psychiatry, 40,* 241–249.

Reiger, D. A. (2000). Community diagnosis counts. *Archives of General Psychiatry, 57,* 223.

Reiger, D. A., Kaelber, C. T., Rae, D. S., Farmer, M. E., Knauper, B., Kessler, R. C., et al. (1998). Limitations of diagnostic criteria and assessment instruments for mental disorders: Implications for research and policy. *Archives of General Psychiatry, 55,* 109–115.

Romano, S. J., & Quinn, L. (2001). Evaluation and treatment of bulimia nervosa. *Primary Psychiatry, 6*(2), 57–62.

Rush, A. J., & Frances, A. (2000). Expert consensus guidelines series: Treatment of psychiatric and behavioral problems in mental retardation. *American Journal of Mental Retardation, 105,* 161–228.

Sadock, B. J., & Sadock, B. J. (2007). *Kaplan & Sadock's synopsis of psychiatry* (10th ed.). Baltimore: Lippincott Williams & Wilkins.

Shaffer, D., Fisher, P., Dulcan, M., Davies, M., Piacentini, J., Schwab-Stone, M. E., Regier, D. A. (1996). The NIMH diagnostic interview schedule for children: Description, acceptability, prevalence rates, and performance in the MECA study. *Journal of the American Academy of Child and Adolescent Psychiatry, 35,* 865–877.

Spitzer, R. (1998). Diagnosis and need for treatment are not the same. *Archives of General Psychiatry, 55,* 120.

Spencer, T., Biederman, J., & Wilens, T. (1999). Attention-deficit/hyperactivity disorder and comorbidity. *Pediatric Clinics of North America, 46,* 573–579.

U. S. Department of Health and Human Services. (2000). *Mental health: A report of the Surgeon General.* Washington, DC: U.S. Department of Health and Human Services.

CHAPTER 15

SLEEP

This chapter addresses sleep issues and disorders commonly encountered by the psychiatric–mental health nurse practitioner (PMHNP). These conditions and clinical problems may co-occur with the disorders already discussed or may present in patients with no other identifiable psychiatric or mental health problems. They also may be frequent findings in primary care settings while working with patients with general medical conditions.

General Considerations

► Must be systematically assessed

► Comparison of present level of sleep to historical baseline

► Can be measured by polysomnography

► Rapid eye movement (REM) alternating with four distinct nonrapid eye movement stages (NREM)

▻ Stage I

▷ NREM

▷ Transitional stage from wakefulness to sleep

▷ 5% of total normal sleep cycle

▻ Stage II

▷ NREM

▷ Specific EEG waveforms

▷ 50% of total sleep cycle

▻ Stages III and IV

▷ NREM

▷ Slow-wave sleep period

▷ Deepest level of sleep

▷ 20%–25% of total sleep cycle.

- Sleep stages organized and sequential during sleep period
  - Stages 3 and 4 tend to occur in first one-third to one-half of sleep period.
  - REM occurs cyclically throughout the night, alternating with NREM on average every 80–100 minutes.
  - REM increases in duration toward morning.
- Sleep patterns varying with age
  - Children and adolescents have large amounts of slow-wave sleep.
  - Sleep continuity and depth decrease with age.
  - Consider age when assessing for sleep–rest problems.
- Sleep patterns varying with medication use
  - Many medications and agents of abuse affect sleep cycle.
  - Assess recent changes in medication or drug use in patient presenting with sleep pattern disturbances.
  - Insomnia

Description

- *Insomnia* is the inability to get the amount of sleep needed to function efficiently during the day.
- It is not a specific disease; commonly associated with several disorders, and commonly occurs with mood disorders.
- It is associated with increased mortality, poor career performance, overeating, and increased hospitalization.

Etiology

- Dysfunction in sleep–wake circuits of the brainstem
- Neurochemical imbalances impinging on these circuits
- May be stress-related in brief episodic insomnia.

Incidence and Demographics

- 35% of Americans have difficulty sleeping.
- 18% of Americans have serious sleep problems.
- 4% of Americans take prescription medications to help them sleep.

Risk Factors

- Age
- Past history of insomnia
- Significant stress

- Forced pattern changes
  - Working alternating shifts
  - Swing-shift work patterns
  - Travel across time zones
- High use patterns of medications, drugs, or substances known to affect sleep cycles
  - Caffeine, other stimulants
  - Alcohol
  - Benzodiazepines (BNZs)

Prevention and Screening
- At-risk family education
- Limits on shift work
- Avoidance of medications known to affect sleep patterns
- Good sleep hygiene patterns
- Avoidance of stimulants late in the day
- Early recognition, intervention, and initiation of treatment
- Routine screening at all healthcare settings

Assessment
- Detailed history of present illness, including time frame, progression, and associated symptoms
- Social history, including present living situation; marital status; occupation; education; and alcohol, tobacco, or illicit drug use
- Medication use, including prescription, over-the-counter, alternative, supplements, and home remedies
- Initial and periodic functional history and assessment

History
- Assess for the following:
  - Sleep–rest patterns
    - Number of hours in usual sleep pattern
    - Initial or middle-phase insomnia; early morning awakening
    - Sleep aids

- Position
  - Pillow
  - Environmental regulation
    - Temperature
    - Sound control
    - Light control
    - Duration of sleep disturbance

▶ Transient insomnia
  - Can be caused by stress, jet lag, or physical environment
  - May last several days
  - Generally can be relieved by exercise, a hot bath, warm milk, and changing bedroom environment.

▶ Short-term insomnia
  - Result of stress, illness, or bereavement
  - May linger for up to 3 weeks

▶ Long-term insomnia
  - Lasts for more than 3 weeks
  - Calls for an extensive diagnostic examination.

▶ Insomnia related to another psychiatric disorder
  - More than 50% of insomnia cases related to primary psychiatric disorder
    - Mood disorders (see Chapter 8)
    - Anxiety disorders (see Chapter 9)
    - Substance-related disorders (see Chapter 12).
    - Attention-deficit hyperactivity disorder (ADHD; see Chapter 14)
  - Early-morning wakefulness a possible sign of depression
  - Sudden, dramatic decrease in sleep a sign of possible mania or schizophrenia
  - Poor sleep a sign of possible obsessive–compulsive disorder
  - Panic and anxiety episodes during sleep a sign of possible panic disorder
  - Alcohol may cause numerous awakenings during the night.

Physical Exam

▶ Nonspecific

▶ Sleep problems often a manifestation of an underlying disorder

▶ Patients with insomnia should have full exam

Mental Status Exam

▶ May have preoccupation or excessive worry about "not getting enough sleep"

▶ Depending on duration of sleep deprivation, many areas of MSE may be affected.

Diagnostic Studies

▶ CBC, chemistry profile, thyroid function tests, ferritin level (if restless legs) and B_{12} level to rule out metabolic causes or unidentified conditions

▶ Drug toxicity screening, if indicated by history

Differential Diagnosis

▶ Cardiac illnesses

▶ Parasomnias

▶ Gastrointestinal disorders

▶ Chronic obstructive pulmonary disease

▶ Medication side effects

▶ Sleep apnea

▶ Restless legs syndrome

▶ Anxiety

▶ Depression

▶ Stress reaction

▶ Active substance abuse

▶ Drug use

    ▹ Caffeine

    ▹ Stimulants

Management

▶ Rule out or treat any conditions that may contribute to current symptom manifestation.

Pharmacologic Treatment

▶ Melatonin is particularly useful to correct sleep onset issues. May be helpful for the person with ADHD

  ▸ Ramelteon (Rozerem)

▶ Benzodiazepine (BNZ) and hypnotics

  ▸ Flurazepam (Dalmane)

    ▹ Long-lasting agent

    ▹ May cause excess drowsiness

    ▹ Avoid in older adults

  ▸ Temazepam (Restoril)

    ▹ Intermediate-acting agent

  ▸ Triazolam (Halcion)

    ▹ Short-acting agent

    ▹ Little to no excess sedation

  ▸ Common side effects

    ▹ Impaired memory

    ▹ Poor learning for new information

    ▹ Efficacy decreases over time

    ▹ Should not be used on a long-term basis or for longer than 2 weeks.

▶ Nonbenzodiazepine hypnotics

    ▹ Zaleplon (Sonata)

    ▹ Zolpidem (Ambien, Ambien CR)

    ▹ Eszopiclone (Lunesta)

▶ Antidepressants

  ▸ Used for sedating properties (off-label use)

    ▹ Amitriptyline (Elavil); generally avoid use in older adults

    ▹ Mirtazapine (Remeron)

    ▹ Trazodone

▶ Eszopiclone (Lunesta) Antidepressants

  ▸ Used for sedating properties (off-label use)

    ▹ Amitriptyline (Elavil); generally avoid use in older adults

    ▹ Mirtazapine (Remeron)

    ▹ Trazaodone

Nonpharmacologic Treatment

- ▶ Sleep hygiene practices
  - ▹ Establish a bedtime routine
  - ▹ Have a regular time to sleep and wake
  - ▹ Avoid computer use 1 hour before bedtime
  - ▹ Never lie in bed for more than 15 minutes if not able to sleep
  - ▹ Reduce stress
  - ▹ Do stress reduction activities before bedtime
  - ▹ Avoid late-in-the-day exercise
  - ▹ Avoid late-in-the-day stimulant use, such as caffeine in coffee
  - ▹ Do not lie in bed other than to sleep (e.g., avoid watching TV in bed)
- ▶ Psychotherapy
  - ▹ Cognitive therapy
- ▶ Relaxation therapies
  - ▹ Abdominal breathing
  - ▹ Progressive muscle relaxation
  - ▹ Meditation
  - ▹ Imaging
  - ▹ Hypnosis
  - ▹ Biofeedback
  - ▹ Stimulus control
  - ▹ Sleep curtailment
  - ▹ Light therapy
- ▶ Somatic and other therapies
  - ▹ Exercise
  - ▹ Warm bath
  - ▹ Warm milk
  - ▹ Change bedroom environment

Special Considerations

- ▶ Insomnia in children
  - ▹ This is most commonly related to stress.
  - ▹ Children with insomnia often have been poor sleepers since birth.
  - ▹ Pharmacologic treatment is not recommended for most children.

▶ Insomnia in older adults

   ▸ If first presentation is in older years, insomnia often is the result of changes in chronobiological rhythms. Older adults often become sleepier early in the evening and wake up early.

   ▸ Sleep latency, decreased REM sleep, and increased sleep fragmentation are common.

▶ Insomnia may be related to the following underlying psychiatric disorders:

   ▸ Mood disorders

   ▸ Anxiety disorders

   ▸ Alzheimer's disease

   ▸ Older adults often manifest confusion and restlessness as aspects of insomnia.

   ▸ A careful, complete assessment is necessary when pharmacological interventions are planned.

CASE STUDY

Mrs. Jones, a 43-year-old receptionist, presents at your clinic with a primary complaint of insomnia. She reports lifelong problems with sleeping that "comes and goes" depending on her stress level and general health. She has been experiencing a 4–5-day period of poor sleeping, reporting only 3–4 hours of sleep and early-morning awakening. She has tried over-the-counter medication and has received no relief. She reports that her health is generally good but states that she is a 2-pack-a-day smoker and has increased her recreational use of alcohol to 1–2 drinks a night in the past few weeks in order to get to sleep.

Her insomnia is now beginning to impair her daily functioning and her interest in social activities. She reports an irritable mood since her sleep has been difficult and problems with memory and concentration in the morning after she has slept poorly. She denies depression or any other mood problem and currently is taking no routine medication. Her physical exam is unremarkable, and routine lab studies, including TSH, CBC, and electrolytes, are all normal.

▶ What is the most likely diagnosis for this patient at this time?

▶ What further assessment would you make?

▶ What treatment would you consider?

▶ Is medication warranted at this time to induce sleep?

REFERENCES

American Psychiatric Association. (2000). *Diagnostic and statistical manual of mental disorders* (4th ed., text rev.). Washington, DC: American Psychiatric Association.

Brown, D. B. (1999). Managing sleep disorders: Solutions in primary care. *Clinical Reviews, 9*(10), 51–69.

Rajput, V., & Johnson, R. (1999). Chronic insomnia: A practical review. *American Family Practice, 11,* 1–6.

Shea, C. A., Pelletier, L., Poster, E. C., Stuart, G. W., & Verhey, M. P. (1999). *Advanced practice nursing in psychiatric mental health care.* St. Louis, MO: Mosby.

CHAPTER 16

VIOLENCE

This chapter deals with the psychiatric–mental health nurse practitioner's (PMHNPs) role in identifying and treating patients who are impacted by domestic violence, sexual assault, or suicide. Assessment of lethality will also be reviewed. These issues may co-occur with the disorders already discussed or may present in patients with no other identifiable psychiatric or mental health problems. They also may be frequent findings in primary care settings while working with patients with general medical conditions.

DOMESTIC VIOLENCE

Description

► *Domestic violence* is physical, emotional, economic, or sexual pain and injury that is intentionally inflicted.

  ▻ The goal of the abuser is to

    ▹ Establish power

    ▹ Manipulate the other person

    ▹ Intimidate the other person

    ▹ Control the other person

Etiology

▶ Characteristics of abusers:

  ▸ Personality disorders

  ▸ Antisocial personality disorder

  ▸ Narcissistic personality disorder

  ▸ Borderline personality disorder

▶ Environmental stressors

  ▸ Financial difficulties

  ▸ Ending of a relationship

  ▸ Unemployment

Incidence and Demographics

▶ Domestic violence is the leading cause of injury to women ages 15–44.

▶ 1 in 4 pregnant women have a history of domestic violence.

▶ 15%–25% pregnant women are physically abused.

▶ 22%–35% of all women seen in emergency rooms experience injuries as a result of domestic violence; 50% of homeless women experience domestic violence.

▶ 63% of males incarcerated between the ages 11–20 have murdered their mother's abuser.

▶ 33% of male abusers are well-educated and include men in professional jobs.

Risk Factors

▶ For abusers:

  ▸ Exposure to violence at an early developmental age

  ▸ Low self-esteem

  ▸ Social isolation

  ▸ Lack of support

  ▸ Cognitive impairment

  ▸ Physical, financial dependency

Prevention and Screening

▶ Public education and awareness

▶ Social programs

▶ At-risk family education

▶ Community education

- Stigma reduction
- Signs and symptoms of illness
- Prevention programs
- Treatment potential for control of symptoms
► Early recognition, intervention, and initiation of treatment
- Routine screening at all healthcare settings

Assessment

► Interview the patient alone who has experienced violence
► Determine primary caregivers, living arrangements, legal custodian, and power of attorney.

History

► Assess for the following:
- Determine recurrent history of medical treatment consistent with abuse:
  ▷ Accidents
  ▷ Fractures
  ▷ Physical injuries
  ▷ Traumas
  ▷ Refusal of ongoing treatment or follow-up
  ▷ Missed medical appointments
- Determine environmental, psychosocial, and financial stressors

Physical Exam

► Monitor nutritional status for dehydration and malnutrition.
► Look for lacerations, bruises, wounds, burns, or fractures.
► Look for poor skin and personal hygiene.

Mental Status Exam

► Findings of traits and behaviors suggestive of experiencing abuse:
- Fearful
- Evasive
- Guarded
- Depressed
- Passive
- Dependent

Diagnostic Studies

▶ None specific to abuse

▶ Determine general health and nutritional status.

Differential Diagnosis

▶ Accidental injuries

▶ Mood disorders (see Chapter 8)

▶ Anxiety disorders (see Chapter 9)

▶ Substance abuse (see Chapter 12)

Management

▶ Most state laws mandate reporting of suspected abuse and neglect of vulnerable populations:

» Elderly people

» People with disabilities

» Children

Pharmacologic Treatment

▶ None specific to condition

Nonpharmacologic Treatment

▶ The safety and medical well-being of the patient experiencing the abuse is most important.

▶ Refer the patient to a domestic abuse shelter when feasible.

▶ Help the patient develop a safety plan

» Assist patient in developing a "code word" for family or other support system as an attempt to inform them that the person is in need of help

» Advise patient to tell one person in his or her support system about the situation

» Advise patient to pack an "emergency bag" and hide it in case of need to quickly leave

» Advise patient to keep the domestic violence hotline and other telephone numbers (e.g., police department, counselor, shelter) in a secure place

▶ Monitor medical status as symptomology presents.

▶ Monitor nutritional status and vital signs.

▶ Suggest psychotherapy to assist in gaining insight and in developing new coping skills.

▶ Suggest hospitalization when in the best interest of the patient

SEXUAL ASSAULT AND ABUSE

Description

► *Sexual assault or abuse* is any sexual act or penetration committed through coercion or physical force.

  ▻ This includes rape, incest, sodomy, oral and anal acts, or use of a foreign object.

  ▻ It is an act of violence and humiliation expressed through sexual means.

  ▻ It is used to express power or anger.

Etiology

► For abusers:

  ▻ Character disorders

  ▻ Behavioral act of violence is reinforcing

► Once done, likely to repeat

  ▻ Social exposure to violence in culture, media, and home

Incidence and Demographics

► Women have a greater incidence of being assaulted than men.

► Sexual assault is the most common form of abuse.

  ▻ Men are more frequently perpetrators than women.

  ▻ The assaults are committed by fathers and stepfathers, uncles, older siblings, and men that women are dating as well as strangers

► Alcohol is involved in 34% of all forcible rapes.

► Only 1 in 4 rapes is reported.

Risk Factors

► For abusers:

  ▻ Substance abuse disorders

  ▻ Psychiatric disorders

  ▻ Divorce

  ▻ Pregnancy

  ▻ Family or personal history of physical or sexual abuse

  ▻ Long-term exposure to violence

  ▻ Social isolation and lack of support systems

  ▻ Environmental stressors such as unemployment or financial difficulty

Prevention and Screening

▶ Public education and awareness campaigns

▶ Community resources and support

▶ Community emergency shelters, help lines, and safe houses

▶ Assertiveness training and self-defense

▶ At-risk family education

▶ Community education

　▹ Prevention programs

▶ Early recognition, intervention, and initiation of treatment

　▹ Routine screening at all healthcare settings

Assessment

▶ Interview patients who have experienced assault alone.

▶ Establish a safe, trusting relationship to promote sharing.

History

▶ Assess for the following:

　▹ Include questions concerning domestic violence in medical history.

　▹ Interview alone and not in presence of family, friend, or partner.

　▹ Interview for social history, including history of living arrangements and relationships.

Physical Exam

▶ Nonspecific

▶ Presentation of traits and behaviors consistent with possibility of having been abused

　▹ Withdrawn

　▹ Frightened appearance

　▹ Hyper-reactive to touch

▶ Associated findings:

　▹ Unexplained bruises, abrasions, cuts, laceration, burns, soft-tissue swellings, and hematomas

　▹ Sexually transmitted infections

　　▷ Genital rash or discharge

　　▷ Rectal tissue swelling or discharge

► Physical signs that are *strongly suggestive of sexual abuse in children:*

  » Lacerations, ecchymosis, and newly healed scars of the hymen or posterior fourchette

  » No hymenal tissue from 3 to 9 o'clock area

  » Healed hymenal transactions, especially in the above area

  » Perianal lacerations

► Remember that any child presenting with concerning physical signs should be evaluated by a sexual abuse expert. A complete history and a sexual abuse examination need to take place.

Mental Status Exam

► Withdrawn

► Frightened

► Anxious

► Scattered appearance

► Hyperreactive to touch

► Dissociative

Diagnostic Studies

► Nonspecific

► Assessment and documentation labs

  » Forensic specimens

  » Pregnancy tests

  » Rectal, throat, and vaginal cultures

  » VDRL, HIV

  » Herpes B, herpes simplex

  » Human papillomavirus

  » Trichomonas vaginalis

Differential Diagnosis

► Accidental injuries

► Consensual sexual activity

► Lichen sclerosis

► Posttraumatic stress disorder

► Anxiety disorder (see Chapter 9)

Management

▶ Use sensitivity and respectful care.

▶ Be aware of legal reporting requirements.

▶ Utilize available community resources.

Pharmacologic Treatment

▶ Emergency contraception

⇒ Diethylstilbestrol (DES), 25 mg b.i.d. for 5 days within 48 hours of incident

⇒ Norgestrel, 0.5 mg, and ethinyl estradiol, 0.05 mg (Ovral), 2 tablets within 72 hours of incident

⇒ Norgestrel, 0.3 mg, and ethinyl estradiol, 0.03 mg (Lo/Ovral), 4 tablets within 72 hours of incident with 4 tablets 12 hours later.

▶ If required, clinical management of anxiety.

Nonpharmacologic Treatment

▶ Ensure safety and well-being.

▶ Ensure confidentiality.

▶ Complete accurate documentation.

▶ Assess for potential suicidal ideation if the patient is showing any depressive symptoms.

▶ Suggest cognitive–behavioral therapy (CBT).

▶ Offer support groups and community resources.

▶ Assist with access to criminal and legal supports.

LETHALITY ASSESSMENT

▶ *Lethality* refers to the likelihood that a person will commit suicide or homicide—referred to as focused violence at the extreme.

▶ *Lethality assessment:* Evaluation, screening, or testing

▶ *Violence:* The behavioral expression of anger, rage, and hostility that is demonstrated by the use of physical force directed toward persons (in case of suicide, toward self) or property.

Violence in School

▶ Serious physical fighting with peers or family members

▶ Severe destruction of property

▶ Severe rage for seemingly minor reasons

▶ Detailed threats of lethal violence

► Possession or use of firearms or other weapons

► Self-injurious behaviors or threats of suicide

► Bullying or being bullied

► When warning signs indicate that danger is imminent, safety must always be the first and foremost consideration. Action must be taken immediately. Immediate intervention by school authorities and possibly law enforcement officers is needed when a child:

  ► Has presented a detailed plan (time, place, method) to harm or kill others, particularly if the child has a history of aggression or has attempted to carry out threats in the past

  ► Is carrying a weapon, particularly a firearm, and has threatened to use it

Suicide: Risk Factors

► Depression

► All antidepressants have black box warning about increased risk of suicide in children, adolescents, and young adults under the age of 24

► Prior suicide attempt

► Family history of mental disorder or substance abuse

► Family history of suicide

► Family violence

► Firearms in the home

► Incarceration

► Males are 5x more likely than females to commit suicide

► White males over age 85 have highest rate of suicide

Suicide: Signs of Imminent Danger

► Threatening to hurt or kill oneself

► Looking for ways to kill oneself (weapons, pills, or other means)

► Talking or writing about death, dying, or suicide

► Has made plans or preparations for a potentially serious attempt

► Alcohol use increases the risk of suicide attempts in persons with ideation.

Homicide: Early Warning Signs

▶ Prior history of threatening or violent behavior

▶ Paranoia or easily panicked behavior

▶ A fascination or preoccupation with weapons, particularly weapons or explosives that could be used for mass destruction, such as semi-automatic guns

▶ Extreme stress from personal problems or a life crisis

▶ Identifying with incidents of workplace violence reported in the media and either condoning or sympathizing with the actions of the persons committing violence

▶ Being a loner with little or no involvement with other employees

▶ Engaging in frequent disputes with supervisors or coworkers

▶ Persistent violation of company policy

▶ Obsessive involvement with one's job, particularly where it occurs with no apparent outside interest

▶ Volatile or violent home or other personal situation that has the potential to bring violence into the workplace

Threats of Violence

▶ Throwing objects

▶ Making a verbal threat to harm another person or destroy property

▶ Making menacing gestures or physical posturing without actually touching the person

▶ Displaying an intense or obsessive romantic interest that exceeds the normal bounds of interpersonal interest

▶ Attempting to intimidate or harass other people

▶ Behavior indicating that the person is significantly out of touch with reality and that he or she may pose a danger either to himself or herself or to others

▶ Volatile or violent personal situations such as found in some custody battles

▶ Alcohol use increases the risk for violence.

▶ Safety is the number one priority and any threatening behavior must be taken seriously.

REFERENCES

American Nurses Association. (2000). *Scope and standards of psychiatric–mental health clinical nursing practice.* Washington, DC: American Nurses Association.

American Psychiatric Association. (2000). *Diagnostic and statistical manual of mental disorders* (4th ed., text rev.). Washington, DC: American Psychiatric Association.

Brown, D. B. (1999). Managing sleep disorders: Solutions in primary care. *Clinical Reviews, 9*(10), 51–69.

Davidson, J. R. (2000). Trauma: The impact of post-traumatic stress disorder. *Journal of Psychopharmacology, 14*(Suppl. 1), 5–12.

Eddy, M. (1999). Insomnia. *American Family Practice, 1,* 11–16.

Edmunds, M. W., Horan, N. M., & Mayhew, M. S. (2000). *Adult nurse practitioner review manual.* Washington, DC: American Nurses Association.

National Center on Sleep Disorders, Research Working Group. (1999). Recognizing problem sleepiness in your patients. *American Family Physician, 15,* 11–13.

Nettina, S. M., & Knudtson, M. (2001). *The family nurse practitioner review manual.* Washington, DC: American Nurses Association.

Rajput, V., & Johnson, R. (1999). Chronic insomnia: A practical review. *American Family Practice, 11,* 1–6.

Shea, C. A., Pelletier, L., Poster, E. C., Stuart, G. W., & Verhey, M. P. (1999). *Advanced practice nursing in psychiatric mental health care.* St. Louis, MO: Mosby.

U. S. Department of Health and Human Services. (2000). *Mental health: A report of the Surgeon General.* Washington, DC: U.S. Department of Health and Human Services.

APPENDIX A

CASE STUDIES DISCUSSION

Chapter 2: Psychiatric–Mental Health Nurse Practitioner Role, Scope of Practice, and Regulatory Process

1. Would Ms. Harris be legally authorized to treat both children and adults?

   The key word here is legally. Professional standards and scope of practice documents suggest what is reasonable and prudent practice. Professional nursing organizations will provide information on what is seen as acceptable educational preparation for practice. However, the individual legislative regulations of each state determine what constitutes legal practice for each individual PMHNP.

2. What regulation, rule, or standard should Ms. Harris consult to determine if she is legally allowed to treat both children and adults?

   The Nurse Practice Act and related legislation of the state in which she practices will delineate the legal boundaries of her practice.

3. What regulation, rule, or standard should Ms. Harris consult to determine if she is legally allowed to treat both physical and psychiatric disorders?

   Professional standards and scope-of-practice documents suggest what is reasonable and prudent practice. Professional nursing organizations provide information and policy statements about what is seen as acceptable practice roles for PMHNPs. The individual legislative regulations of each state determine what constitutes legal practice for each individual PMHNP.

4. What is the role of professional psychiatric nursing organizations in assisting Ms. Harris to determine the scope of practice that is appropriate for her as a new graduate?

   Professional nursing organizations provide information and policy statements about what is seen as acceptable practice roles for PMHNPs.

5. Is Ms. Harris able to treat the client if he is not consenting to care?

   Any client, including a psychiatric client, has the right to refuse treatment, and Ms. Harris is legally and ethically bound to honor that right.

6. What legal standards must be met if she is to involuntarily treat this client?

   Ms. Harris must meet the legal standard in the state where she practices to treat the client against his or her wishes. This usually entails performing the legal task of committing a client and, in most states, ensuring that the following criteria are met:

   - **Individual has a diagnosed psychiatric disorder**
   - **Individual is unaware or unwilling to accept the nature and severity of disorder**
   - **Treatment is likely to improve functioning**
   - **Individual is harmful to self or others as a consequence of the disorder.**

7. Is the inclusion of a durable power of attorney an appropriate strategy in relapse planning for this client?

A durable power of attorney allows individuals to choose, when they are healthy, an individual to act on their behalf should they become unable to make their own health care decisions. Because this client has a chronic illness that has the potential to render him unable to make his own healthcare decisions, a durable power of attorney document should be part of relapse planning.

8. What quality indicators should be considered in planning his care with the client?

Standardized client assessment and rating scales, evidence-based standards of care, and measures of quality, including client and family satisfaction measures should be considered.

9. What risk management and liability issues should Ms. Harris consider?

Adhere to standards and scope of practice and identify factors specific to this client that increase liability exposure.

Chapter 3. Theoretical Basis of Care

1. Chronologically, what stage of development should Thomas be experiencing?

Adolescence

2. What are the tasks of this stage?

Identity vs. role confusion

3. How would you assess the actual developmental issues that he is experiencing?

Assess the degree of development of his personal sense of identity.

4. What factors do you need to consider to determine if he is experiencing normative or non-normative behaviors?

The PMHNP must have an awareness of the normal milestones of development and the behaviors that indicate failure of developmental stages. Client's history and behaviors are then matched to the known norm for comparison.

5. What characteristic do you as the PMHNP need to display to establish a therapeutic relationship with him?

Genuineness, acceptance, nonjudgmental attitude, authenticity, empathy, and respect professional boundaries.

6. What would be the goal of continued work with Thomas?

    Assisting the individual to establish insight into behaviors and to increase range and maturity of coping behaviors.

7. If you were to start therapy with him, what kind of therapy would you consider?

    Options depend on factors such as the client's goals, motivation, past experiences with counseling, expectations for therapy, and resources.

8. Would you consider him to have a mental illness?

    Mental illness can be defined as any disruption in the usual constitutions of mental health. Mental illness assumes an underlying psychopathology and can be defined as a clinically significant behavioral/psychological syndrome or pattern that occurs in an individual and that is associated with persistent distress or disability or with a significant increased risk of death, pain, disability, or an important loss of freedom. Mr. Jones appears to be experiencing mental health concerns but does not, based on available data, fit the definition of mental illness.

Chapter 4: Neuroanatomy, Neurophysiology, and Behavior

1. Are the symptoms described by Ms. Franklin consistent with a psychiatric disorder?

    More assessment would be needed to determine this, but they may be consistent with an anxiety or mood disorder.

2. Do psychiatric disorders run in families, as Ms. Franklin believes?

    Most psychiatric illnesses have been shown to have, in part, a genetic link and, therefore, do tend to run in families.

3. Do the symptoms as described by Ms. Franklin link with any known neuroanatomical or neurophysiologic deficit?

    Ms. Franklin's symptoms are consistent with excessive levels of norepinephrine.

4. Is a brain scan warranted for Ms. Franklin?

    No. There is insufficient data to warrant the cost of such a procedure at this time.

5. Can the risk of Ms. Franklin's children developing psychiatric disorders be determined?

    Yes, but only if Ms. Franklin is diagnosed as experiencing an actual psychiatric illness. Once this is determined, the genetic risk to her children can be identified through the use of such things as concordant rate tables.

CASE STUDIES DISCUSSION **401**

Chapter 5: Assessment of Acute and Chronic Disease States

1. What additional assessments would you make at this time?

   Physical assessment, mental status exam, and diagnostic and lab testing.

2. What specific diagnostic and laboratory tests would you order, and why?

   To evaluate the possibility of a psychiatric disorder, a thyroid panel should be obtained, because symptoms of thyroid disorder can mimic symptoms of depressive disorders. Electrolyte panel and CBC may be indicated as well for similar reasons. If there are any other clinical indications, a drug screening may be indicated.

3. What, if any, specific physical findings would you look for?

   The presence of the physical findings suggestive of mood disorders and inconsistent with any other specific physical disorder.

4. What communication strategies would you use to facilitate assessment of this patient?

   Broad opening statements, accepting, exploring, and clarifying.

5. What milieu considerations would precede your interactions with her?

   Patient comfort level, low sensory stimulus area, private but safe area, with access to supplies or other staff if needed.

Chapter 6: Pharmacological Principles

1. What is your biggest pharmacological concern at this point with the combination of medication the client is being prescribed?

   The SSRI is potentially increasing the concentration of the TCA to possibly toxic blood levels.

2. What would be your plan of action?

   Check a blood level of amitriptyline and decrease the dosage. Afterward, consider tapering the client off the TCA.

3. What pharmacokinetics should you keep in mind when treating older adults?

   Elderly people have greater body fat content, and because psychotropic drugs are lipophilic, they have an increased risk of toxicity. They also have decreased gastric acid secretion, which can slow the absorption of medications. Older people metabolize drugs slowly, which also can predispose them to toxicity. They are more prone to anticholinergic toxicity and orthostatic hypotension.

Chapter 7: Nonpharmacological Principles

1. What cognitive and behavioral techniques would be helpful for Judy?

   First, identify the negative thoughts and distortions (core beliefs) using a thought record, then use thought-stopping and cognitive restructuring to change the negative thoughts, which will result in a behavioral and emotional change.

2. What type of distortions does Judy have?

   Catastrophic thinking and all-or-nothing distortions

Chapter 8: Depressive Disorders, Grief and Bereavement States, and Bipolar Disorders

1. What is the most probable diagnosis?

   This client's presentation is consistent with the symptoms of major depression.

2. What further assessment is needed?

   Ensure that the client meets the DSM-IV criteria for major depression. Complete physical assessment and use common symptom rating scale such as Beck's Depression Inventory or Zung's Depression Self Rating Scale. Complete assessment for any other physical health states.

3. What target symptoms does the client display that are consistent with the probable diagnosis?

   Depressed mood most of the day, nearly every day, lack of energy, suicidal ideation, MSE findings consistent with MDD.

4. What medications would be considered?

   SSRIs often are considered the first-line agents for the treatment of MDD.

5. If the client had psychotic features with her depression, how would this change the treatment plan?

   Clinical management often includes the short-term use of an antipsychotic agent to control psychotic symptoms. If used, an atypical antipsychotic is usually best tolerated.

CASE STUDIES DISCUSSION **403**

6. How would the plan differ if the client had a heart condition and was taking no other medications?

    Look at issues of compatibility of the various pharmacological agents that the client may be placed on, ensure that the medications used to treat the MDD did not have significant risk of adverse cardiac side effects, ensure that appropriate and complete patient teaching occurred.

Chapter 9: Anxiety Disorders

1. What is the most likely diagnosis?

    Panic disorder; also must be assessed for mood disorder.

2. How will you separate comorbidity from complications of current diagnosis?

    Perform a complete assessment on the client, including physical examination, MSE, and lab studies. The client's current medications should be examined, and the chronology of symptoms should be compared to any changes in his health status.

3. What medication adjustments would you make?

    Consider changing the client's antidepressant medication. Decision should be based on results of complete assessment, final diagnostic impressions, and input from the client and his family. Long-term use of a potentially addictive drug such as Valium needs to be examined carefully.

4. How will you address the family issues?

    Several approaches might be appropriate, including using psychoeducation for the family, providing supportive counseling, or involving the family in family therapy are possible strategies.

5. How often will you plan to see the client?

    The client should be seen frequently until symptoms are stable. Seeing the client weekly initially is ideal. If medication adjustments have been made, the client should return for evaluation at intervals consistent with the pharmacodynamics of the medication for the PMHNP to assess the effects of medication treatment.

Chapter 10: Schizophrenia and Other Psychotic Disorders

1.   What is the top priority for the PMHNP?

     To help the client develop a plan that addresses his multiple health needs and that he feels he can comply with and manage with some assistance from the PMHNP.

2.   What medications are reasonable to consider for the client at this time?

     Given his young age and probable lifelong need for medication, the atypical class of antipsychotics is most indicated, but his medications will need to be managed carefully given his history of diabetes.

3.   What is the relationship between his diabetes and schizophrenia?

     Both disorders are well known to produce concerns with compliance, have multiple complications, and affect many areas of a patient's life. Diabetes is a common comorbid disorder with schizophrenia, complicating the clinical management of patients with both disorders.

4.   How will his co-morbid illness affect your care planning?

     The client's diet, weight management, exercise, and activity tolerance all must be considered in planning care for this client. Both disorders are chronic in nature, and long-term planning will need to consider relapse prevention and crisis care.

5.   What routine ongoing monitoring will he require?

     The PMHNP needs to be alert and monitor the client for common complications of both disorders. The PMHNP needs to be able to separate clinical findings of both disorders and be aware of the complex interplay of the two disorders on the functioning of the client.

Chapter 11: Delirium, Dementia, and Other Cognitive Disorders

1.   What is the probable diagnosis at this time?

     Although complete assessment needs to be done, given client's family history and current clinical presentation, dementia must be considered.

2.   What further assessment is needed?

     Full physical exam, MSE, diagnostic and lab tests, determination of memory and cognitive functioning of the patient.

3. What role does the medication taken by the patient play in decision making?

Consider effects of Pravachol and kava kava use on current clinical presentation because they can cause confusion and memory problems in some clients. Timeline of symptoms should be compared to medication use history.

4. Would you include the family at this time in the care planning?

Although the client's wishes should be honored, involvement of the family may decrease the client's concerns and increase support and assistance during this difficult time for her.

5. Are medications indicated at this time?

Only once diagnostic clarity is reached. At that time, if dementia is the diagnosis, the use of cholinesterase inhibitor such as Aricept may be indicated. Discontinuation of kava kava is indicated as well.

6. What steps would you take to reduce the client's discomfort as she discusses her concerns?

Pay attention to milieu considerations, allow the client to ventilate concerns, provide information to reduce anxiety, and use therapeutic communication strategies.

Chapter 12: Substance-Related Disorders

1. What is the primary healthcare concern of this client?

Although the client has multiple health needs, her current noncompliance and self-medication with alcohol are of primary concern.

2. Is her use of potentially addictive prescription drugs warranted?

Although the client has a significant wound, and the probability is that she is in pain, her reliance on potentially addictive drugs is of concern, and alternative treatments should be considered.

3. What further assessment should be considered?

The client's psychiatric history and family history should be established. The reason she has frequently changed providers should be explored. The client's social supports and her substance use/abuse history should be assessed as well.

4. If the client is unwilling to participate in further assessment, how will you deal with her health needs?

Careful establishment of a rapport with this client will increase the likelihood of engaging her in treatment. The principles of therapeutic relationship building must be utilized, and careful use of therapeutic communication will increase the likelihood that she will remain in treatment.

Chapter 13: Personality Disorders

1. What is the most probable diagnosis for this client?

    Schizotypal personality disorder.

2. What further assessment should occur?

    A complete assessment of the client should occur, including a physical exam, full MSE, and diagnostic and lab studies. In addition, a full history of this presentation and the health habits of the client are needed.

3. If the client desires no treatment, should the PMHNP attempt to follow up with him?

    Personality disorders are chronic conditions with recurrent behaviors. The PMHNP should work on the development of a therapeutic relationship with the client to work toward assisting the client to identify his psychiatric health needs and to assist him to optimize his daily social and occupational functioning.

4. What treatment should be suggested at this time?

    Personality disorders most often are treated with nonpharmacological interventions such as psychotherapy.

Chapter 14: Disorders of Childhood and Adolescence

1. What is the most accepted theory of etiology regarding ADHD?

    Polygenic deficits leading to problems with executive functioning and abnormalities of fronto–subcortical pathways, especially with dopamine and norepinephrine functioning.

2. What is the empirical database for dietary treatment in clients with ADHD?

    Empirical evidence suggests no association between dietary alteration and improvement in symptoms of ADHD.

3. What is the natural course of this illness? Is it likely that the son's symptoms will improve as he ages?

    Hyperactivity symptoms tend to improve as children age, but inattentive symptoms may persist into adulthood.

CASE STUDIES DISCUSSION **407**

4. What are the other issues to consider regarding the parent's request to keep confidential the concerns that they are expressing?

Treatment of ADHD requires significant family involvement. Parental counseling to deal with issues often is very helpful. In addition, parents are an integral aspect of the behavioral therapy commonly used to treat ADHD symptoms. Working with the parents is an essential role for the PMHNP.

Chapter 15: Sleep

1. What is the most likely diagnosis for this client at this time?

Transient insomnia.

2. What further assessment would you make?

Identify life stressors, complete full psychiatric assessment, and identify any other mental health needs.

3. What treatment would you consider?

Assist the client in managing her sleep; use effective sleep hygiene strategies; encourage change in diet, reduction of smoking, and use for alcohol for sleep induction.

4. Is medication warranted at this time to induce sleep?

Short-term use of sleep induction medications such as Remeron or Elavil would provide relief with little risk to the client and may help her reduce current reliance on alcohol.

APPENDIX B

REVIEW QUESTIONS

410 PSYCHIATRIC-MENTAL HEALTH NURSE PRACTITIONER REVIEW MANUAL, 3RD EDITION

1. The purpose of the American Nurses Association's *Scope and Standards of Psychiatric–Mental Health Clinical Nursing Practice* is to

    A. Define the role and actions for the NP
    B. Establish the legal authority for the prescription of psychotropic medications
    C. Define the legal statutes of the role of the PMHNP
    D. Define the differences between the physician role and the NP role

2. Primary prevention care practices are an essential aspect of the PMHNP role. Which of the following is the best example of a primary prevention care strategy for community behavioral health?

    A. Aftercare program for chronically mentally ill clients recently discharged from the hospital
    B. Court-ordered counseling for abusive parents
    C. 24-hour crisis hotlines
    D. Parenting skills classes for pregnant adolescents

3. The trend in legal rulings on cases involving mental illness over the past 25 years has been to

    A. Encourage juries to find defendants not guilty by reason of insanity
    B. Protect the individual's freedoms or rights when he or she is committed to a mental hospital
    C. Place increasing trust in mental health professionals to make good and ethical decisions
    D. Decrease the "red tape" associated with commitments so that commitments are faster and easier

4. Mr. Smithers, an involuntarily hospitalized patient experiencing psychotic symptoms, refuses to take any of his ordered medication because he believes "Jesus Christ told me I am the prophet and must fast for a year." Your actions should be based on your knowledge that

    A. Psychiatric clients cannot refuse treatment
    B. Psychiatric clients don't always know what's good for them
    C. Psychiatric clients can refuse treatment
    D. Psychiatric clients cannot be trusted to make good healthcare decisions and, therefore, the nurse's best clinical judgment should guide actions

5. Which of the following statements best reflects the difference between the nurse–client relationship (N–C) and a social relationship?

   A. In the N–C relationship, the primary focus is on the client and his needs.

   B. Goals in the N–C relationship are deliberately left vague and unspoken so that the client can work on any issue.

   C. In the N–C relationship, the nurse is solely responsible for making the relationship work.

   D. In the N–C relationship, there is no place for social interaction.

6. A community has an unusually high incidence of depression and drug use among the teenage population. The public health nurses decide to address this problem, in part, by modifying the environment and strengthening the capacities of families to prevent the development of new cases of depression and drug use. This is an example of

   A. Primary prevention

   B. Secondary prevention

   C. Tertiary prevention

   D. Protective factorial prevention

7. Mrs. Kemp is voluntarily admitted to the hospital. After 24 hours, she states she wishes to leave because "this place can't help me." The best nursing action that reflects the legal right of this client is

   A. Discharge the client

   B. Explain that the client cannot leave until you can complete further assessment

   C. Allow the client to leave but have her sign forms stating she is leaving against medical advice

   D. Immediately start the paperwork to commit the client and to allow you to treat her against her wishes

8. In forming a therapeutic relationship with clients, the PMHNP must consider developing many characteristics that are known to be helpful in relationship-building. These characteristics include all of the following *except*:

   A. Genuineness

   B. Acceptance

   C. Authenticity

   D. Accuracy in assessment

9. The *DSM-IV-TR* provides for holistic client assessment by using a multiaxial assessment format. The general medical conditions experienced by a client that may influence treatment of his or her psychiatric disorders are coded on which of the five axes of the *DSM*?

    A. Axis I

    B. Axis II

    C. Axis III

    D. Axis IV

10. Mrs. French has been in individual therapy for 3 months. She has shown much growth and improvement in her functioning and insight and is to discontinue services within the next few weeks. In the next session, after you discuss service termination, she suddenly begins to demonstrate the original symptoms that had brought her to treatment initially. She is now hesitant to discharge, wants to continue services, and is displaying an increase in regressive defense mechanisms. The best explanation of Mrs. French's behavior is:

    A. An exacerbation of her symptoms related to stress

    B. The normal cyclic nature of chronic mental health symptoms

    C. A sign of normal resistance to termination seen in the termination phase of therapy

    D. A sign of pathological attachment to the therapist that must be addressed

11. A client is displaying low self-esteem, poor self-control, self-doubt, and a high level of dependency. These behaviors indicate developmental failure of which of the following stages of development:

    A. Infancy

    B. Early childhood

    C. Late childhood

    D. School age

12. Mr. Thompson has been forgetful lately, for example, forgetting where he has placed his keys or what time appointments are scheduled, and he has stated that he thinks these are just random behaviors that have no particular meaning. Which Freudian-based psychodynamic principle assumes that all behavior and actions are purposeful?

    A. Pleasure principle

    B. Psychic determinism principle

    C. Reality principle

    D. Unconsciousness principle

REVIEW QUESTIONS 413

13. An example of a mature, healthy defense mechanism is

    A. Denial

    B. Rationalization

    C. Repression

    D. Suppression

14. Mr. Johnson is a 54-year-old client you have been seeing for several weeks in therapy. While discussing his current concerns of marital stress, he lies on the floor and assumes the fetal position. This is most likely an example of

    A. Immature regressive defense mechanism

    B. Denial of reality

    C. Immature fantasy defense mechanism

    D. Repressive behavior

15. Defense mechanisms are best viewed as a function of the ego

    A. To alert us to harm and danger

    B. To alert us to problems

    C. Used to resolve a conflict

    D. Used to protect the id

16. A man thinks to himself that his wife is really ugly as he sees her at the breakfast table one morning. He doesn't tell her his thinking because he doesn't want to hurt her feelings. Later in the day he gets a sudden unexplainable urge to send his wife flowers. The best explanation for his unconscious action is:

    A. Undoing

    B. Suppression

    C. Denial

    D. Repression

17. A woman is the only survivor of a fire that kills her two housemates. As the PMHNP caring for her, you ask her how she is doing, and she replies, "I don't remember a thing about the fire." The best explanation of this is

    A. Undoing

    B. Suppression

    C. Denial

    D. Repression

18. A woman is the only survivor of a fire that kills her two housemates. As the PMHNP caring for her, you ask her how she is doing, and she replies, "You must have the wrong client. I wasn't in any fire." The best explanation of this is

    A. Undoing

    B. Suppression

    C. Denial

    D. Repression

19. A woman is the only survivor of a fire that kills her two housemates. As the PMHNP caring for her, you ask her how she is doing and she replies, "I don't want to talk about it. It hurts too much to think about my friends." The best explanation of this is

    A. Undoing

    B. Suppression

    C. Denial

    D. Repression

20. The role of neurotransmitters in the central nervous system is to function as

    A. A communication medium

    B. A gatekeeper for transmissions

    C. A building block for amino acids

    D. A agent to break down enzymes

21. Serotonin is produced in which of the following locations:

    A. Locus ceruleus

    B. Nucleus basalis

    C. Raphi nuclei

    D. Substantia nigra

22. Dopamine is produced in which of the following locations:

    A. Locus ceruleus

    B. Nucleus basalis

    C. Raphi nuclei

    D. Substantia nigra

23. A client presents with complaints of changes in appetite, feeling fatigued, problems with sleep–rest cycle, and changes in libido. The neuroanatomical area of the brain responsible for the normal regulation of these functions is the

    A. Thalamus

    B. Hypothalamus

    C. Limbic system

    D. Hippocampus

24. In considering whether or not to order an MRI of the head for a client, which of the following would be a contraindication to this diagnostic test?

    A. Prosthetic limb

    B. History of head trauma

    C. Pacemaker

    D. Pregnancy

25. The primary excitatory neurotransmitter is

    A. GABA

    B. Serotonin

    C. Dopamine

    D. Glutamate

26. A client who is experiencing difficulties with working memory, planning and prioritizing, insight into his problems, and impulse control presents for assessment. In planning his care, the PMHNP should apply his or her knowledge that these symptoms represent problems with the

    A. Frontal lobe

    B. Temporal lobe

    C. Parietal lobe

    D. Occipital lobe

27. The concept of target symptom identification is best explained as

    A. Identification of the major clinical presentation of the client

    B. Identification of specific, precise, and individualized symptoms reasonably expected to improve with medication

    C. Identification of the secondary messenger system syndrome

    D. Intentional modulation of synaptic pathways

416 PSYCHIATRIC-MENTAL HEALTH NURSE PRACTITIONER REVIEW MANUAL, 3RD EDITION

28. The goal of the psychiatric assessment process performed by the PMHNP is to

    A. Gain an understanding of the life experiences of the client
    B. Correctly diagnose the client
    C. Identify the mental health needs of the client
    D. Be able to communicate with other staff about the client's health needs

29. Mr. Johnson is a newly admitted client to an inpatient psychiatric hospital. The PMHNP on call at the facility plans to perform the initial intake assessment and diagnostic process. Mr. Johnson asks to please talk in his room because, he says, "People make me nervous." His room is at the end of the hallway and is the farthest away from the nursing station. The PMHNP's action should be based on awareness that the best location to do the assessment is

    A. In Mr. Johnson's room, because it is least noisy and most comfortable for him, thus facilitating data collection
    B. In the dayroom, which is full of people, to observe his interactions with other individuals
    C. In a quiet place, but public enough to get assistance with client care should it be required during the assessment
    D. In the treatment room with the door closed, a neutral location

30. Which communication technique is the PMHNP using in the following situation? Client: "Sorry I was late. I didn't realize what time it was." PMHNP: "This is the third time now that you have been late for our sessions. I am wondering how committed you are to our working on your problems."

    A. Theming
    B. Recognizing
    C. Validating
    D. Sequencing

31. In assessing a client, you ask him the meaning of the proverb "People who live in glass houses shouldn't throw stones." He replies, "Because it will break the windows." The correct interpretation of this findings is

    A. Client has a probable mood disorder
    B. Client has a probable anxiety disorder
    C. Client has limited intellectual ability
    D. Unable to interpret the finding without knowing the client's age

32. The PMHNP is planning to work with a client using an individual therapy model of care. During the first session, the client makes the following statement: "This is the third time my son has run away. I've grounded him, taken away his bike, even tried cutting of his allowance and locking him in his room. What should I do now?" The most therapeutic response for the PMHNP to make is

    A. "I wonder if locking him in his room was abusive?"

    B. "Maybe that depends on what you are trying to accomplish."

    C. "Perhaps talking to his friends and teachers would help."

    D. Remain silent

33. A client says to the PMHNP, "Some days life is just not worth it. All my wife and I ever do is fight and scream. Things at home would be calmer and simpler if I just wasn't there anymore." The most therapeutic response for the PMHNP to make is

    A. "Do you mean that you are thinking about leaving your wife and moving out?"

    B. "Tell me what you mean by 'it would be simpler if you just weren't there anymore.'"

    C. "So you are thinking suicide might be an option for you?"

    D. Remain silent

34. Mrs. Shea has come to the mental health center seeking treatment for depression. She has a history of a suicide attempt by overdose 1 month ago. She was started on imipramine (TCA) after that event but stopped taking the medication 1 week later because it "did no good." The PMHNP meets with Mrs. Shea to plan care with her. Which of the following is the most appropriate initial action?

    A. Asking Mrs. Shea how to help her

    B. Providing client teaching about the long time frame for TCAs to work

    C. Contracting with Mrs. Shea for 6 sessions of individual therapy

    D. Providing Mrs. Shea with feedback about how suicide might affect her family

35. As the PMHNP treating Mrs. Shea, what is your primary concern about continued treatment on imipramine, a tricyclic antidepressant?

    A. Tricyclic antidepressants are lethal in overdose

    B. Tricyclic antidepressants may take 2 to 4 weeks to achieve therapeutic action.

    C. Tricyclic antidepressants can cause QTc interval prolongation.

    D. Tricyclic antidepressants have anticholingeric side effects, dry mouth, weight gain, constipation, and blurred vision.

418 PSYCHIATRIC-MENTAL HEALTH NURSE PRACTITIONER REVIEW MANUAL, 3RD EDITION

36. A client comes into the clinic with a longstanding history of depression and chronic renal failure. He is on an antidepressant and a diuretic and complains of increased depression, mild confusion, irritability, and overall apathy from being too tired to do anything. The best initial PMHNP action to take at this time is

    A. Readjust his dose of antidepressant medication to better capture symptoms

    B. Change him to another antidepressant for better symptom control

    C. Obtain a serum calcium level

    D. Obtain a serum magnesium level

37. Sarah presents for her initial intake appointment with complaints of depression. She is being treated for hypertension and asthma by her primary care provider. Knowing that certain medications can cause or exacerbate depression, you obtain a complete medication history. Which of the following medications is known to exacerbate or cause depression?

    A. Omeprazole

    B. Propranolol

    C. Levothyroxine

    D. Clarithromycin

38. When treating older adults, you should keep in mind that they are more sensitive to issues of drug toxicity because of which of the following reasons?

    A. Decreased body fat

    B. Increased liver capacity

    C. Decreased protein binding

    D. Increased muscle concentration

39. Which known teratogenic effects can be caused by the common psychotropic medications divalproex and lithium?

    A. Divalproex—Epstein anomaly; lithium—cleft palate

    B. Lithium—Epstein anomaly; divalproex—spina bifida

    C. Divalproex—limb malformations; lithium—seizure disorder

    D. Lithium—spina bifida; divalproex—mental retardation

40. The study of what the body does to drugs is called

    A. Pharmacodynamics

    B. Pharmacology

    C. Pharmacokinetics

    D. Distribution

41. Your client Sam is being treated for panic disorder with agoraphobia. He currently is being prescribed paroxetine (Paxil CR; 37.5 mg q.d.) and clonazepam (Klonopin; 0.5 mg q.d. p.r.n.). He has been on clonazepam for 2 years and admits to needing 4 pills to achieve the same effect that 1 pill initially produced. This is possibly an example of which process?

    A. Kindling

    B. Addiction

    C. Tolerance

    D. Potency

42. Group therapy would be beneficial because it:

    A. Increases social skills

    B. Is cost effective

    C. Enables participants to acquire the curative factors

    D. All of the above

43. You are using Beck's cognitive–behavioral therapy and know that this will help the client:

    A. Recognize and change his or her automatic thoughts

    B. See reality as you see it

    C. Change his or her reality by changing his or her environment

    D. Recognize and accept that automatic thoughts suggest delusional thinking

44. When working with a dysfunctional family, you find that the father Jim worries excessively and is resistant to change. You give Jim a paradoxical directive to worry extremely well for 1 hour per day, knowing that he will likely be noncompliant, and thus change will occur. With this technique, you are using which type of therapy?

    A. Experiential therapy

    B. Structural therapy

    C. Strategic therapy

    D. Solution-focused therapy

45. Homeostasis in a family refers to:

    A. Choices a family makes to keep the peace

    B. Balance or stability that the family returns to despite its dysfunction

    C. Need for change and balance in a family

    D. Calm in a family that returns after a crisis

46. In an attempt to bring the client toward the goal he or she is working on, you ask the client, "If a miracle were to happen tonight while you slept, and you awoke in the morning and the problem no longer existed, how would you know, and what would be different?" This technique is used in which type of therapy?

    A. Behavioral therapy

    B. Solution-focused therapy

    C. Adlerian therapy

    D. Existential therapy

47. Ms. Thomas has been diagnosed with MDD and is placed on fluoxetine 20 mg for her depression. For the PMHNP to effectively monitor this client's use of the medication, which of the following actions should be part of ongoing care?

    A. Use of a standardized rating scale of depression

    B. Monitoring for potential abuse of the medication

    C. Monitoring of baseline labs of renal functioning

    D. Monitoring for potential cardiac side effects

48. The SSRI class of antidepressants is considered the first-line drug of choice for depression for which of the following reasons:

    A. Need to stair step initial dosages

    B. Sedating and calming effect of the medication

    C. Safe use in suicidal overdose clients

    D. Ability to obtain therapeutic serum drug levels

49. A 23-year-old female is brought into the ER after attempting suicide by cutting her wrists. Which nursing action by the PMHNP would be of highest priority initially?

    A. Assess her coping behaviors

    B. Assess her current level of suicidality

    C. Take her vital signs

    D. Assess her health history

APPENDIX C

ANSWERS TO THE REVIEW QUESTIONS

1. **Correct Answer: A.** The ANA's Scope and Standards of Psychiatric–Mental Health Clinical Nursing Practice defines the role and actions of the nurse practitioner.

2. **Correct Answer: D.** Information reduces incidence of disease.

3. **Correct Answer: B.** Identifies the trend of ensuring the protection of individual civil liberties for psychiatric clients.

4. **Correct Answer: C.** As with any client, psychiatric clients can refuse treatment unless a legal process resulting in a mandatory court order for treatment has been obtained.

5. **Correct Answer: A.** Social relationships are mutual interpersonal relationships in which the needs of both parties are addressed. The N–C relationship is most concerned with meeting the needs of the client.

6. **Correct Answer: A.** This action focuses on interventions designed to reduce the incidence of new cases of disease.

7. **Correct Answer: B.** Almost every state allows for a brief period of detainment to assess a client for dangerousness to self or others before allowing the client to leave a hospital setting, even if the admission was voluntary.

8. **Correct Answer: D.** Although an important aspect of the PMHNP role, accuracy in assessment does not in and of itself facilitate relationship building.

9. **Correct Answer: C.** Medical conditions are coded on Axis III.

10. **Correct Answer: C.** Clients frequently display resistance and regression at the termination of a meaningful therapeutic process. The PMHNP is responsible for planning an effective termination and monitoring clients during the termination period.

11. **Correct Answer: B.** These signs indicate developmental failure of early childhood.

12. **Correct Answer: B.** The psychic determinism principle states that all behavior has purpose and meaning, often unconscious in nature, and that no behaviors occur randomly or by coincidence.

13. **Correct Answer: D.** Suppression is the only defense mechanism listed in which the client channels conflicting energies into growth-promoting activities.

14. **Correct Answer: A.** Immature regressive defense mechanism is a return to a behavior common to an earlier stage of development.

15. **Correct Answer: C.** Defense mechanisms are a function of the ego used to resolve a conflict.

16. **Correct Answer: A.** His urge to buy flowers after thinking his wife ugly is an example of undoing his earlier thoughts.

17. **Correct Answer: D.** Repression is the unconscious placement of thought content into the unconscious to avoid dealing with the conflict.

18. **Correct Answer: C.** Denial is the unconscious refusal to accept the reality of some fact or detail to avoid dealing with the conflict.

19. **Correct Answer: B.** Suppression is the conscious, intentional refusal to think about a conflictual issue or event.

20. **Correct Answer: A.** Neurotransmitters in the central nervous system function as a communication medium.

21. **Correct Answer: C.** Serotonin is produced in the raphi nuclei.

22. **Correct Answer: D.** Dopamine is produced in the substantia nigra.

23. **Correct Answer: B.** Appetite, sleep, and libido are regulated by the hypothalamus.

24. **Correct Answer: C.** A client with a pacemaker should not receive an MRI of the head.

25. **Correct Answer: D.** Glutamate is the primary excitatory neurotransmitter.

26. **Correct Answer: A.** Problems with working memory, planning and prioritizing, insight into problems, and impulse control indicate a problem in the frontal lobe.

27. **Correct Answer: B.** Target symptom identification is the identification of specific, precise, and individualized symptoms reasonably expected to improve with medication—it must have the target symptoms identified.

28. **Correct Answer: C.** Although diagnosis is an important aspect of the assessment process, the assessment ultimately should identify the needs of the client.

29. **Correct Answer: C.** One PMHNP role is to control the milieu as an aspect of assessment, so the PMHNP should choose a quiet place that is public enough to get assistance with patient care should it be required during the assessment.

30. **Correct Answer: B.** This exchange is an illustration of the technique of recognizing.

31. **Correct Answer: D.** The answer demonstrates concrete thought processes, which are normal in individuals younger than age 12 but are abnormal after age 12. To interpret the finding, the PMHNP must know the age of the client.

32. **Correct Answer: B.** This response will be the most therapeutic in moving forward with the client.

33. **Correct Answer: B.** This response is the most therapeutic, without influencing the client's thought process.

424 PSYCHIATRIC-MENTAL HEALTH NURSE PRACTITIONER REVIEW MANUAL, 3RD EDITION

34. **Correct Answer: A.** Asking the client how to help is an aspect of assessment—all other answers are aspects of interventions, which are not initial actions of the PMHNP.

35. **Correct Answer: A.** Energy lifts before mood, and tricyclic antidepressants can be fatal in OD and for patients at high risk for suicide. No more than 1 week of prescription should be provided. This patient recently overdosed and, given ongoing depression, is at risk for another OD.

36. **Correct Answer: D.** Client symptoms are consistent with low levels of magnesium, which needs to be evaluated.

37. **Correct Answer: B.** Beta blockers can cause or exacerbate depression.

38. **Correct Answer: C.** Elderly people usually have decreased protein levels. Most psychotropic medications are highly protein-bound. It is the unbound (free) concentration of the drug that is active; the bound concentration of the drug is inert. Thus, with decreased protein available for binding, there exists more free (active) drug, which then predisposes elderly people to toxicity.

39. **Correct Answer: B.** Lithium—Epstein anomaly can be cause by lithium and spina bifida can be caused by divalproex.

40. **Correct Answer: C.** Pharmacokinetics is the study of what the body does to drugs.

41. **Correct Answer: C.** Tolerance means needing more to achieve the same effect.

42. **Correct Answer: D.** Group therapy is beneficial because it increases social skills, is cost effective, and enables participants to acquire the curative factors.

43. **Correct Answer: A.** Cognitive–behavioral therapy helps clients recognize and change their automatic thoughts.

44. **Correct Answer: C.** Paradoxical directives are used in strategic therapy.

45. **Correct Answer: B.** Homeostasis is balance or stability that the family returns to despite its dysfunction.

46. **Correct Answer: B.** Miracle questions are used in solution-focused therapy.

47. **Correct Answer: A.** The use of a standardized rating scale will allow the PMHNP to monitor the level of client symptoms and to evaluate the efficacy of the medication.

48. **Correct Answer: C.** SSRIs are considered first-line for depressions because of safe use in suicidal overdose clients.

49. **Correct Answer: C.** The PMHNP needs to ensure that her suicide attempt has not led to medical instability.

INDEX

A

Abdomen, 88–89
Abnormal Involuntary Movement Scale
    (AIMS), 118, 120t
Absorption, drug, 133
Abuse
    child, 89
    sexual, 389–392
Access to care model, 115
Accreditation, 15
Accredited Commission for Nursing
    Education (ACNE), 15
Acetylcholine
    explanation of, 62
    function of, 64t
    psychiatric disorders and, 62t
Active listening, 73
Acupressure, 151
Acupuncture, 151
Addiction, 306, 310, 317. *See also* Substance-
    related disorders
ADHD (Parent and Teacher Scales), 121t
Admission, to treatment facility, 22
Adolescents. *See also* Children
    Asperger syndrome in, 354–356
    assessment of, 341–342
    attention-deficit hyperactivity disorder in,
        348–354
    autism spectrum disorder in, 359–362
    bipolar disorder in, 203
    conduct disorder in, 345–348
    eating disorders in, 362–368
    exercise recommendations for, 115
    gender-based screening for, 110–111
    mental retardation in, 368–372
    oppositional defiant disorder in, 343–345
    patient history for, 80–81
    Rett syndrome in, 357–359
    therapeutic care planning for, 342
Adoption studies, 67
Adrenergic medications, 319
Advance directives, 26
Adverse treatment effects, 120t
Advocacy, patient, 22, 23
Aggression-turned-inward theory, 159
Aging. *See* Older adults
Agonist effect, 135
Agoraphobia, 227–228. *See also* Anxiety
    disorders

Alanine aminotransferase, 106
Alcohol use. *See also* Substance-related
    disorders; Substance use/abuse
    assessment for, 122t, 312–315, 314t, 316t
    incidence of, 307–308
    inpatient detoxification programs for, 321
    pregnancy and, 308
    withdrawal from, 317–318
Alcohol Use Disorders Identification Test -
    Consumption (AUDIT-C), 122t
Alzheimer's disease. *See also* Dementia
    assistance in coping with, 110
    dementia and, 289
    insomnia and, 282
    pharmacologic treatment for, 296
Amino acids, 62
Amygdala, 59
Anal stage, 47t
Analysis of variance (AQNOVA), 33
Anger patients with, 77
Anhedonia, in depressive disorders, 164
Anorexia nervosa. *See also* Eating disorders
    assessment of, 364–365
    diagnostic studies for, 366
    explanation of, 362
Antagonist effect, 135
Anticraving medications, 319, 320t
Antidepressants
    for autism spectrum disorder, 362
    classes of, 171–172
    miscellaneous, 178t
    monoamine oxidase inhibitors, 61, 139t,
        171, 175–176, 177t
    norepinephrine dopamine reuptake
        inhibitors, 171
    selective serotonin reuptake inhibitors,
        139t, 171, 172, 173t, 219
    serotonin agonist and reuptake inhibitors,
        172
    serotonin norepinephrine reuptake
        inhibitors, 171
    for sleep disorders, 380
    target symptoms for, 170, 171t
    tricyclic antidepressants, 171, 173–174,
        175t, 220
    variations among, 172
Antipsychotics
    atypical, 259, 260t–262t
    for autism spectrum disorder, 362

commonly used, 138t
for schizophrenia, 138t, 258–269,
	260t–263t, 266t, 267t
side effects of, 264–265, 267t, 268, 296
typical, 263, 266t
Antiseizure medications, 319
Antisocial personality disorder, 333, 334t
Anxiety
in children, 242–243
description of, 211–212
levels of, 211, 212t, 213
pathological levels of, 216
Anxiety disorders
agoraphobia as, 227–228
assessment of, 77, 123t, 215–218
in children, 221, 233, 235–236, 240,
	242–243
description of, 213
differential diagnosis and, 218, 219t
etiology for, 213–214
follow-up for, 222–223
generalized anxiety disorder as, 240–243
incidence and demographics for, 215
nonpharmacologic treatment for, 221,
	226, 231
obsessive–compulsive disorder as, 233–
	236
panic disorder as, 223–226
pharmacologic treatment for, 139t, 219–
	221, 221t, 226, 228, 231, 296
posttraumatic stress disorder as, 236–240
prevention of and screening for, 215
risk factors for, 215
social anxiety disorder as, 231–232
special considerations for, 221–222
specific phobias as, 228–231
Anxiolytics, 139t
Aromatherapy, 152
Aspartate, 62
Aspartate amino transferase, 106–107
Asperger syndrome, 354–356
Assertive community treatment (ACT), 268
Assessment. *See also specific disorders*
considerations for, 72–73
differential diagnosis and, 112–114
gender-based, 110–112
health behavior guidelines and, 114–116
Mental Status Examination and, 89–90,
	91t, 92–93, 92t

Mini-Mental Status Exam and, 94–95
Montreal Cognitive Assessment and
	Short Portable Mental Status
	Questionnaire and, 95–110
spiritual needs and, 77
therapeutic communication principles
	and, 116–117
Assessment components
abdomen as, 88–89
back as, 87
breasts as, 88
coordination and fine-motor skills as, 84
ears as, 87
eyes as, 86–87
head, skin and nails as, 86
heart as, 88
history as, 78–81
indicators of child abuse as, 89
motor functions as, 85
musculoskeletal system as, 89
neck as, 87
neurological exam as, 82–84
neurological soft signs as, 85
nose and sinuses as, 87
physical exam as, 82–89
sensory functions as, 85
thorax and lungs as, 88
vital signs as, 85–86
Assessment tools
characteristics of, 120t–130t
diagnostic, 117–119
function of, 118
screening, 117
Astereognosis, 255
Attention deficit disorder (ADD), 139t
Attention-deficit hyperactivity disorder
	(ADHD)
assessment of, 121t, 349–351
comorbidities and, 354
description of, 348
differential diagnosis and, 351
etiology of, 348–349
follow up for, 354
incidence and demographics of, 349
nonpharmacologic treatment for, 353–354
pharmacologic treatment for, 139t, 351,
	352t, 353–354
prevention of and screening for, 349
risk factors for, 349

Autism spectrum disorder (ASD)
    Asperger syndrome and, 355
    assessment of, 360–361
    description of of, 359
    differential diagnosis and, 361
    etiology of, 359
    incidence and demographics for, 359–360
    nonpharmacologic treatment for, 362
    pharmacologic treatment for, 362
    prevention of and screening for, 360
    risk factors for, 360
Autonomic nervous system, 56
Avoidant personality disorder, 335, 336t
Axon, 60

B

Back, 87
Bandura, Albert, 52
Barnes Akathisia Rating Scale (BARS), 120t
Basal ganglia, 59
Beck, Aaron, 144, 159
Beck Anxiety Inventory (BIA), 123t
Beck Depression Inventory (BDA), 125t, 136
Becker, Marshall, 51
Behavioral therapy
    for anxiety disorders, 221
    for conduct disorder, 348
    explanation of, 144
    for substance-related disorders, 319
Belladonna, 153
Benzodiazepines (BNZs)
    for anxiety disorders, 220, 296
    description of, 139t
    for sleep disorders, 380
Binge eating disorder, 362. *See also* Eating
    disorders
Biofeedback, 151–152
Biologically based therapies, 150–151
Biological preventative factors, 25
Biological risk factors, 25
Biological theories
    bipolar disorder and, 193
    depressive disorders and, 160–162
    of personality disorders, 330
    substance abuse and, 306
Biopsychosocial framework of care, recovery
    and, 41–42
Bipolar disorder (BD)
    in adolescents, 203

    assessment of, 194–197
    description of, 192–193
    differential diagnosis and, 198
    etiology for, 193
    follow-up for, 203
    incidence and demographics for, 193
    management of, 198–203
    nonpharmacologic treatment for, 202
    pharmacologic treatment for, 138t, 199–
        200, 200t, 201t
    prevention of and screening for, 194
    risk factors for, 193
Black cohosh, 153
Body mass index (BMI), 86
Borderline personality disorder, 333, 334t
Bowen, Murray, 148
Brain/brain function
    brain stem and, 59–60
    cerebrum and, 57–59
    gray matter and, 56
    neurophysiology and, 60–64
    outermost surface of, 57
    schizophrenia and, 250
    substance use and, 306–307
    white matter and, 56
Brain imaging
    of children with autism, 359
    depressive disorders and, 161
    functional, 65
    structural, 65
    structural and functional, 66
Brain injury. *See* Traumatic brain injury (TBI)
    associated with military action
Brainstem, 59–60
Brain tissue, 56–57
Breasts, 88
Brief Psychiatric Rating Scale (BPRS), 129t,
    136
Brief psychotic disorder, 277–278
Brief therapy, 181
Bright Futures, 110
Bulimia nervosa. *See also* Eating disorders
    assessment of, 364, 365
    diagnostic studies for, 366–367
    explanation of, 362
    medications for, 367

C

CAGE, 118, 308, 309t
CAGE-AID, 122t
Calcium, 98–100
Caring theory, 52
Carrier proteins, 135
Case management, 23
Case studies, 35–36, 53, 68, 130, 141, 154,
    206–207, 243–244, 280, 303, 323–
    324, 372, 382
Catecholamine. *See* Dopamine
Catnip, 153
Cell body, neuron, 56, 60
Central nervous system (CNS), 56
Cerebellum, 59
Cerebral cortex, 58
Cerebrum
    basal ganglia in, 59
    brainstem and, 59–60
    cerebral cortex in, 58
    function of, 57
    limbic system in, 58–59
    lobes in, 57–58
Certification, 16–17
Certification examination
    creating study plan for, 4–5
    facts about, 9–10
    preparation for, 1–3
    resources for, 10
    strategies prior to, 6–7
    test-taking strategies for, 7–9
Chamomile, 153
Child abuse, 89. *See also* Violence
Children. *See also* Adolescents
    anxiety disorders in, 221, 233, 235–236,
      240
    anxiety in, 242–243
    Asperger syndrome in, 354–356
    assessment of, 76, 341–342
    attention-deficit hyperactivity disorder in,
      348–354
    autism spectrum disorder in, 359–362
    conduct disorder in, 345–348
    delirium in, 289
    dementia in, 298
    developmental and social history for,
      80–81
    dysthymic disorder in, 188
    eating disorders in, 362–368

exercise recommendations for, 115
gender-based screening for, 110–111
insomnia in, 381
major depressive disorder in, 182
mental retardation in, 368–372
mental status examination for, 342
obsessive–compulsive disorder in, 233,
    235–236
oppositional defiant disorder in, 343–345
personality disorders in, 338
posttraumatic stress disorder in, 240
Rett syndrome in, 357–359
schizophrenia in, 271
speech assessment in, 342
substance abuse in, 322
therapeutic care planning for, 342
thought process in, 342
Children's Yale-Brown Obsessive Compulsive
    Scale (CY-BOCS), 128t
Chloride, 103–104
Cholinergics, 62
Cholinesterase inhibitors, 296
Chromosomes, 67
Chronobiological theory, 162
Clinical Institute Withdrawal Assessment of
    Alcohol Scale, Revised (CIWA-Ar),
    130t, 318
Clinical Institute Withdrawal Assessment of
    Alcohol Scale (CIWA), 118
Clinical Opiate Withdrawal Scale (COWS),
    130t
Cluster A personality disorders, 329t, 332
Cluster B personality disorders, 329t, 330t,
    333
Cluster C personality disorders, 329t, 334–
    335, 336t
Cognitive–behavioral therapy (CBT), 181,
    301, 301t
Cognitive disorders. *See also specific disorders*
    delirium as, 284–289
    dementia as, 289–298
    description of, 283
    etiology for, 283
    traumatic brain injury as, 298–302
Cognitive function
    assessment tools for, 124t
    traumatic brain injury and, 298, 299t, 300,
      301, 301t
Cognitive theory, 49–50, 159–160

Cognitive therapy, 144
Commission on Collegiate Nursing Education
    (CCNE), 15
Commitment, involuntary, 21–22
Communication. *See* Therapeutic
    communication
Communities, health determinants and, 26
Competency, elements of, 21
Complementary and alternative therapies
    (CAMs)
    origins of, 150
    types of, 150–154
Computed tomography (CT), 65
Concrete operations stage, 49
Conduct disorder
    assessment of, 346–347
    description of, 345
    differential diagnosis and, 347–348
    etiology of, 345
    incidence and demographics for, 346
    management of, 348
    prevention of and screening for, 346
    risk factors for, 346
Confidentiality
    exceptions to guaranteed, 18
    principles of, 21
Conflict, defense mechanisms and, 48
Conflict of interest (COI), 116–117
Confrontation, 73
Connors Rating Scales - Revised (CRS-R),
    121t
Conservation, 50
Coordination, 84
Cornell Scale for Depression in Dementia
    (CCSD), 125t
Corpus striatum, 59
Countertransference, 43–44
CRAFFT, 118, 122t
Cranial nerves, 82–83
Credentialing, 16
Creutzfeldt-Jakob disease, 290–291
Crisis management planning, for
    schizophrenic individuals, 268–269
Critical thinking, 24
Cultural competencies
    assessment and, 75–76
    forensics and corrections and, 30–31
    homeless individuals and, 27–28
    migrant and seasonal farm workers and,

    28–29
    sexual orientation and, 29–30
Cultural differences
    in anxiety manifestation, 212
    assessment and, 75–76
    health determinants and, 26
    health influences and determinants and,
      26–27
    manifestations of depression and, 157
Culturally competent care, 26
Culture, 75
Cyclothymic disorder, 204–206

D

Data, collateral sources of, 76
Defense mechanisms, 48, 49t
Delirium. *See also* Cognitive disorders
    assessment of, 285–287
    description of, 284
    differential diagnosis and, 287
    incidence and demographics for, 284
    nonpharmacologic treatment for, 288
    pharmacologic treatment for, 287, 288
    prevention of and screening for, 285
    risk factors for, 284
    special considerations for, 288–289
Delirium tremens (DTs), 318
Delusional disorder, 275–277
Delusions
    assessment of, 275
    in schizophrenia, 253
    types/subtypes of, 92, 276
Dementia. *See also* Cognitive disorders
    assessment of, 292–295
    description of, 289
    differential diagnosis and, 295
    etiology for, 291
    forms of, 289–291
    HIV-related, 290, 297–298
    incidence and demographics for, 292
    nonpharmacologic management of,
      297–298
    pharmacologic treatment for, 295–297
    prevention of and screening for, 292
    risk factors for, 292
    special considerations for, 298
Dementia of Alzheimer's type (DAT), 289
Dendrites, 56, 60
Deontological theory, 20

Dependent personality disorder, 335, 336t
Depolarization, 60
Depressive disorders. *See also* Major
depressive disorder (MDD)
assessment tools for, 125t–127t
medications that induce, 140t
pharmacologic treatment for, 139t, 170–179, 297
suicide risk in, 181–182
Descriptive statistics, 33
deShazer, Steve, 149
Detoxification agents, 318
Developmental history, 80
Developmental stages, 110–112
Developmental theories, 45
Dexamethasone suppression test (DST), 161
Diagnostic and Statistical Manual of Mental Disorders (DSM-IV-TR) (American Psychiatric Association)
application of, 114
classification schema in, 43t
diagnostic criteria for personality disorders in, 328, 329t
diagnostic criteria for schizophrenia in, 253
explanation of, 42
substance use and, 113
Diagnostic and Statistical Manual of Mental Disorders (DSM-V) (American Psychiatric Association), 42
Diagnostic tools, 117–118
Dialectical behavioral therapy, 144
Differential diagnosis. *See also specific disorders*
anxiety disorders and, 198, 218, 219t, 225–2256
depression and, 168
explanation of, 112
function of, 112
grief/bereavement and, 191
schizophrenia and, 257–258
steps in, 113–114
Disability, assessment tools for, 127t
Disclosure
benefits of, 20–21
of disability, 20
ethics of provider, 20
risk of, 20
Disease prevention strategies

immunizations and, 108–109
implementation of, 109–110
Distribution, drug, 133–134
DNA, 67
Domestic violence. *See also* Violence
assessment of, 387
description of, 385
etiology of, 386
incidence and demographics for, 386
management of, 388
nonpharmacologic treatment for victims of, 388
prevention of and screening for, 386–387
risk factors for, 386
Donabedian model, 34
Dopamine
antipsychotics and, 259, 263–265, 267t
electroconvulsive therapy and, 179
explanation of, 61, 62t, 63t
function of, 63t, 161
impaired neuronal communication and, 250
psychiatric disorders and, 62t, 171, 259
Durable power of attorney for health care, 26
Dysidiadochokinesia, 255
Dysthymic disorder
assessment of, 187
clinical management of, 188–189
description of, 186
incidence and demographics for, 186
prevention of and screening for, 186
risk factors for, 186

E

Ears, 87
Eating disorders
assessment of, 363–366
description of, 362
diagnostic studies for, 366–367
differential diagnosis and, 367
etiology of, 363
forms of, 362
incidence and demographics for, 363
nonpharmacologic treatment for, 367–368
pharmacologic treatment for, 367
prevention of and screening for, 363
risk factors for, 363
EEG, 66
Ego, 47–48

Ego-dystonic behavior, 328
Ego-syntonic behavior, 327–328
Electroconvulsive therapy (ECT), 179–180
Electrolytes, 98
Electronic health records, function of, 18
Elimination, drug, 134
Emancipated minors, 18
Empowerment, of patients, 115
Endocrine dysfunction, depressive disorders
    and, 160–161
Environment, health determinants and, 27
Enzymes, drug metabolism and, 135
Epidemiology, 71
Epinephrine, 61
Erikson, Erik, 45
Ethical issues
    in decision-making, 19, 20
    disclosure by providers as, 20
    for nurse practitioners, 19
    in research, 34
Evidence-based practice, 31
Evoked potentials testing, 66
Excitatory response, 135
Exercise
    benefits of, 114
    monitoring intensity of, 115
    patient teaching regarding, 114–115
    recommendations for, 115
Existential therapy, 144
Experiential therapy, 149
External validity, 33
Extrapyramidal motor system, 59
Extrapyramidal side effects (EPSE)
    medications to treat, 264, 267t
    in schizophrenic patients, 259, 263t, 264
Eye movement desensitization and
    reprocessing (EMDR), 145
Eyes, 83, 86–87

F

Facilitative communication techniques, 73
Fairbairn, Ronald, 158
Families
    health determinants and, 26
    of individuals with substance abuse
        problems, 321–322
    of individuals with traumatic brain injury,
        302
    of individual with attention-deficit

hyperactivity disorder, 353–354
Family history
    elements of, 80
    explanation of, 66
Family studies, 67
Family systems theory, 147–148
Family system therapy, 148
Family therapies
    for depressive disorders, 181
    family systems concepts in, 147–148
    types of, 148–150
Family tree, 66
Fetal alcohol syndrome, 308, 369
Fine-motor skills, 84
First-pass metabolism, 134
Fish oil, 153
Fissures, brain, 56
Ford, Loretta C., 15
Forensic knowledge base, 30–31
Formal operations, 50
Frankl, Viktor, 144
Free thyroxine T4, 96
Freud, Sigmund, 46, 47t, 143, 159, 213
Frontal lobe, 57
Functional imaging, 65

G

GABA
    explanation of, 62
    function of, 64t
    psychiatric disorders and, 62t
Galactorrhea, 88
Gamma gludamyl transpeptidase, 107–108
Gender-based screening, 110–112
Gender identity, 29
Generalized anxiety disorder (GAD)
    assessment of, 240–242
    description of, 240
    differential diagnosis and, 242
    incidence and demographics for, 240
    nonpharmacologic treatment for, 242
    pharmacologic treatment for, 242
    risk factors for, 240
    special considerations for, 242–243
Genes, 67, 68
Gene therapy, 67
Genetic counseling, 66
Genetic terms, 67
Genetic testing, 68

Genomics, 66–67
Geriatric Depression Scale (GDS), 125t
Ginkgo, 153
Ginseng, 153
Glia, 60
Global Assessment of Functioning (GAF), 118
Glutamate, 62, 64t
Glycine, 62
Gray matter, 56
Grief/bereavement
    assessment of, 190–191
    description of, 189–190
    differential diagnosis and, 191
    etiology for, 190
    follow-up for, 192
    incidence and demographics for, 190
    management of, 191–192
    prevention of and screening for, 190
    risk factors for, 190
    special considerations for, 192
Group therapy
    for depressive disorders, 181
    explanation of, 146
    phases in, 146–147
    for schizophrenia, 268
Gryri, 56
Guided imagery, 150

H

Haley, Jay, 149
Half-life, 134
Hallucinations, in schizophrenia, 253
Hamilton Anxiety Scale (HAM-A), 123t
Hamilton Rating Scale for Depression
    (HAM-D), 125t
Health, cultural influences on, 26–27
Health belief model, 51
Health care delivery systems, 35
Health Information Technology for Economic
    and Clinical Health Act (HITECH)
    of 2009, 18
Health policy, nurse practitioners and, 23–24
Health promotion, 24
Heart, 88
Herbal products/supplements, 152–153
Hierarchy of needs theory, 50–51
HIPAA, privacy protections under, 18
History of present illness (HPI), 79
Histrionic personality disorder, 334t

HIV-related dementia, 290, 297–298
HLA-B*1502, 68
Homelessness, 27–28
Homicide, 394
HOPE questions, 77
Human Genome Project, 67
Humanistic therapy, 145
Huntington's disease, 291
Hypemagnesemia, 103
Hyperactivity, 350. *See also* Attention-deficit
    hyperactivity disorder (ADHD)
Hypercalemia, 99–100
Hyperkalemia, 105
Hypernatremia, 101
Hyperthyroidism, 97–98
Hypnotics, for sleep disorders, 380
Hypocalcemia, 99
Hypomagnesemia, 102
Hypomania, 127t–128t
Hyponatremia, 101
Hyporkalemia, 105
Hypothalamic-pituitary-adrenal axis (HPA),
    depressive disorders and, 160–161
Hypothalamus, 59
Hypothyroidism, 97

I

Id, 47
Illness management recovery (IMR), 269
Immunizations, 108–109
Impulsivity, 350. *See also* Attention-deficit
    hyperactivity disorder (ADHD)
Incarcerated individuals, 30–31
Incidence rate, 71
Indole. *See* Serotonin
Inferential statistics, 33–34
Informed consent, 18, 19
Inhibitory response, 135
Insomnia, 376, 378. *See also* Sleep issues/
    disorders
Institutional review boards (IRBs), 34
Internal validity, 33
Interpersonal theory, 50, 52, 214
Interpersonal therapy, 145
Interventions, effectiveness of, 32f
Interviews
    cultural considerations and, 75, 76
    fundamentals of, 72
    location for, 74

Inverse agonist effect, 135
Involuntary admission, 22
Involuntary commitment, 21–22

K

Kiddie Schedule for Affective Disorders and
  Schizophrenia (Kiddie-SADS), 127t
Klerman, Gerald L., 145

L

Lamictal, 86
Latency stage, 47t
Lazarus, Arnold, 144
Leadership, nurse practitioners and, 23
Learned helplessness-hopelessness theory, 160
Left hemisphere, brain, 57
Leininger, Madeline, 52
Lethality assessment, 392–394
Lewy body disease, 291
Licensure, 16
Liebowitz Social Anxiety Scale - Child/
  Adolescent Version (LSAS-CA),
  123t
Limbic system, 58–59
Linehan, Marsha, 144
Lithium, 199, 200t
Liver function tests, 106
Living wills, 26
Lungs, 88

M

Macrobiotics, 154
Magnesium, 101–103
Magnetic resonance imaging (MRI), 65
Magnetoencephalography (MEG), 66
Major depressive disorder (MDD). *See also*
  Depressive disorders
  assessment of, 163–169
  in children, 182
  clinical management of, 170
  comorbidities and, 179
  description of, 158
  etiology for, 158–162
  follow-up care practices for, 183–185
  incidence and demographics for, 162–163
  indications for consults, referrals or
    hospitalizations for, 181–182

nonpharmacologic management of,
  179–181
in older adults, 183
pharmacologic management of, 170–179
prevention of and screening for, 163
psychotic features with, 179
risk factors for, 163
Malpractice, negligence as proof of, 21
Malpractice insurance, 21
Mania
  assessment tools for, 127t–128t
  medications that induce, 140t
Maslow, Abraham, 50
Massage, 153
Mean, 33
Meaning, effectiveness of, 32f
Medication
  for sexual assault victims, 392
Medications. *See also specific disorders; specific
    medications*
  adrenergic, 319
  anticraving, 319, 320t
  antiseizure, 319
  for anxiety disorders, 139t, 219–221, 221t,
    226, 228, 231, 235, 239, 242
  for attention-deficit hyperactivity
    disorder, 139t, 351, 352t,
    353–354
  for autism spectrum disorder, 362
  for bipolar disorder, 138t, 199–200, 200t,
    201t
  for delirium, 287, 288
  for dementia, 295–297
  for depressive disorders, 139t, 170–179,
    297
  for eating disorders, 367
  management process for, 136–137
  for mental retardation, 371
  for personality disorders, 336–337
  pharmacodynamics and, 135
  pharmacokinetics and, 133–134
  psychiatric disorders, 138t–139t, 258–268
  for schizophrenia, 138t, 258–269,
    260t–263t, 266t, 267t
  for sleep disorders, 380
  for substance-related disorders, 318–319,
    320t, 321
  terminology related to, 135
  that induce altered mood states, 140t, 169

for traumatic brain injury, 300–301
Meditation, 150
Medulla, 59
Melatonin, 153, 380
Mellow, June, 11
Memory impairment, 293
Mental health promotion, 24
Mental retardation
    assessment of, 369–371
    description of, 368
    etiology of, 368–369
    incidence and demographics for, 369
    nonpharmacologic treatment for, 372
    pharmacologic treatment for, 371
    risk factors for, 369
Mental status examination (MSE). *See also*
    specific disorders
    for children and adolescents, 342
    delusions and, 92
    function of, 89, 90
    structured data set of, 93
    thought disorder and, 90, 92t
    thought processes and, 90, 91t
Mentoring, 22
Messenger RNA, 67
Metabolism, drug, 134
Midbrain, 59
Migrant workers, 28–29
Milieu therapy, 269
Military-related injury. *See* Traumatic brain
    injury (TBI) associated with
    military action
Mind–body interventions, 150
Mini-Mental Status Exam (MMSE), 94–95,
    124t, 293
Minuchin, Salvador, 148
Moles, cancerous, 86
Monoamine oxidase inhibitors (MAOIs), 61,
    139t, 171, 175–176, 177t
Montreal Cognitive Assessment (MoCA),
    95–110, 124t, 293
Mood Disorder Questionnaire (MDQ), 128t,
    136
Mood disorders. *See also* Bipolar disorder
    (BD); Depressive disorders; Grief/
    bereavement; Major depressive
    disorder (MDD)
    overview of, 157
    pharmacologic treatment for, 138t–139t

sadness and, 157–158
screening tools for, 136
Motor skills fine, 84
Musculoskeletal system, 89

N

Narcissistic personality disorder, 334t
National Center for Complementary and
    Alternative Medicine (NCCAM),
    150
National Center for Cultural Competence
    (Georgetown University), 75
Neck, 87
Negligence, 21
Nervous system
    central, 56
    components of, 56
    function of, 55
    peripheral, 56
Neuroadaptation, substance use and, 307
Neuroanatomy, 56–60. *See also* Brain/brain
    function
Neurobiological theory
    anxiety disorders and, 214
    neuroadaptation and, 307
    reinforcement and, 306–307
Neuroimaging, 65, 66
Neuroleptic malignant syndrome (NMS), 265
Neurological examination, 82–84
Neurological soft signs, 85
Neurons, 56, 60, 61
Neuropeptides, 62, 62t
Neurophysiology, 60–64. *See also* Brain/brain
    function
Neurotransmitters
    categories of, 61–62
    depressive disorders and, 161
    function of, 61, 63t–64t
    personality disorders and, 330
    psychiatric disorders and, 62t
    recovery and degradation of, 63
Nonbenzodiazepine anxiolytics, 220–221,
    221t
Nonpharmacologic treatment
    for anxiety disorders, 221, 226, 231, 232,
        235, 239, 242
    for Asperger syndrome, 356
    for attention-deficit hyperactivity
        disorder, 353–354

for bipolar disorder, 202
complementary and alternative therapy
    as, 150–154
for delirium, 288
for dementia, 297–298
for domestic violence victims, 388
for eating disorders, 367–368
family therapy as, 147–150
group therapy as, 146–147
individual therapy as, 143–145
interpersonal therapy as, 145
issues related to, 143
for major depressive disorder, 179–181
for mental retardation, 372
for personality disorders, 337
for schizophrenia, 258–259, 268–269
for sexual assault victims, 392
for sleep disorders, 380–381
for substance-related disorders, 321–322
for traumatic brain injury, 301–302, 301t
Norepinephrine
explanation of, 61
function of, 63t
psychiatric disorders and, 62t
Norepinephrine dopamine reuptake
    inhibitors (NDRIs), 171
Nose, 87
Nurse practitioners. *See also* Psychiatric–
    mental health nurse practitioners
    (PMHNPs)
admissions criteria and, 22
commitment process and criteria and,
    21–22
competency issues and, 21
core competencies of, 12–13
cultural competencies of, 27–31
disclosure issues and, 20–21
ethical behavior for, 19
health policy and, 23–24
historical background of, 15
legal considerations for, 21
mentoring of, 22
patient advocacy and, 22
public health principles and, 24–27
research utilization and, 31
responsibilities of, 17–20
role of, 15–17
scholarly activities of, 22
specialty competences for, 13–14
Nursing theories, 52

O

Obesity, health risks of, 270
Object loss theory, 158–159
Object permanence, 49
Obsessive–compulsive disorder (OCD)
    assessment of, 128t, 233–235
    description of, 233
    incidence and demographics for, 233
    risk factors for, 233
Obsessive–compulsive personality disorder,
    335, 336t
Occipital lobe, 58
Older adults
    antipsychotics in, 135, 296
    anxiety in, 212
    assessment of, 76
    cognitive disorders in, 283, 284, 289
    delirium in, 284, 289
    depressive disorder in, 183
    gender-based screening for, 111, 112
    grief/bereavement in, 192
    insomnia in, 381
    obsessive–compulsive disorder in, 236
    schizophrenia in, 271
    substance abuse in, 322
Omega-3 fatty acids, 152
Opiod neuropeptides, 62t, 64t
Oppositional defiant disorder (ODD), 343–
    345
Oral stage, 47t
Orem, Dorothy, 52

P

Panic disorder. *See also* Anxiety disorders
    with agoraphobia, 227
    assessment of, 223–225
    description of, 223
    differential diagnosis and, 225–226
    nonpharmacologic treatment for, 226
    pharmacologic treatment for, 226
    special considerations for, 226
Paraphrasing, 73
Parasympathetic nervous system, 56
Parietal lobe, 58
Partial agonist effect, 135
Patient advocacy, 22, 23
Patient-centered care model (PCC), 115–116
Patient Health Questionnaire (PHQ-2), 126t

Patient Health Questionnaire (PHQ-9), 126t
Patient history
    for children and adolescents, 80–81
    during crisis period, 81
    elements of, 78–81
Pearson's r correlation, 34
Pedigree, 66
Peplau, Hildegard, 11, 52
Peptides, 64t. *See also* Opiod neuropeptides
Peripheral edema, 88
Peripheral nervous system (PNS), 56
Personality, 327–328
Personality disorders
    assessment of, 331–335, 336t
    categories of, 329t, 332–335, 332t, 334t,
        336t
    description of, 328–329
    differential diagnosis and, 336
    etiology of, 329–330
    follow-up for, 338
    incidence and demographics for, 331
    nonpharmacologic treatment for, 337
    pharmacologic treatment for, 336–337
    prevention of and screening for, 331
    risk factors for, 331
    special considerations for, 338
Phallic stage, 47t
Pharmacodynamics, 133, 135. *See also*
        Medications
Pharmacogenomics, 68
Pharmacokinetics. *See also* Medications
    alterations in, 134
    elements of, 133–135
    explanation of, 133
Pharmacology. *See also* Medications
    considerations related to, 140
    explanation of, 133
Phenotype, 67
Phobias. *See* Anxiety disorders; Social anxiety
        disorder; Specific phobias
Phototherapy, 181
Physical examination, 82–89. *See also specific
        disorders*
Physical exercise. *See* Exercise
Piaget, Jean, 49
Pick's disease, 290
Polytherapy, 318–319
Pons, 59
Population genetics, 67

Positive and Negative Syndrome Scale
        (PANSS), 129t, 136
Positron emission tomography (PET), 66
Posttraumatic stress disorder (PTSD)
    assessment of, 237–239
    description of, 236–237
    nonpharmacologic treatment for, 239
    pharmacologic treatment for, 239
    risk factors for, 237
    special considerations for, 240
Potassium, 104–105
Potency, drug, 135
Preoperational stage, 49
Prevalence rate, 71–72
Preventive factors, 25
Primary prevention, 24
Probability, 34
Psychiatric disorders
    age of onset for, 45, 46t
    among incarcerated individuals, 30–31
    assessment of (*See* Assessment)
    classification of, 42, 43
    insomnia related to, 378, 382
    nature of symptom presentation in, 77–78
    neurotransmitters and, 62t
    pharmacologic treatment for, 138t–139t
    statistics for, 71–72
    substance use and, 307
    therapeutic communication
        considerations for, 73–77
Psychiatric history, 78, 79
Psychiatric interviewing, 72
Psychiatric–mental health nurse practitioners
        (PMHNPs). *See also* Nurse
        practitioners
    assessment role of (*See* Assessment;
        Assessment tools)
    foundational theories supporting role of,
        46–52
    nursing theories and, 52–53
    origins of, 11
    pharmacological management role of,
        136–141
    relationship formation between patients
        and, 72–73
    research utilization by, 31
    specialized content for, 13–14
Psychiatric nursing, 11
Psychiatry, 19

Psychic determinism, 46
Psychoanalytical theory, 46
Psychoanalytical therapy, 143
Psychodynamic theories
    anxiety disorders and, 213
    explanation of, 46–49
    major depressive disorder and, 158–159
    of personality disorders, 329–330
    substance abuse and, 306
Psychological preventative factors, 25
Psychological risk factors, 25
Psychosexual stages of development, 47
Psychosis
    assessment of patients with, 78
    assessment tools for, 129t
Psychotic disorders. *See also* Schizophrenia
    description of, 247
    symptoms associated with, 247–248, 248t
Psychotropic medications
    older adults and, 135
    weight gain and, 86
Public health principles, 24–27
p value, 34

Q

Quality improvement, 34
Quick Inventory of Depressive
    Symptomatology (QIDS), 126t

R

RADS (child), 127t
RADS -2 (Reynolds Adolescent Depression
    Inventlry), 127t
Rapid eye movement (REM), 375, 376
Recovery, 41–42
Reflective practice, 24
Reflexes, 82–83
Reflexology, 153
Reinforcement, substance abuse and, 306–307
Religion, spirituality vs., 77
Reminiscence therapy, 147
Repolarization, 60
Research
    dissemination of, 33
    donabedian model, 34
    interpretation of, 33–34
    population genetics, 67
    quality improvement, 34
    utilization of, 31, 33

Reticular formation system, brain, 59
Rett syndrome, 357–359
Reuptake pumps, 135
Reversibility, 49
Right hemisphere, brain, 57
Risk assessment, 25, 31. *See also* Suicide risk
Risk factors, 25, 67. *See also specific disorders*
Risk management, 25
Rogers, Carl, 145

S

Sadness, 157–158. *See also* Depressive
    disorders; Major depressive
    disorder (MDD)
Sam-e, 152
Satir, Virginia, 149
Schizoaffective disorder, 274–275
Schizophrenia. *See also* Psychotic disorders
    assessment of, 252–257
    comorbidities and, 269
    crisis management planning for relapse
        issues in, 268–269
    description of, 249
    differential diagnosis and, 257–258
    etiology of, 249–250
    follow-up for, 271–272
    incidence and demographics for, 250–251
    nonpharmacologic treatment for, 268–269
    overview of, 247
    pharmacologic treatment for, 138t, 258–
        269, 260t–263t, 266t, 267t
    prevention of and screening for, 251–252
    risk factors for, 251
    special considerations for, 269–271
    substance abuse and, 307
    subtypes of, 254, 255t
    symptom clusters for, 252, 253t
Schizophreniform disorder, 272–274
Scholarly activities, 22
School violence, 392–393
Scope of practice, 17
Screening tools. *See also* Assessment tools
    explanation of, 117, 118
    for mood disorders, 136
SDS Zung Self-Rating Depression, 126t
Seasonal farm workers, 28–29
Secondary prevention, 24–25
Selective serotonin reuptake inhibitors
    (SSRIs)

for anxiety disorders, 219
for depressive disorders, 171, 172, 173t
description of, 139t
Self-awareness, 117
Self-disclosure, 117
Self-efficacy/social learning theory, 52
Self-system, 50
Seligman, M., 160
Sensorimotor stage, 49
Sensory functions, 85
Serotonin, 61, 64t
Serotonin agonist and reuptake inhibitors
(SARIs), 172
Serotonin norepinephrine reuptake inhibitors
(SNRIs), 171
Sexual assault/abuse
assessment of victims of, 390–391
description of, 389
differential diagnosis and, 391
etiology of, 389
incidence and demographics for, 389
nonpharmacologic treatment for victims
of, 392
pharmacologic treatment for victims of,
392
prevention of and screening for, 390
risk factors for, 389
Sexual behavior, 30
Sexual identity, 29
Sexual orientation, 29–30
Shapiro, Francine, 145
Shared psychotic disorder (Folie á deux),
278–279
Sheehan Disability Scale (SDS), 127t
Short Portable Mental Status Questionnaire
(SPMSQ), 95–110, 124t
Short-term insomnia, 378
Silence, 73
Silver, Henry K., 15
Single photon emission computer tomography
(SPECT), 66
Sinuses, 87
Sleep, general considerations related to,
375–376
Sleep hygiene, 380–381
Sleep issues/disorders
description of, 376
etiology for, 376
incidence of, 376

Sleep/sleep disorders
assessment of, 377–379
differential diagnosis and, 379
medications for, 380
nonpharmacologic treatment for, 380–381
prevention of and screening for, 377
risk factors for, 376–377
special considerations for, 381–382
Social anxiety disorder, 231–232
Social history, 80
Social preventative factors, 25
Social risk factors, 25
Sodium, 100
Solution-focused therapy, 149–150
Somatic nervous system, 56
Specific phobias
assessment of, 229–230
description of, 228
nonpharmacologic treatment for, 231
pharmacologic treatment for, 230
risk factors for, 228–229
Spirituality, religion vs., 77
Spiritual needs, 77
Stages of human development (Erikson), 45,
45t
Standard deviation, 33
Standards of practice, 17
State statutes, 15–16
Statistics
descriptive, 33
inferential, 33–34
Statutory law, 16
Steady state, 134
Stevens-Johnson syndrome, 86
Stimulants, 139t
Strategic therapy, 149
Structural and functional imaging, 66
Structural family therapy, 148–149
Structural imaging, 65
Substance, 306
Substance abuse treatment facilities, 307
Substance-related disorders
assessment of, 118, 122t, 309–316
description of, 305–306
differential diagnosis and, 316–317
etiology of, 306–307
incidence and demographics for, 307–308
management of, 317–322
nonpharmacologic treatment for, 321–322

pharmacologic treatment for, 318–319, 320t, 321
    prevention of and screening for, 308–309, 309t
    risk factors for, 308
    special considerations for, 322
Substance use/abuse
    anxiety disorders and, 239, 242
    assessment tools for, 118, 122t
    in children, 322
    cognitive disorders and, 283–285, 287, 291, 292
    diagnosis of, 113
    incidence of, 307–308
    maternal, 249
    medications that cause false positive for, 141t
    in older adults, 322
    overview of, 305
    reinforcement and, 306–307
    risk factors for, 308
    schizophrenia and, 249, 257, 269
    withdrawal symptoms and, 311, 312
Suicide Probability Scale (SPS), 129t
Suicide risk
    assessment tools for, 129t
    depressive disorders and, 166, 167, 167t, 181–182
    factors for, 392
    schizophrenia and, 270
    substance use and, 270, 300
    traumatic brain injury and, 300
Sulci, 56
Sullivan, Harry Stack, 50, 214
Superego, 48
Suspiciousness, 77
Symptom presentation, 77–78
Synapse, 60, 61
Synaptic cleft, 60

T

Tachyphylaxis, 135
Tardive dyskinesia (TD), 264–265
Team leadership model, 23
Teleological theory, 20
Temporal lobe, 58

Tertiary prevention, 25
Thalamus, 59
Theory of cultural care, 52
Theory of self care, 52
Therapeutic communication
    elements of, 73–74
    principles of, 116–117
    techniques for, 73, 74t
Therapeutic index, 135
Therapeutic nurse–patient relationship, 43–44, 44t
Therapeutic nurse–patient relationship theory/interpersonal theory, 52
Therapy. *See also specific therapies*
    for anxiety disorders, 221
    for children and adolescents, 342, 345, 348
    complementary and alternative, 150–154
    for depressive disorders, 181
    family, 147–150
    group, 146–147
    individual, 143–145
    interpersonal, 145
    for schizophrenia, 258–259
Thorax, 88
Thyroid function tests, 95–98
Thyroid-stimulating hormone, 96–97
Tolerance, drug, 135
Transcranial magnetic stimulation (TMS), 180
Transference, 43
Transient insomnia, 378
Transtheoretical model of change, 51
Traumatic brain injury (TBI) associated with military action
    assessment of, 299–300, 299t
    description of, 298
    differential diagnosis and, 300
    etiology for, 298
    follow-up for, 302
    incidence and demographics for, 298
    nonpharmacologic treatment for, 301–302
    pharmacologic treatment for, 300–301
    prevention of and screening for, 298–299
    risk factors for, 298
    special considerations for, 302
Treatment. *See* Medications; Pharmacology

Treatment-directed tools, 118
Tricyclic antidepressants (TCAs)
    for anxiety disorders, 220
    for depressive disorders, 171, 173–174,
        175t
    description of, 139t
Tryptophan, 152
t test, 33
Twin studies, 67, 249

U

Unipolar affective disorders, 139t

V

Vagal nerve stimulation (VNS), 180
Valerian, 153
Validity, 33
Vanderbilt ADHD Parent and Teacher, 121t
Variance, 33
Vascular dementia (VD), 289–290
Violence. *See also* Child abuse
    domestic, 385–388
    lethality assessment for, 392–394
    school, 392–393
    sexual assault and abuse as, 389–392
    threats of, 394
Virtue ethics, 20
Vital signs, 85–86
Vitamin E, 152

W

Watson, Jean, 52
White matter, 56
Withdrawal symptoms, substance use/abuse
    and, 311, 312

Y

Yale-Brown Obsessive Compulsive Scale
    (YBOCS), 128t
Yalom, Irvin, 146
Yoga, 150, 154
Young Mania Rating Scale (YMRS), 128t

ABOUT THE AUTHORS

Kathryn Johnson, MSN, PMHNP-BC, PMHCNS-BC, is board certified as both an Adult Psychiatric and Mental Health Clinical Nurse Specialist and Adult Psychiatric Mental Health Nurse Practitioner. Kathryn has more than 38 years of psychiatric nursing experience and holds a master's degree in Adult Psychiatric and Mental Health Nursing from Wayne State University, Detroit, Michigan. She has done post-graduate coursework at the University of California San Francisco, where she is an Associate Clinical Professor. Kathryn is in private practice in Santa Cruz, California. Her areas of clinical interest include the psychopharmacologic treatment of adults and adolescents with mood, anxiety, attention and thought disorders. She is also experienced in the treatment of women who have perinatal mood and anxiety disorders and in adults who have been traumatized as children.

Dawn Vanderhoef, PhD, DNP, PMHNP-BC, PMHCNS-BC, has 18 years of experience working as a psychiatric nurse, 12 of those as an advanced practice psychiatric mental health nurse practitioner. Her experience is in both the inpatient and outpatient psychiatric mental health setting, treating patients across the lifespan. In addition to direct patient care experience, she has taught in master's and doctoral nursing programs, with a focus on psychiatric nursing. During her 8 years of academic experience, she have taught students from a wide variety of professional backgrounds, some were new to psychiatric mental health nursing and others who already had a master's or doctoral degree in a related field.

Made in the USA
Middletown, DE
23 June 2015